KLINE'S

Neuro-Ophthalmology

REVIEW MANUAL

EIGHTH EDITION

KLINE'S

Neuro-Ophthalmology

REVIEW MANUAL

EIGHTH EDITION

ROD FOROOZAN, MD
Associate Professor
Department of Ophthalmology
Baylor College of Medicine
Houston, Texas

MICHAEL S. VAPHIADES, DO
Professor
Department of Ophthalmology
University of Alabama School of Medicine
Birmingham, Alabama

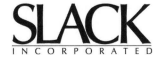
SLACK
INCORPORATED

www.Healio.com/books

ISBN: 978-1-63091-427-1

The procedures and practices described in this publication should be implemented in a manner consistent with the professional standards set for the circumstances that apply in each specific situation. Every effort has been made to confirm the accuracy of the information presented and to correctly relate generally accepted practices. The authors, editors, and publisher cannot accept responsibility for errors or exclusions or for the outcome of the material presented herein. There is no expressed or implied warranty of this book or information imparted by it. Care has been taken to ensure that drug selection and dosages are in accordance with currently accepted/recommended practice. Off-label uses of drugs may be discussed. Due to continuing research, changes in government policy and regulations, and various effects of drug reactions and interactions, it is recommended that the reader carefully review all materials and literature provided for each drug, especially those that are new or not frequently used. Some drugs or devices in this publication have clearance for use in a restricted research setting by the Food and Drug and Administration or FDA. Each professional should determine the FDA status of any drug or device prior to use in their practice.

Any review or mention of specific companies or products is not intended as an endorsement by the author or publisher.

Although Lanning Kline, MD is a member of the Board of Directors of the American Board of Ophthalmology (ABO), this work and its content shall not be marketed or construed as board preparatory material and the views expressed herein do not necessarily reflect those of the American Board of Ophthalmology. Furthermore, though he served as the lead editor in previous editions of this work, Dr. Kline played no role in the creation of the present Eighth Edition.

SLACK Incorporated uses a review process to evaluate submitted material. Prior to publication, educators or clinicians provide important feedback on the content that we publish. We welcome feedback on this work.

Published by: SLACK Incorporated
                  6900 Grove Road
                  Thorofare, NJ 08086 USA
                  Telephone: 856-848-1000
                  Fax: 856-848-6091
                  www.Healio.com/books

Contact SLACK Incorporated for more information about other books in this field or about the availability of our books from distributors outside the United States.

Library of Congress Cataloging-in-Publication Data

Names: Foroozan, Rod, author. | Vaphiades, Michael S., author.
Title: Kline's neuro-ophthalmology review manual / Rod Foroozan, Michael S.
  Vaphiades.
Other titles: Neuro-ophthalmology review manual
Description: 8th edition. | Thorofare, NJ : Slack Incorporated, 2017. |
  Preceded by Neuro-ophthalmology / Lanning B. Kline, Rod Foroozan, Frank J.
  Bajandas. 7th ed. c2013. | Includes bibliographical references and index.
  Identifiers: LCCN 2017034709 (print) | LCCN 2017035286 (ebook) | ISBN
  9781630914288 (epub) | ISBN 9781630914295 (web) | ISBN 9781630914271
  (paperback)
Subjects: | MESH: Eye Diseases | Eye--innervation | Eye Manifestations |
  Neurologic Manifestations | Nervous System Diseases--complications |
  Handbooks
Classification: LCC RE725 (ebook) | LCC RE725 (print) | NLM WW 39 | DDC
  617.7--dc23
LC record available at https://lccn.loc.gov/2017034709

Printed in the United States of America.

Last digit is print number: 10 9 8 7 6 5 4 3 2 1

Dedication

This manual is dedicated to Dr. Lanning Kline, a great mentor and even better friend to both of us. Dr. Kline's dedicated service to this manual over the last 35 years has resulted in several editions, each more comprehensive than the previous, yet without sacrificing the concept of a "review manual." We also would like to recognize David Fisher for his many years of work on the illustrative material in this manual.

CONTENTS

ABOUT THE AUTHORS

Rod Foroozan, MD is a neuro-ophthalmologist at the Baylor College of Medicine, Department of Ophthalmology in Houston, TX. He graduated from Albert Einstein College of Medicine in New York City, NY and completed his residency and fellowship at Wills Eye Hospital in Philadelphia, PA. He has written and lectured on a number of topics in neuro-ophthalmology and is the editor of the *International Ophthalmology Clinics.*

Michael S. Vaphiades, DO completed his residency training in neurology at Loyola University Chicago in Illinois and his neuro-ophthalmology fellowship at Michigan State University in East Lansing, MI. He is certified by the American Board of Psychiatry and Neurology and the United Council for Neurologic Subspecialties in neuroimaging. He is a tenured full professor in the Department of Ophthalmology, Neurology and Neurosurgery and Chief of the Neuro-Ophthalmology and Electrophysiology Services at the University of Alabama at Birmingham. He is also the chair of the neuro-ophthalmology section of the One Network for the American Academy of Ophthalmology. Dr. Vaphiades has well over 100 peer-reviewed publications, has given multiple presentations, and has garnered multiple awards including 2 Secretariat Awards and a Senior Achievement Award from the American Academy of Ophthalmology. He has been married for 25 years to his wife, Ann, an accomplished fine artist. They have 2 children, Alyssa and Samantha. Alyssa is an award-winning photographer and Samantha is pursuing a career in veterinary medicine. He dedicates this book to them.

Contributing Authors

Jason J. S. Barton, MD, PhD, FRCPC (Chapter 18)
Professor, Marianne Koerner Chair in Brain
  Diseases, Canada Research Chair
Departments of Medicine (Neurology), Ophthal-
  mology and Visual Sciences, Psychology
University of British Columbia
Vancouver, British Columbia, Canada

John E. Carter, MD (Chapter 15)
Neuro-ophthalmology
The University of Texas Health Science Center
San Antonio, Texas

Richard H. Fish, MD, FACS (Chapter 17)
Retina Consultants of Houston
Clinical Associate Professor
Houston Methodist Hospital
Weill Cornell Medical College
Clinical Associate Professor
Department of Ophthalmology
Baylor College of Medicine
Houston, Texas

*Christopher A. Girkin, MD, MSPH, FACS
  (Chapter 18)*
EyeSight Foundation of Alabama Chair, UAB
  Callahan Eye Hospital
Department of Ophthalmology
University of Alabama at Birmingham
Birmingham, Alabama

Saunders L. Hupp, MD (Chapter 14)
Vision Partners
Clinical Professor
Department of Neurology
University of South Alabama
Mobile, Alabama

Angela R. Lewis, MD (Chapter 19)
Christie Clinic
Department of Ophthalmology
Savoy, Illinois

Jennifer T. Scruggs, MD (Chapter 14)
Private Practice
Little Rock, Arkansas

Mark F. Walker, MD (Chapters 2, 3)
Associate Professor, Neurology
Case Western Reserve University
Cleveland VA Medical Center
Cleveland, Ohio

Milton F. White Jr, MD (Chapter 16)
Deceased

PREFACE

This review manual originated with Frank Bajandas, MD. Like me, he completed a fellowship in neuro-ophthalmology at the Bascom Palmer Eye Institute, Miami, FL. He began his practice in San Antonio, TX, and decided to transform the notes he had taken during fellowship into a "nuts and bolts" manual for what is often considered a daunting subspecialty. Appropriately, he dedicated this publication to 3 of his mentors at the Eye Institute: Joel Glaser, J. Lawton Smith, and Robert Daroff. In 1981, Frank tragically died in a motor vehicle accident. I had met Frank on one occasion and spoke at the time of revising the book.

It has been a privilege over the past 35 years to update *Neuro-Ophthalmology Review Manual* with the help of a number of colleagues. The First Edition was composed of 11 chapters filling 131 pages, and by the Seventh Edition, contained 20 chapters and 288 pages. I made certain the manual remained true to Frank's initial goal: a summary of the most important clinical aspects of neuro-ophthalmology simplified (but not overly so), schematic illustrations, and material relevant to everyday practice.

Two new editors, Rod Foroozan and Michael S. Vaphiades, will continue this tradition with the Eighth Edition of the manual. We hope that the reader continues to find *Neuro-Ophthalmology Review Manual* a user-friendly resource and that Frank Bajandas would be pleased with our efforts!

Lanning B. Kline, MD
Professor
Department of Ophthalmology
University of Alabama School of Medicine
Birmingham, Alabama

CHAPTER 1

Visual Fields

ROD FOROOZAN, MD AND MICHAEL S. VAPHIADES, DO

I. **TRAQUAIR'S DEFINITION OF THE VISUAL FIELD**
   A. Island of vision in a sea of blindness (Figure 1-1). The peak of the island represents the point of highest acuity—the fovea—while the "bottomless pit" represents the blind spot—the optic disc

II. **FOR CLINICAL TESTING, THE VISUAL FIELD CAN BE DIVIDED INTO 2 AREAS (FIGURE 1-2)**
   A. Central: 30-degree radius
   B. Peripheral: beyond 30 degrees

III. **VISUAL FIELD TESTING**
   A. Stimuli: testing the island of vision at various levels requires targets that vary in the following:
      1. Size
      2. Luminance
      3. Color
   B. Background luminance: at 31.5 asp (apostilb), the fovea has the highest sensitivity; able to detect the dimmest and smallest targets
   C. Field testing methods
      1. Can be examined with Amsler grid, confrontation techniques, kinetic perimetry, automated perimetry
      2. Amsler grid: useful in detecting subtle central and paracentral scotomas. When held at one-third of a meter from the patient, each square subtends 1 degree of visual field
      3. Confrontation techniques
         a. Quick screen for hemianopia and altitudinal defects
         b. Nonquantitative; requires practiced examiner
         c. Many significant neurologic field defects can be found with simple confrontation techniques
         d. The best technique of finger-counting fields evaluates both sides of the vertical meridian with care taken not to move the fingers in various quadrants since many patients with a damaged occipital lobe can still appreciate motion in the blind field (Riddoch phenomenon)

Foroozan R, Vaphiades MS. *Kline's Neuro-Ophthalmology Review Manual, Eighth Edition (pp 1-53).* © 2018 SLACK Incorporated.

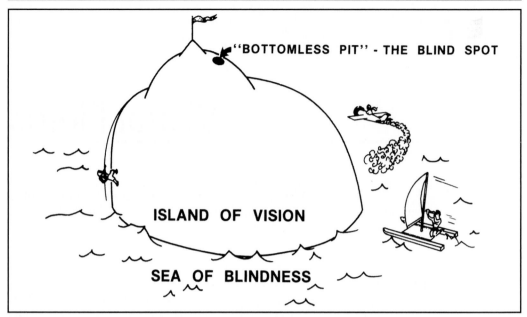

Figure 1-1. Traquair's definition of the visual field—island of vision in a sea of blindness.

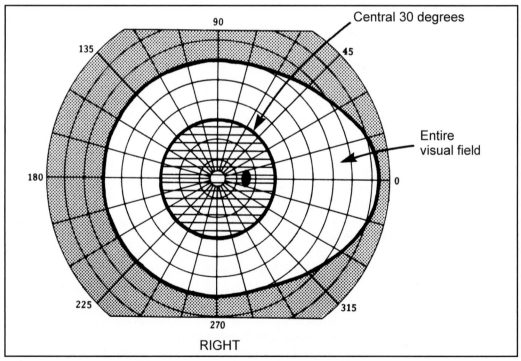

Figure 1-2. Central visual field (30-degree radius) can be tested with automated perimetry, while the entire visual field requires a different algorithm or use of manual perimetry.

e. Procedure (Figure 1-3)
   i. One eye of the patient is occluded
   ii. The patient is then asked to look at the examiner's nose while maintaining steady fixation. The test distance should be approximately 1 meter between patient and examiner
f. Finger counting is then carried out in the 4 quadrants: superior temporal, interior temporal, inferior nasal, and superior nasal. Between 1 and 5 fingers are presented and the number varied. The fingers are presented in a static fashion 20 and 30 degrees from fixation
g. Double simultaneous stimulation (Oppenheim test). The same number of fingers are simultaneously presented on each side of the vertical meridian with careful monitoring of the patient's fixation. Parietal lobe lesions can result in visual field inattention to simultaneous targets even when individually presented targets can be identified
h. Hemifield comparison. Again with controlled fixation, both hands are held on either side of the vertical meridian and the patient is asked to compare their appearance (ie, one "clearer" or "darker" than the other). The patient is always asked to point to the abnormal hand to reduce confusion. If, for example, the hand in the patient's temporal field appears dimmer, then both hands are again presented in the temporal field above and below the horizontal, and the patient is asked to identify the clearer of the two, allowing definition of whether the defect is denser above or below
i. The same procedure is carried out in the other eye

4. Kinetic perimetry (Figure 1-4)
   a. Moving stimulus is used
   b. Both size and luminance of stimulus may be altered
   c. Map the contours of the island of vision at different levels, resulting in one isopter for each level tested
   d. Evaluation of the entire visual field
   e. Particularly helpful in detecting the following:
      i. Ring scotoma (retinitis pigmentosa)
      ii. Nasal step (glaucoma)
      iii. Temporal crescent (occipital lobe)
      iv. Nonorganic field loss (see Chapter 17)
   f. Disadvantages
      i. Variable reproducibility
      ii. Dependent on skill of perimetrist
      iii. Perimetrist bias may affect results
   g. Can be performed with some automated perimeters

5. Static perimetry (see Figure 1-4)
   a. Stimulus location fixed
   b. Stimulus size standardized
   c. Vary stimulus luminance to assess light sensitivity at various points in visual field
   d. Standard automated perimetry is now the most widely used form of perimetry (Figure 1-5)
   e. Advantages include standardized test strategies, well-established normative database for comparison, careful monitoring of fixation behavior, computerized storage of all data

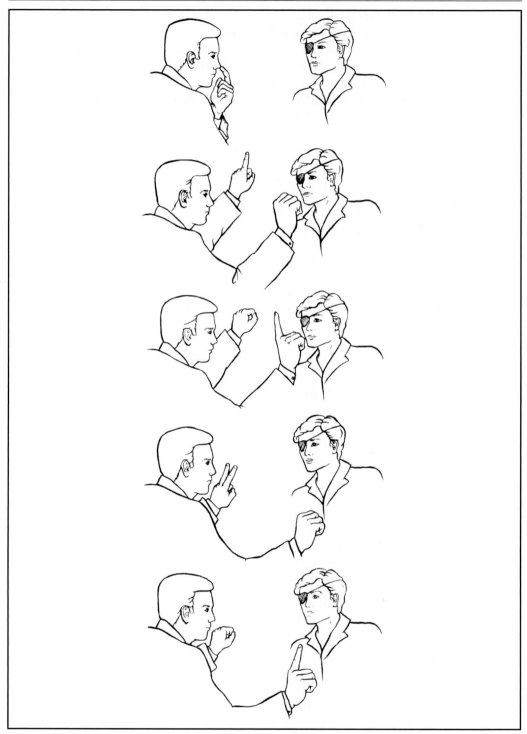

Figure 1-3. Confrontation visual field technique.

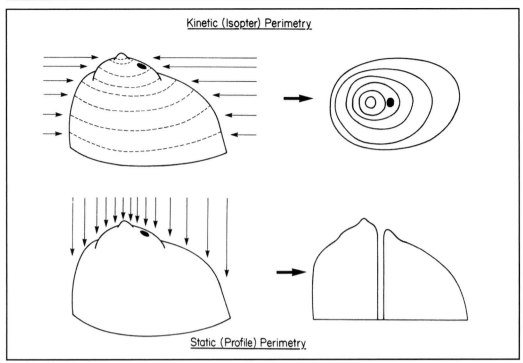

Figure 1-4. Kinetic perimetry: each set of target size-color-intensity and background illumination determines a different level of the island being tested and results in a different oval-shaped cross-section or isopter; note the 6 isopters at the right, the result of testing 6 levels of the island. Static perimetry: the target is held stationary at different points along the selected meridians; the intensity of the target is slowly increased until it is detected by the patient; the intensity required determines the upper level (the greatest sensitivity) of the island at this point.

6. Factors affecting visual field testing:
   a. Testing conditions: background luminance, stimulus size, stimulus deviation, stimulus spectral composition
   b. Physiologic: refractive error, pupil size, ptosis, media opacities, age
   c. Attention: fatigue, practice/learning effects
   d. Response errors: fixation instability, testing artifacts (eg, lens rim obstruction, misalignment)
   e. Criteria for unreliable visual field: fixation losses $\geq 20\%$; false-positive or false-negative rate $\geq 33\%$

IV. **ANATOMY OF THE VISUAL PATHWAYS (FIGURE 1-6)**
   A. The visual field and retina have an inverted and reversed relationship. Relative to the point of fixation, the upper visual field falls on the inferior retina (below the fovea), lower visual field on the superior retina, nasal visual field on the temporal retina, and temporal visual field on the nasal retina
   B. Nasal fibers of ipsilateral eye cross in the chiasm and join uncrossed temporal fibers of the contralateral eye → optic tract → synapse in lateral geniculate nucleus (LGN) → optic radiation → terminate in the visual cortex (V1, area 17) of the occipital lobe
   C. Inferonasal retinal fibers decussate in the chiasm and travel anteriorly in the contralateral optic nerve before passing into the optic tract. They form "Wilbrand knee"
   D. While the presence of Wilbrand knee has been challenged,[1] it still appears to have clinical relevance[2]

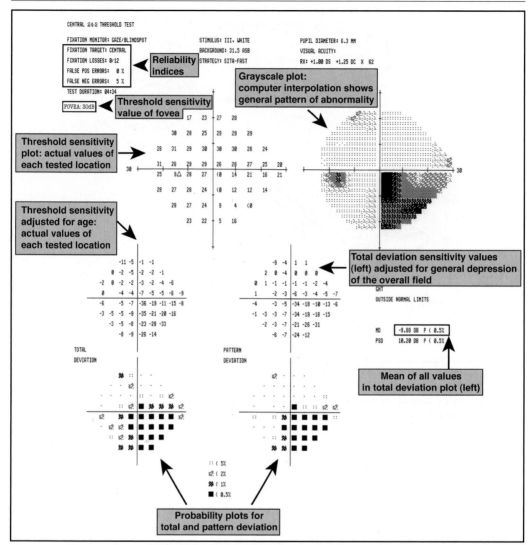

Figure 1-5. Printout of Humphrey 24-2 (which extends to 30 degrees nasally but to 24 degrees superiorly, temporally, and inferiorly) automated static perimetry program, with explanation of statistical analysis, grayscale, and probability plots.

E. Lower retinal fibers and their projections lie in the lateral portion of the optic tract and ultimately terminate in the inferior striate cortex on the lower bank of the calcarine fissure. Upper retinal fibers project through the medial optic tract and ultimately terminate in the superior striate cortex

F. LGN. Visual information from the ipsilateral eye synapses in layers 2, 3, 5; from contralateral in layers 1, 4, 6. Macular vision is subserved by the hilum and peripheral field by the medial and lateral horns

G. The central (30 degrees) visual field occupies a disproportionately large area (68% to 83%) of the visual cortex. The vertical hemianopic meridians are represented along the border of the calcarine lips, while the horizontal meridian follows the contour of the base of the calcarine fissure (Figure 1-7)

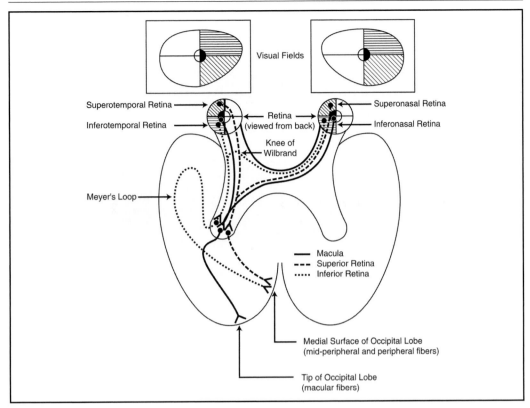

Figure 1-6. Anatomy of visual pathways.

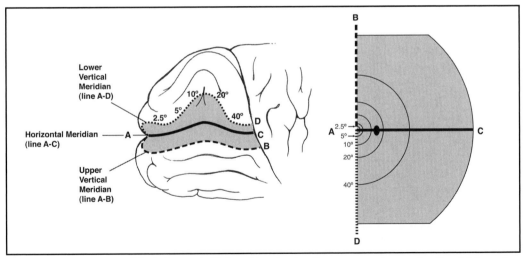

Figure 1-7. Medial view of the left occipital lobe with calcarine fissure opened, exposing the striate cortex. Dashed and solid lines represent coordinates of the visual field.

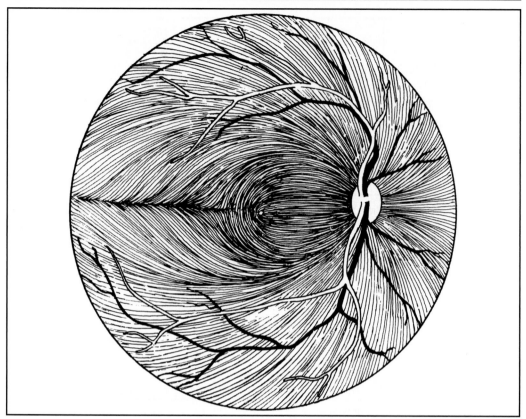

Figure 1-8. Nerve fiber pattern of the retina.

V.   INTERPRETATION OF VISUAL FIELD DEFECTS

A.   Ten key points to remember:
1.   Optic nerve-type field defects
2.   "Rules of the road" for the optic chiasm
3.   Optic tract—LGN defects
4.   Superior-inferior separation in the temporal lobe
5.   Superior-inferior separation in the parietal lobe
6.   Central homonymous hemianopia
7.   Macular sparing
8.   Congruity
9.   Optokinetic nystagmus (OKN)
10. Temporal crescents

B.   Optic nerve-type field defects
1.   Retinal nerve fibers enter the optic discs in a specific manner (Figure 1-8)
2.   Nerve fiber bundle (NFB) defects are of the following 3 main types:
   a.   Papillomacular bundle: macular fibers that enter the temporal aspect of the disc. A defect in this bundle of nerve fibers results in one of the following:
      i.   Central scotoma (Figure 1-9): a defect covering central fixation
      ii. Cecocentral scotoma (see Figure 1-9): a central scotoma connected to the blind spot (cecum)

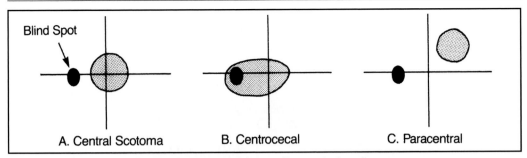

Figure 1-9. Field defects due to interruption of the papillomacular bundle.

iii. Paracentral scotoma (see Figure 1-9): a defect of some of the fibers of the papillomacular bundle lying next to, but not involving, central fixation

b. Arcuate NFB: fibers from the retina temporal to the disc enter the superior and inferior poles of the disc (see Figure 1-8). A defect of these bundles may cause one of the following:

  i. Arcuate scotoma or defect (Figure 1-10): due to involvement of arcuate NFBs

  ii. Seidel scotoma (see Figure 1-10): a defect in the proximal portion of the NFB, causing a comma-shaped extension of the blind spot

  iii. Nasal step (see Figure 1-10): a defect in the distal portion of the arcuate NFB. Since the superior and inferior arcuate bundles do not cross the horizontal raphe of the temporal retina, a nasal step defect respects the horizontal (180-degree) meridian

  iv. Isolated scotoma within arcuate area (see Figure 1-10): defect of the intermediate portion of the arcuate NFB

c. Nasal NFBs: fibers that enter the nasal aspect of the disc course in a straight (nonarcuate) fashion. The defect in this bundle results in a wedge-shaped temporal scotoma arising from the blind spot and does not necessarily respect the temporal horizontal meridian (see Figure 1-10)

3. Lesions at or behind the chiasm tend to cause hemianopic field defects originating from the point of fixation and respecting the vertical meridian

4. Optic nerve lesions cause field defects corresponding to 1 of the 3 major NFB defects described previously. NFB defects originate from the blind spot, not from the fixation point, and do not respect the vertical meridian but do respect the nasal horizontal meridian

5. The key question, therefore, in a patient with a quadrantic field defect is: does the field defect go to fixation or to the blind spot (Figure 1-11)?

6. Additional clinical findings supporting the diagnosis of optic neuropathy as the cause of the field defect include the following:

a. Decreased visual acuity: patients with isolated retrochiasmatic lesions do not have decreased visual acuity unless the lesions are bilateral, then the visual acuities will be equal; if a patient has hemianopic field defects with unequal visual acuities, then look for a lesion around the chiasm (affecting the optic nerves asymmetrically)

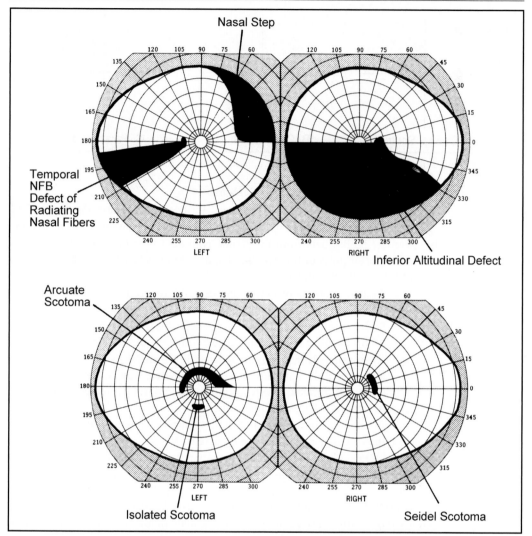

Figure 1-10. Composite diagram depicting different optic nerve-type field defects.

    b.   Patients with decreased (or suspected decreased) visual acuity can be further tested with the following:

        i.   Light-brightness comparison (eye with optic neuropathy will see the light as "less bright")

        ii.   Color perception comparison (color plates or Mydriacyl [tropicamide] bottle cap; eye with optic neuropathy will have diminished color perception)

        iii.   Light-stress recovery time (eye with maculopathy will have delayed recovery visual acuity after bleaching with light)

        iv.   Relative afferent pupillary defect test (RAPD) or "swinging flashlight" (see Chapter 8)

        v.   Tests i through iv may help in distinguishing cases of decreased visual acuity due to macular disease from those due to optic nerve disease

        vi.   Visual-evoked potentials (VEPs)

        vii.   Ophthalmoscopic evidence of optic disc abnormality (eg, pallor, cupping, drusen)

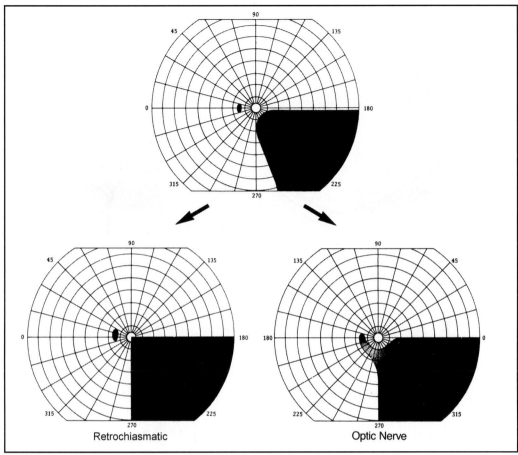

Figure 1-11. The key question in a patient with a quadrantic visual field defect: does the field defect go to fixation (retrochiasmatic lesion) or to the blind spot (optic nerve lesion)?

7. Rarely, optic nerve disease (compression, demyelination) may cause a monocular temporal hemianopia (RAPD present as well). Lesion is posterior enough to disrupt ipsilateral crossing nasal fibers but too anterior to affect contralateral ones. Must distinguish from nonorganic visual field loss (see Chapter 17, IV, A on page 238)

C. "Rules of the road" for the optic chiasm

1. Three rules describe the course of major fiber bundles in the chiasm:

   a. The nasal retinal fibers (including the nasal half of the macula) of each eye cross in the chiasm to the contralateral optic tract. Temporal fibers remain uncrossed. Thus, a chiasmal lesion tends to cause a bitemporal hemianopia due to interruption of decussating nasal fibers (Figure 1-12)

   b. Lower retinal fibers project through the optic nerve and chiasm to lie laterally in the tracts; upper retinal fibers will lie medially (there is a 90-degree rotation of fibers from the nerves through the chiasm into the tracts)

   c. Inferonasal retinal fibers cross into the chiasm and cross anteriorly approximately 4 mm in the contralateral optic nerve (Wilbrand knee) before turning back to join uncrossed inferotemporal temporal fibers in the optic tract (junctional scotoma). Existence of Wilbrand knee is controversial (see page 5, IV, D)

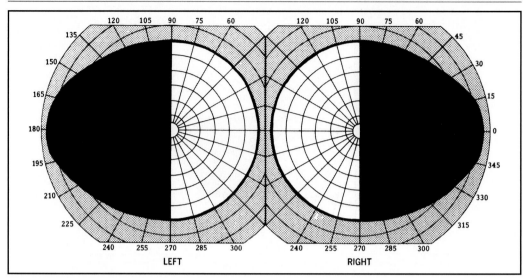

Figure 1-12. Bitemporal hemianopia due to interruption of decussating nasal fibers in the chiasm.

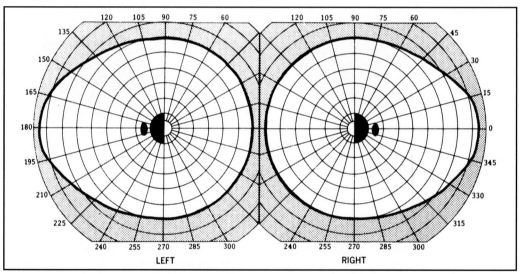

Figure 1-13. A chiasmal lesion may affect only the decussating nasal-macular fibers, resulting in a central bitemporal hemianopia. Therefore, a complete visual field evaluation of a patient suspected of a chiasmal lesion must include examination of the central field.

2. "Macular" crossing fibers are distributed throughout the chiasm and, if primarily affected, cause a "central" bitemporal hemianopia (Figure 1-13)
3. If a patient comes in with poor vision in the left eye, the important eye for visual examination is the right due to involvement of Wilbrand knee. The lesion is now intracranial at the junction of the left optic nerve and chiasm. The field defects constitute a junctional scotoma (Figure 1-14)

D. Optic tract—LGN defects
1. All retrochiasmatic lesions result in a contralateral homonymous hemianopia
2. Congruity describes incomplete homonymous hemianopic defects that are identical in all attributes: location, shape, size, depth, slope of margins

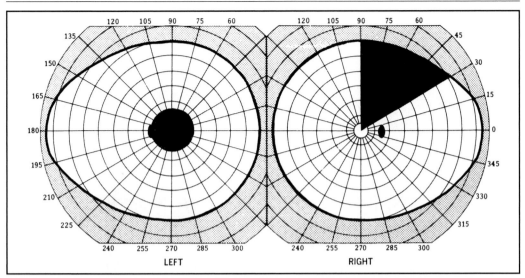

Figure 1-14. Junctional scotoma: a central scotoma in one eye with a superior-temporal defect in the fellow eye indicates a lesion at the junction of the optic nerve (left eye in this case) and the chiasm.

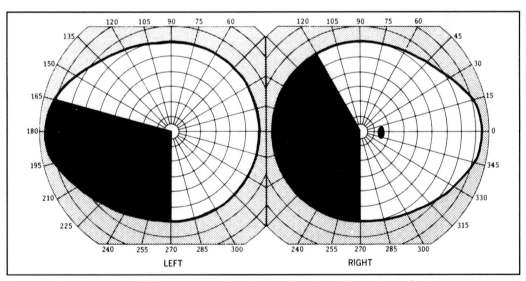

Figure 1-15. Incongruous left homonymous hemianopia due to a right optic tract lesion.

3. **Remember:** the more posterior (toward the occipital cortex) the lesion in the post-chiasmal visual pathways, the more likely the defects will be congruous, although one series showed lesion site was not accurately predicted by the congruity of the field defect

4. In the optic tracts and LGN, nerve fibers of corresponding points (retinal positions of the 2 eyes that image the same position in visual space) do not yet lie adjacent to one another. This leads to incongruous visual field defects (Figure 1-15)

5. In the LGN, afferent fibers are organized into alternating layers; crossed fibers terminate in layers 1, 4, 6 and uncrossed in 2, 3, 5

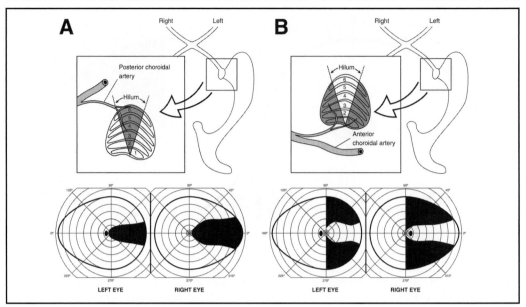

Figure 1-16. (A) Posterior choroidal artery (branch of posterior cerebral artery) occlusion leads to homonymous horizontal sectoranopia. (B) Anterior choroidal artery (branch of internal carotid artery) occlusion causes sector-sparing homonymous hemianopia.

6. Criteria for optic tract syndrome
   a. Incongruous homonymous hemianopia
   b. Bilateral retinal nerve fiber layer (NFL) atrophy or optic (occasionally "bow-tie") atrophy (see Chapter 10, III, G and Figure 10-2 on page 165)
   c. Pupillary abnormalities
      i. RAPD: on the opposite side of the lesion (eye with temporal field loss)
      ii. Wernicke pupil: light stimulation of a "blind" retina causes no pupillary reaction, while light projected on an "intact" retina produces normal pupillary constriction
      iii. Behr pupil: anisocoria with larger pupil on the side of hemianopia; probably does not exist
7. LGN field defect
   a. Visual information from ipsilateral eye synapses in layers 2, 3, 5; from contralateral in layers 1, 4, 6. Macular vision is subserved by the hilum and peripheral field by the medial and lateral horns
   b. Types of defects:
      i. Incongruous homonymous hemianopia
      ii. Unique sector and sector-sparing defects due to dual blood supply of LGN from anterior and posterior choroidal arteries (Figure 1-16)
E. Superior-inferior separation in the temporal lobe
   1. Inferior fibers (ipsilateral inferotemporal fibers and contralateral inferonasal fibers) course anteriorly from the lateral geniculate body into the temporal lobe, forming Meyer loop approximately 2.5 cm (range 2.4 to 2.8 cm) from the anterior tip of the temporal lobe. They are anatomically separated from the superior retinal fibers, which course directly back in the optic radiations of the parietal lobe (see Figure 1-6)
   2. Inferior "macular" fibers do not cross as far anteriorly in the temporal lobe

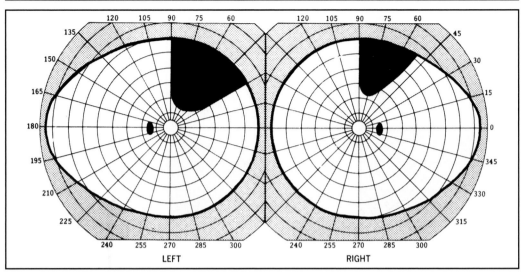

Figure 1-17. Anterior temporal lobe lesion of Meyer loop produces incongruous, midperipheral and peripheral-contralateral, homonymous, superior ("pie in the sky") quadrantanopia. This is an example of a patient with a left temporal lobe lesion.

    3. Anterior temporal lobe lesions tend to produce midperipheral and peripheral contralateral homonymous superior quadrantanopia ("pie in the sky" field defect; Figure 1-17)

    4. More extensive temporal lobe lesions may cause field defects that extend to the inferior quadrants, but hemianopia will be "denser" superiorly

F. Superior-inferior separation in the parietal lobe

    1. Superior fibers (ipsilateral superotemporal fibers and contralateral superonasal fibers) course directly through the parietal lobe to lie superiorly in the optic radiation

    2. Inferior fibers course through the temporal lobe (Meyer loop) and lie inferiorly in the optic radiation

    3. Thus, there is "correction" of the 90-degree rotation of the visual fibers that occurs through the chiasm into the tracts

    4. Parietal lobe lesions tend to affect superior fibers first, resulting in contralateral inferior homonymous quadrantanopia (Figure 1-18) or a homonymous hemianopia "denser" inferiorly (Figure 1-19)

    5. Two signs described with parietal lobe lesions:

        a. Spasticity of conjugate gaze: tonic deviation of eyes to the side opposite a parietal lesion during an attempt to produce Bell phenomenon (see Chapter 2)

        b. OKN asymmetry: evoked nystagmus is dampened when stimuli are moved in the direction of the damaged parietal lobe (see page 21, V, J)

G. Central homonymous hemianopia

    1. In the visual cortex, the macular representation is located on the tips of the occipital lobes

    2. The macular representation is separated from the cortical representation of the midperipheral and peripheral visual fields. These fibers terminate on the medial surface of the occipital lobes (see Figure 1-6)

    3. A lesion affecting the tip of the occipital lobe tends to produce a central homonymous hemianopia (Figure 1-20)

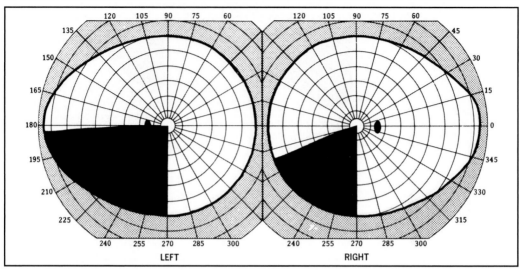

Figure 1-18. Parietal lobe lesions tend to affect the inferior, contralateral visual field quadrants first. This is an example of a patient with a right parietal lobe lesion.

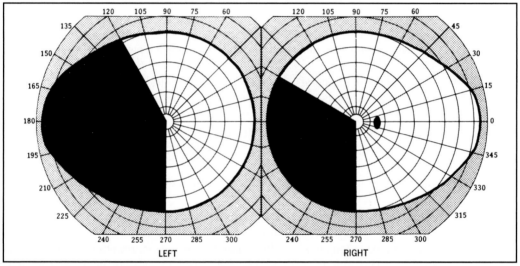

Figure 1-19. Incongruous left homonymous hemianopia.

H. Macular sparing
   1. The macular area of the visual cortex is a watershed area with respect to blood supply (Figure 1-21)
      a. The "macular" visual cortex is supplied by terminal branches of posterior and middle cerebral arteries
      b. The visual cortex subserving the midperipheral and peripheral field is supplied only by the posterior cerebral artery. The area is supplied by a more proximal (not a terminal) vessel
      c. Therefore, when there is obstruction of flow through the posterior cerebral artery, ipsilateral macular visual cortex may be spared because of blood supply provided by the terminal branches of the middle cerebral artery. This may be an explanation for "macular sparing"

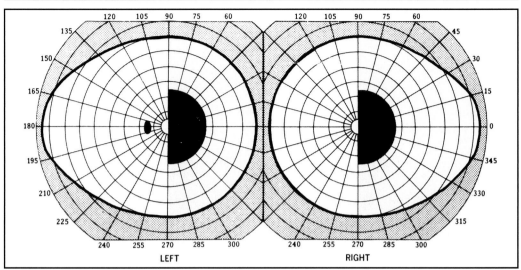

Figure 1-20. A lesion affecting only the tip of the occipital lobe produces a defect of only the central homonymous hemifields. This is an example of a patient with a left occipital tip lesion.

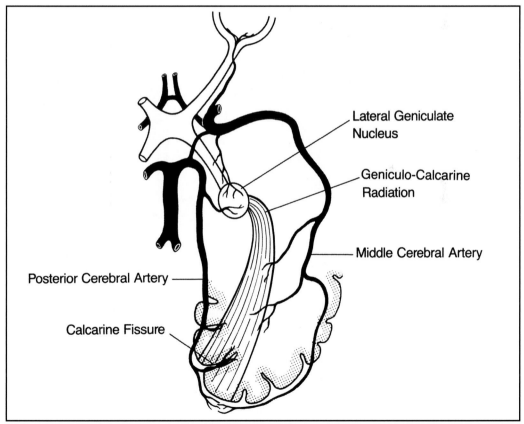

Figure 1-21. The tip of the occipital lobe, where the macular or central homonymous hemifields are represented, is supplied by terminal branches of the middle and posterior cerebral arteries; it is referred to as a *watershed area*. The medial surface of the occipital lobe is supplied by more proximal (not terminal) branches of the posterior cerebral artery.

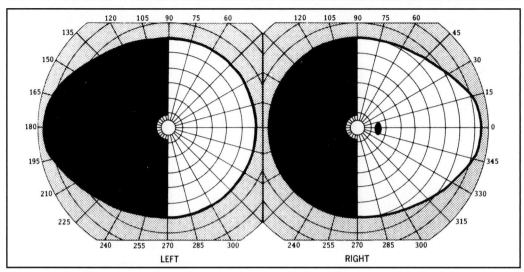

Figure 1-22. Left homonymous hemianopia with "sparing" of the left half of the macular field of each eye.

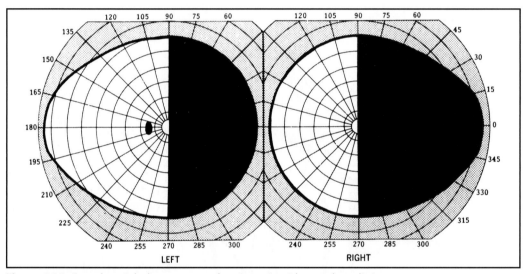

Figure 1-23. Complete right homonymous hemianopia with macular splitting.

    d.   However, when there is a generalized hypoperfusion state (eg, intraoperative hypotension), the first area of the visual cortex to be affected is that supplied by terminal branches—the macular visual cortex—resulting in a central homonymous hemianopia (see Figure 1-20)

  2. In order to qualify as "macular sparing," at least 5 degrees of the macular field must be spared in both eyes on the side of the hemianopia (Figure 1-22)

  3. Macular sparing may at times be an artifact of testing. The patient may shift fixation, anticipating the appearance of the test object

  4. If a patient with a complete homonymous hemianopia is found to have sparing of the macula, then he or she is most likely to have an occipital lobe lesion. However, the majority of patients with occipital lobe lesions demonstrate a splitting of the macula (Figure 1-23); therefore, macular sparing is helpful only if present

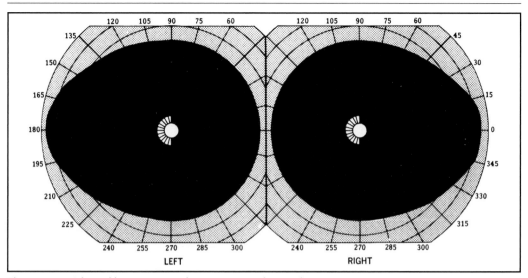

Figure 1-24. Bilateral homonymous hemianopia with macular sparing.

5.   Bilateral homonymous hemianopia with macular sparing produce constricted visual fields (with normal fundi; Figure 1-24). The differential diagnosis of constricted visual fields also includes the following:
  a.   Nonorganic visual field loss
  b.   Glaucoma
  c.   Optic disc drusen
  d.   Postpapilledema optic atrophy
  e.   Retinitis pigmentosa
6.   Items b through e listed above all have abnormal fundi and should be easily diagnosed. Differential from nonorganic field loss requires fields done at 1 and 2 meters (Figure 1-25)

I.   Congruity
1.   Homonymous hemianopic field defects are said to be congruous when the defect is not complete (ie, does not occupy the entire half of the field) and the defect extends to the same angular meridian in both eyes (Figure 1-26; the hemianopic defect extends to the 137-degree meridian in each eye)
2.   Complete homonymous hemianopia (see Figure 1-23) cannot be categorized as "congruous" because it is complete
3.   Figure 1-27 shows an example of incongruity; the hemianopia of the left eye extends to the 160-degree meridian while the hemianopia of the right eye extends to the 115-degree meridian
4.   Optic tract lesions tend to produce markedly incongruous field defects
5.   The more congruous a homonymous hemianopia, the nearer the lesion will be to the occipital cortex (ie, more posterior in the visual pathways)
6.   Congruity is due to the fact that a lesion affects nerve fibers from corresponding retinal points that lie adjacent to one another
7.   One series showed that lesion site did not predict congruity of the visual field defect and called this concept into question

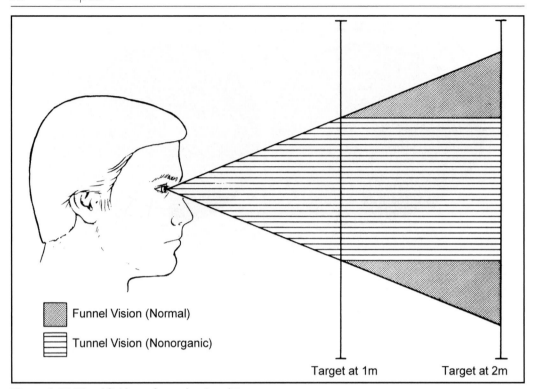

Figure 1-25. Visual fields performed at 1 and 2 meters.

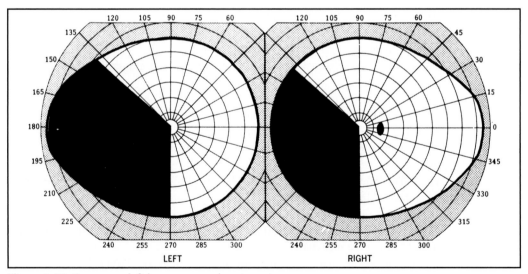

Figure 1-26. Congruous left homonymous hemianopia.

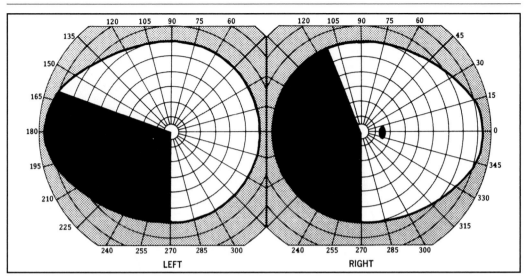

Figure 1-27. Incongruous left homonymous hemianopia.

J. OKN
1. The precise pathways of the optokinetic system are unknown in humans but may share pathways carrying smooth pursuit commands. This pathway extends from the visual association areas (18 and 19) to the horizontal gaze center in the pons (see Chapter 2)
2. The pathway in the left visual association area will terminate in the left pontine gaze center, resulting in pursuit movement of the eyes to the left. Similarly, the pathway originating in the right cerebral hemisphere generates pursuit eye movements to the right
3. A patient with a purely occipital lobe lesion (even if resulting in a complete homonymous hemianopia) will have no difficulty with pursuit, since the pathways begin more anteriorly. OKN response will be symmetric
4. A patient with homonymous hemianopia due to a parietal lobe lesion will have deficient pursuit eye movements to the side of the lesion, resulting in asymmetric OKN. The OKN will be decreased when the drum is rotated toward the side of the lesion
5. Patients with homonymous hemianopia due to an optic tract, temporal lobe, or purely occipital lobe lesion will have symmetric OKN to both sides
6. Cogan dictum
a. Homonymous hemianopia + asymmetric OKN—probably parietal lobe lesion; most likely mass
b. Homonymous hemianopia + symmetric OKN—probably occipital lobe lesion; most likely vascular infarction
K. Temporal crescents
1. When we fixate with both eyes and achieve fusion of the visual information gained by both eyes, there is superimposition of the corresponding portions of the visual fields: the central 60-degree radius of field in each eye
2. There remains, in each eye, a temporal crescent of field for which there are no corresponding visual points in the other eye (Figure 1-28)

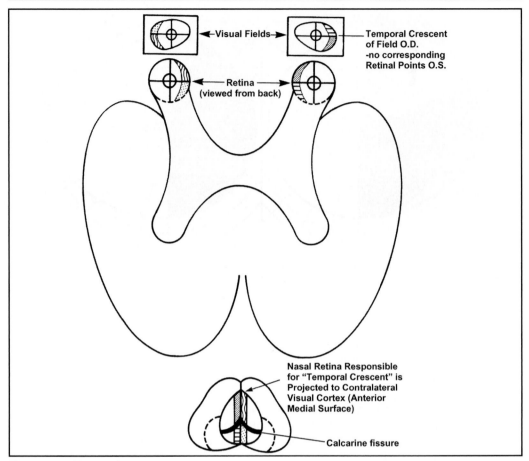

Figure 1-28. Temporal crescents.

3. This temporal crescent of field, perceived by a nasal crescent of retina, is represented in the contralateral visual cortex in the most anterior portion of the medial surface of the occipital lobe (along the calcarine fissure)

4. Representation of the temporal crescent occupies < 10% of total surface area of striate cortex

5. If a patient is found to have a homonymous hemianopia with sparing of the temporal crescent (Figure 1-29), then he or she probably has an occipital lobe lesion since this is the only site where the temporal crescent of fibers are separated from the other nasal fibers of the contralateral eye

VI. **SPECIAL VISUAL FIELD CASES**

A. Pseudobitemporal hemianopia

1. Field defects that do not respect the vertical meridian, but rather "slope" across it (Figure 1-30)

2. Causes include the following:

a. Uncorrected refractive errors (myopia, astigmatism)

b. Tilted optic discs

c. Enlarged blind spots in papilledema

d. Large central or centrocecal scotomas

e. Sectoral retinitis pigmentosa (mainly in nasal quadrants)

f. Overhanging eyelid tissue

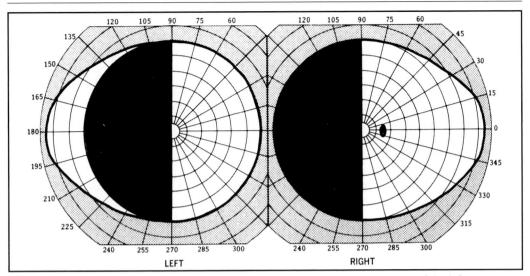

Figure 1-29. Left homonymous hemianopia with sparing of the temporal crescent of the left eye.

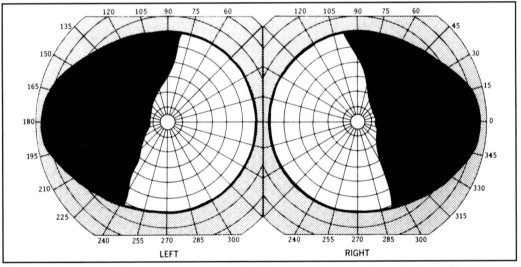

Figure 1-30. Pseudobitemporal hemianopia. Field defects do not respect the vertical meridian.

B. Binasal hemianopia
1. Most nasal field defects are due to arcuate scotomas
2. Rarely, true unilateral or bilateral nasal hemianopia may occur with defects having no arcuate connection to the blind spot and, to some extent, respecting the vertical meridian
3. Never as a result of chiasmal compression
4. May be due to pressure on the temporal aspect of the optic nerve and the anterior angle of the chiasm or near the optic canal; in these locations, a lesion may affect only temporal retinal fibers. The fibers cannot be selectively obstructed in the lateral chiasm
5. Cause includes aneurysm, tumor (pituitary adenoma), vascular infarction

C.   Monocular temporal hemianopia
1.   Rare manifestation of visual pathway damage
2.   May be seen with compressive lesion (pituitary tumor, meningioma, craniopharyngioma), optic disc anomaly (dysversion, optic nerve hypoplasia), or optic neuritis
3.   In all cases, an RAPD is present with or without optic disc pallor
4.   If RAPD absent, consider nonorganic cause (see Chapter 17)
5.   Attributed to involvement of ipsilateral optic nerve close enough to the chiasm to impair crossing nasal fibers but too anterior to affect crossing nasal retinal fibers from the contralateral eye
D.   Big blind spot syndrome
1.   Sudden onset of temporal scotoma centered on the physiologic blind spot in one or both eyes
2.   Often accompanied by photopsia or scintillations in the blind spot
3.   Predilection for females
4.   Associated with a variety of disorders, including some of the white dot syndromes (multiple evanescent white dot syndrome [MEWDS], multifocal choroiditis [MFC], acute zonal occult outer retinopathy [AZOOR], acute macular neuroretinopathy [AMN])
5.   Optic disc may appear normal or mildly swollen
6.   The involved eye may have a mild vitritis
7.   Optical coherence tomography (OCT): disruption of the photoreceptor inner/outer segment junction
8.   Full-field and multifocal electroretinography (ERG) abnormalities may be found
9.   Etiology: transient peripapillary or diffuse photoreceptor dysfunction of unknown cause

Visual Field Quiz

1. Test yourself in the interpretation of the following hypothetical cases (Exercises 1 to 50).
2. Unless stated otherwise, assume that the visual fields have been evaluated with either manual perimetry (using the same stimulus and testing conditions for each eye) or with an automated technique.
3. Describe and categorize the visual field defects and suggest the probable localization and possible causes of the lesion(s).
4. Develop a systematic approach that includes a review of the "Ten Key Points to Remember."
5. Remember the significance of altered visual acuities (see page 9, V, B, 6).
6. To help avoid confusing the right and left eyes (and hence nasal and temporal fields), the field of the right eye (which should have the blind spot to the right of fixation) should be placed page right and the field of the left eye (which should have the blind spot to the left of fixation) page left. Initially examine both fields simultaneously to look for a pattern. While looking at a single field in isolation, it may be helpful to occlude your fellow eye (ie, when examining the field of the right eye, occlude your left eye) and imagine yourself having the field defect in the same location.
7. Congruity may be difficult to determine with automated fields (most often evaluating the central 10 to 30 degrees) as the full extent of the field is not typically tested. For example, when a complete hemianopia is noted to 30 degrees on the right side of both visual fields, the fields may look congruous but may be incongruous in the periphery outside of 30 degrees.

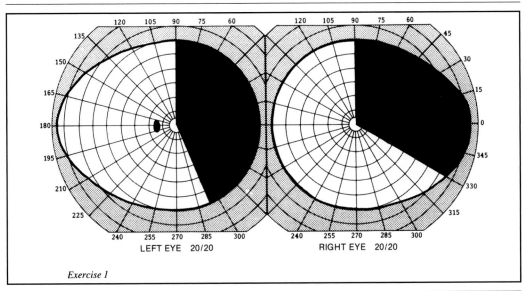

Exercise 1

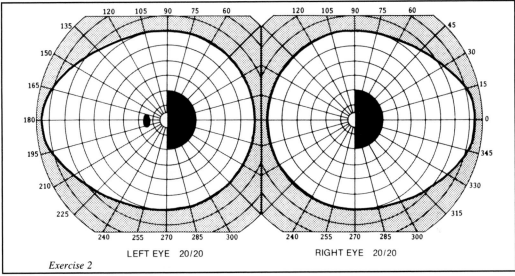

Exercise 2

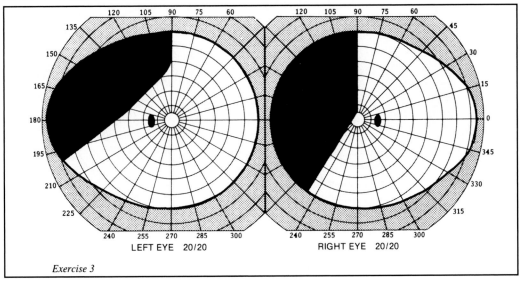

Exercise 3

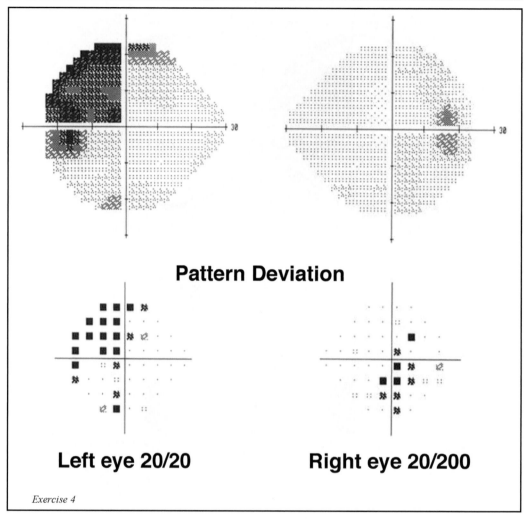

Pattern Deviation

Left eye 20/20

Right eye 20/200

Exercise 4

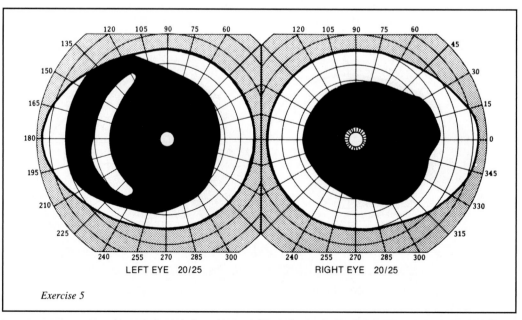

LEFT EYE   20/25

RIGHT EYE   20/25

Exercise 5

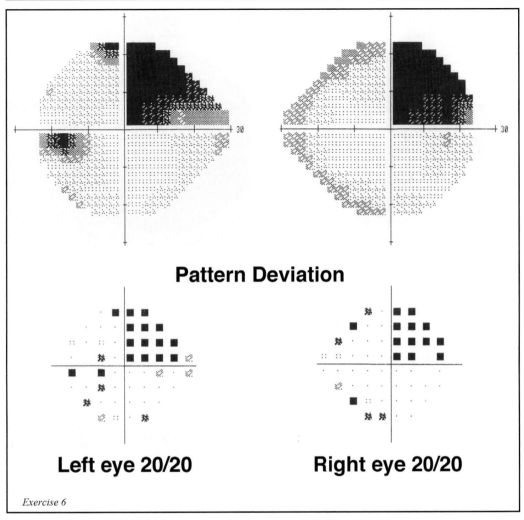

Pattern Deviation

Left eye 20/20

Right eye 20/20

Exercise 6

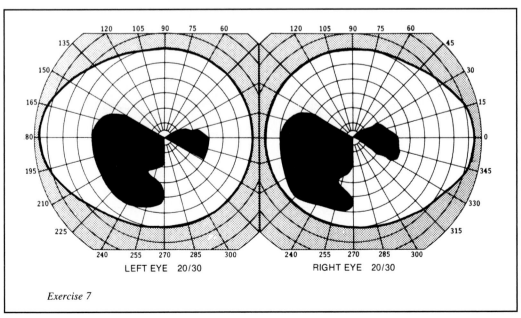

LEFT EYE   20/30

RIGHT EYE   20/30

Exercise 7

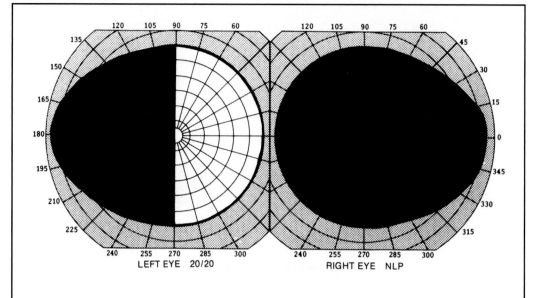

Exercise 8

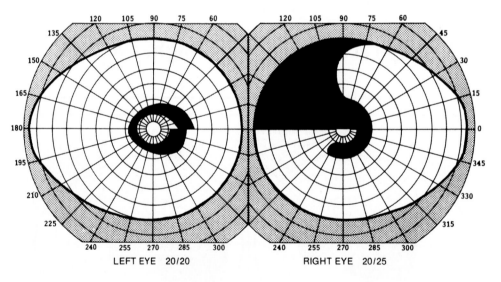

Exercise 9

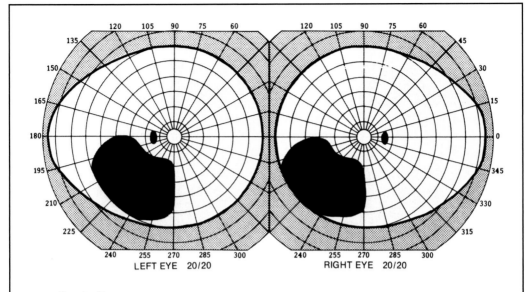

LEFT EYE   20/20   RIGHT EYE   20/20

Exercise 10

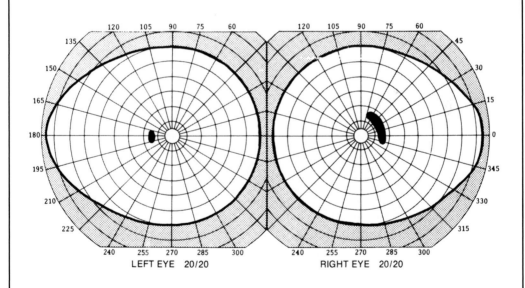

LEFT EYE   20/20   RIGHT EYE   20/20

Exercise 11

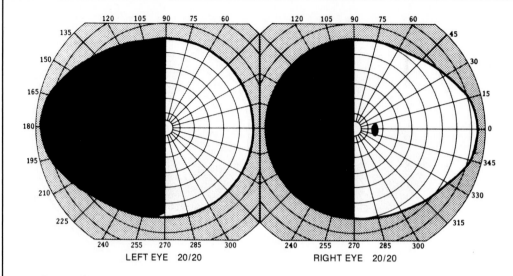

LEFT EYE   20/20   RIGHT EYE   20/20

Exercise 12

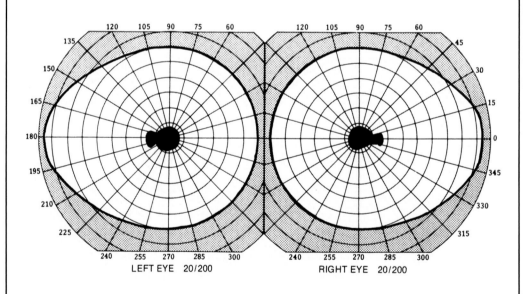

LEFT EYE   20/200   RIGHT EYE   20/200

Exercise 13

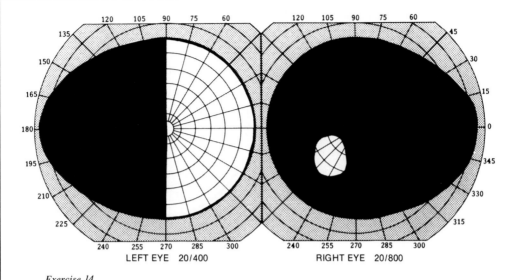

LEFT EYE   20/400   RIGHT EYE   20/800

Exercise 14

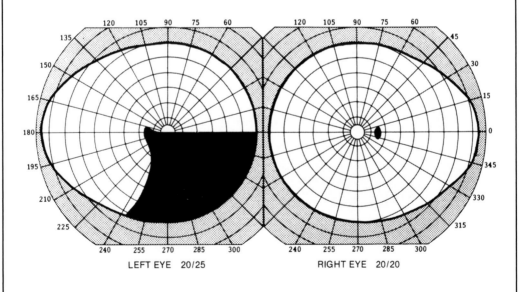

LEFT EYE   20/25   RIGHT EYE   20/20

Exercise 15

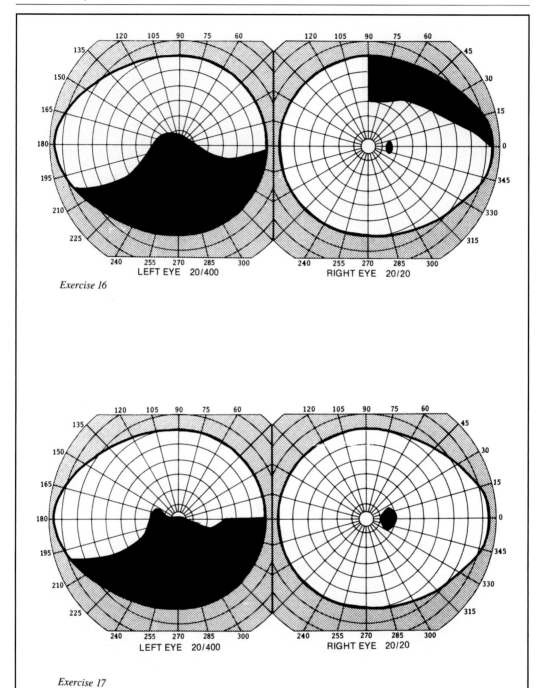

Exercise 16

LEFT EYE   20/400

RIGHT EYE   20/20

Exercise 17

LEFT EYE   20/400

RIGHT EYE   20/20

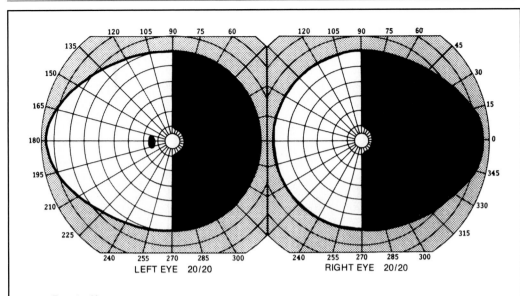

LEFT EYE   20/20   RIGHT EYE   20/20

Exercise 18

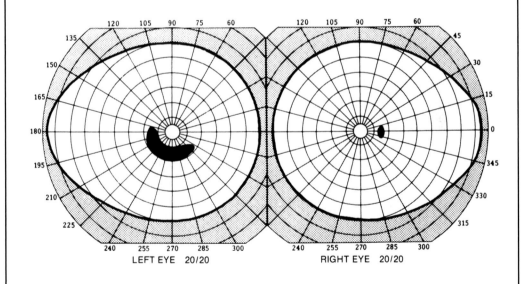

LEFT EYE   20/20   RIGHT EYE   20/20

Exercise 19

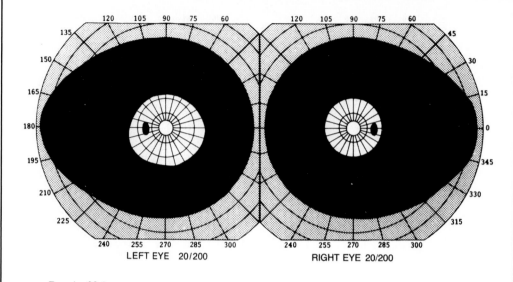

Exercise 20-A

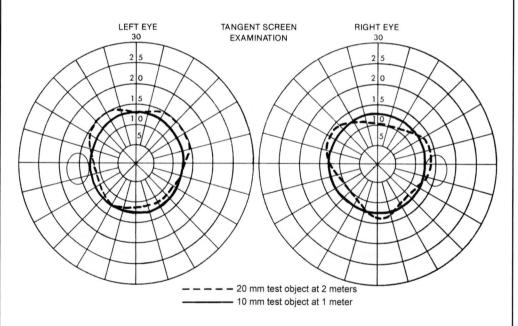

Exercise 20-B

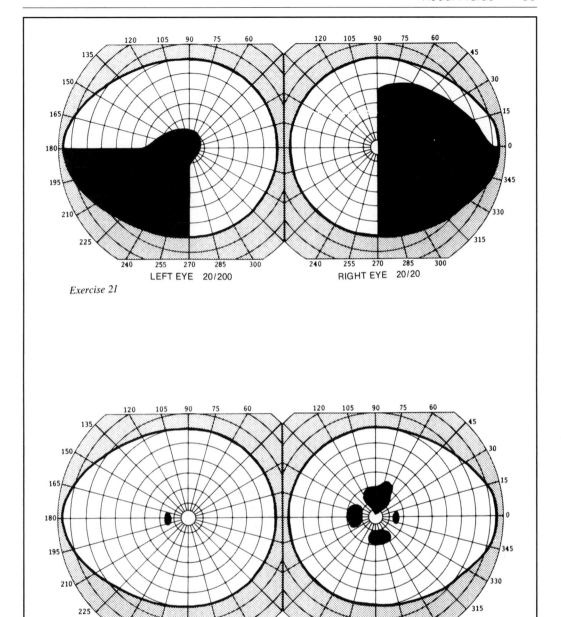

Exercise 21

LEFT EYE   20/200   RIGHT EYE   20/20

LEFT EYE   20/20   RIGHT EYE   20/400

Exercise 22

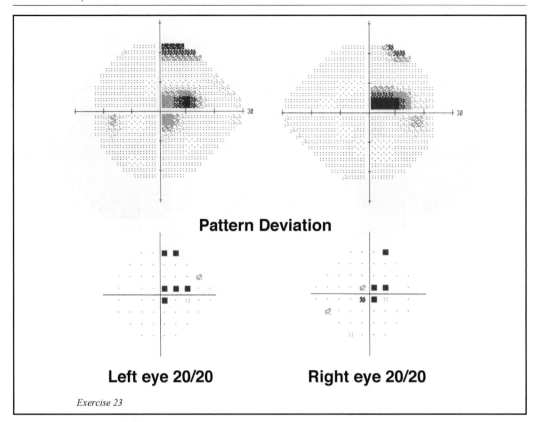

Pattern Deviation

Left eye 20/20   **Right eye 20/20**

Exercise 23

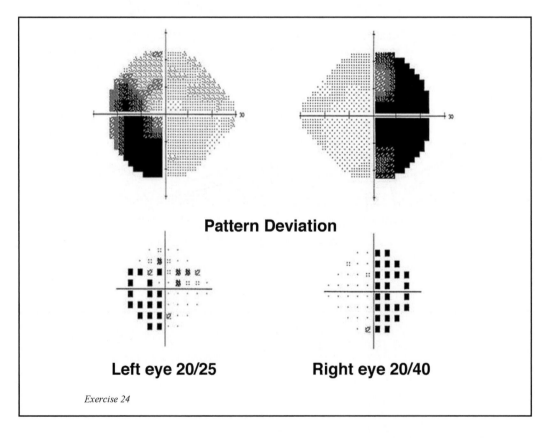

Pattern Deviation

Left eye 20/25   **Right eye 20/40**

Exercise 24

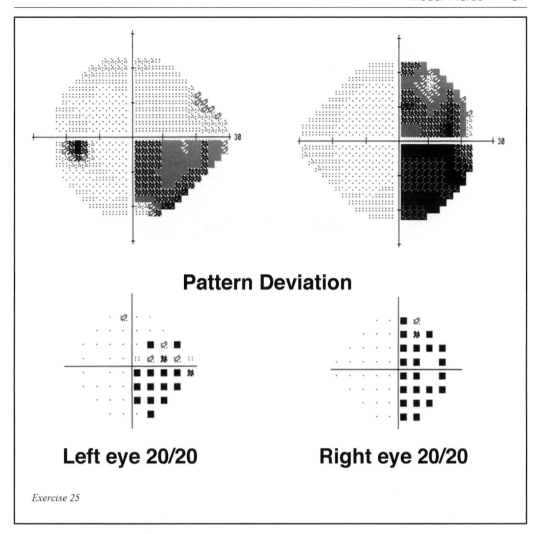

Pattern Deviation

Left eye 20/20

Right eye 20/20

Exercise 25

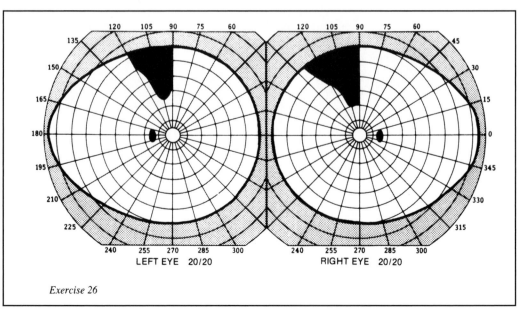

LEFT EYE   20/20

RIGHT EYE   20/20

Exercise 26

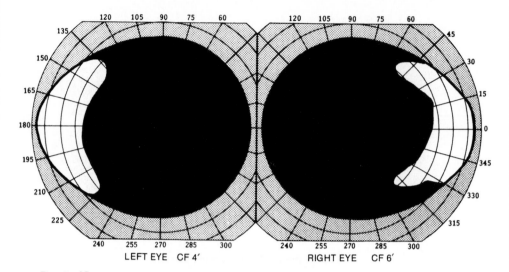

Exercise 27

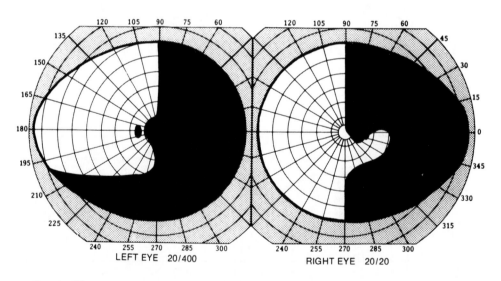

Exercise 28

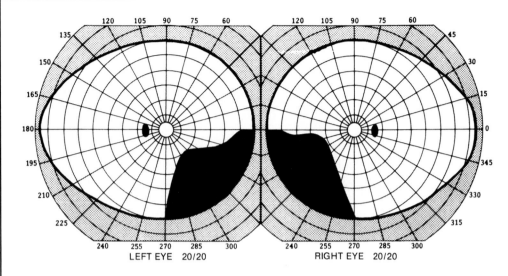

Exercise 29

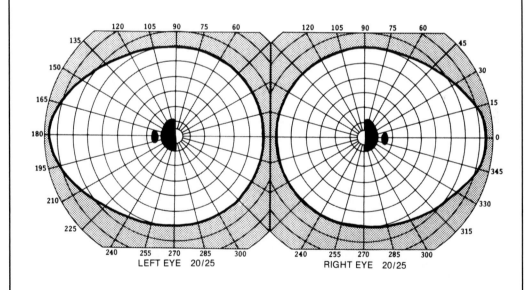

Exercise 30

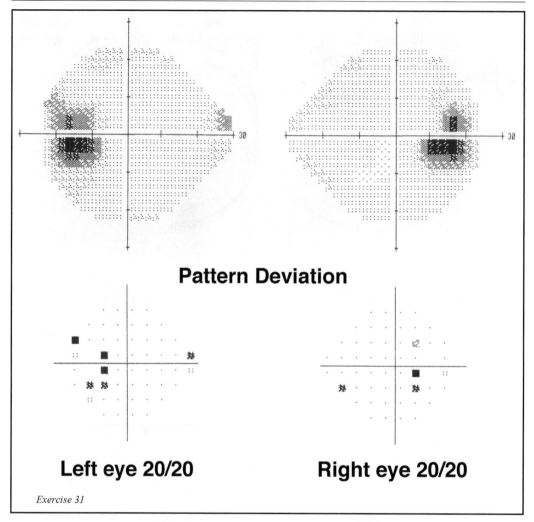

Pattern Deviation

Left eye 20/20   **Right eye 20/20**

Exercise 31

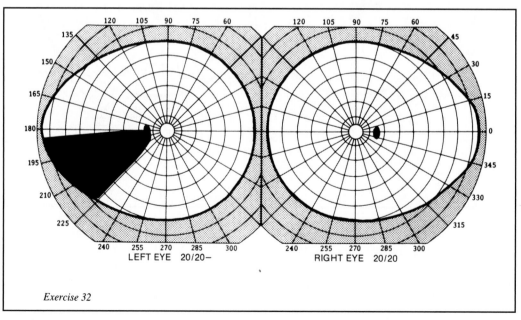

LEFT EYE   20/20−   RIGHT EYE   20/20

Exercise 32

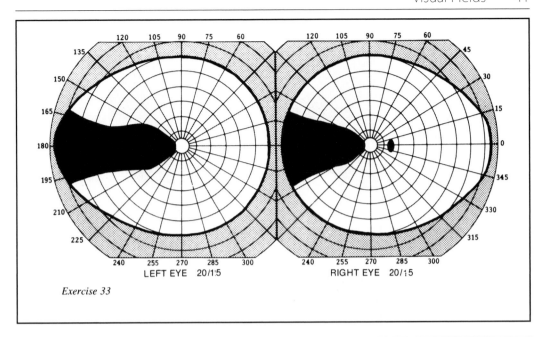

Exercise 33

LEFT EYE   20/15   RIGHT EYE   20/15

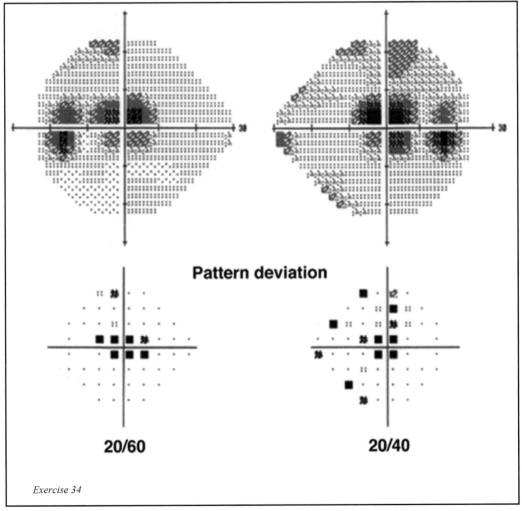

Pattern deviation

20/60   20/40

Exercise 34

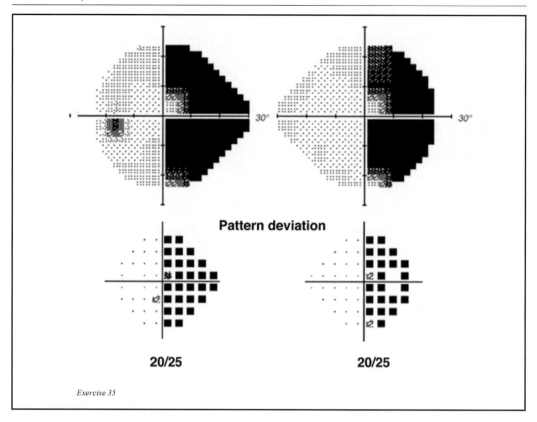

Pattern deviation

20/25   20/25

Exercise 35

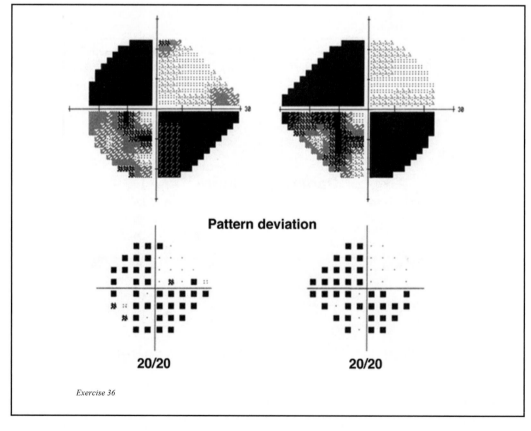

Pattern deviation

20/20   20/20

Exercise 36

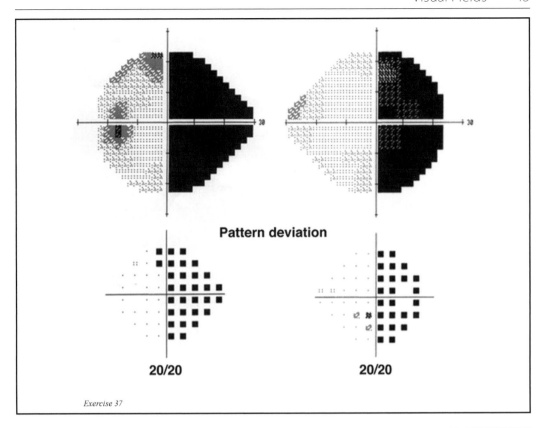

Pattern deviation

20/20   20/20

Exercise 37

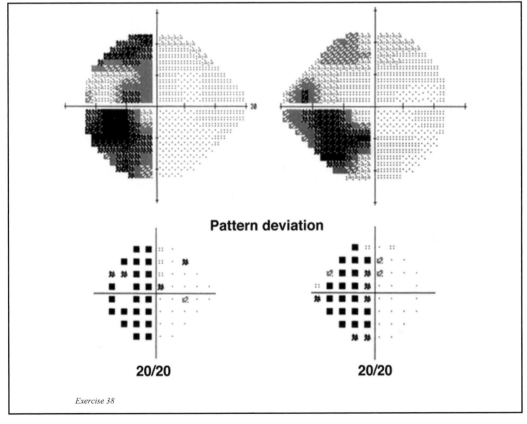

Pattern deviation

20/20   20/20

Exercise 38

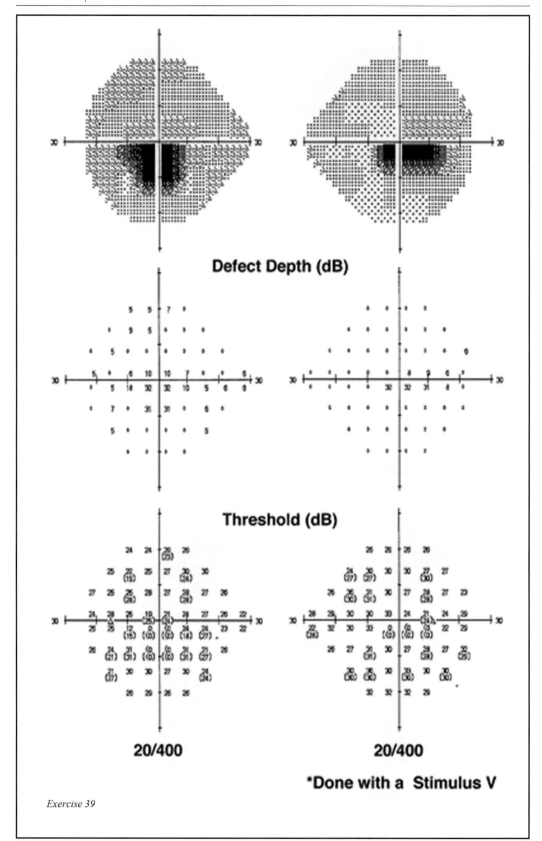

Defect Depth (dB)

Threshold (dB)

20/400

20/400

*Done with a Stimulus V

Exercise 39

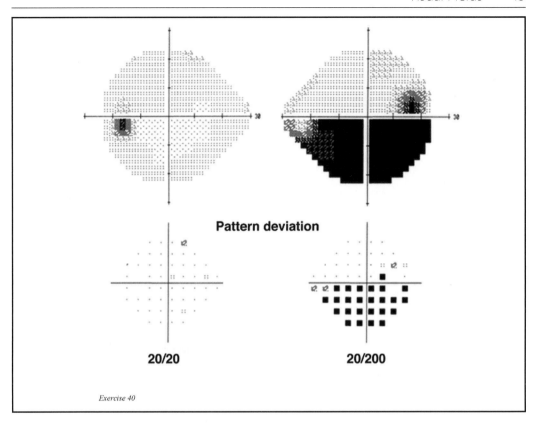

Pattern deviation

20/20   20/200

Exercise 40

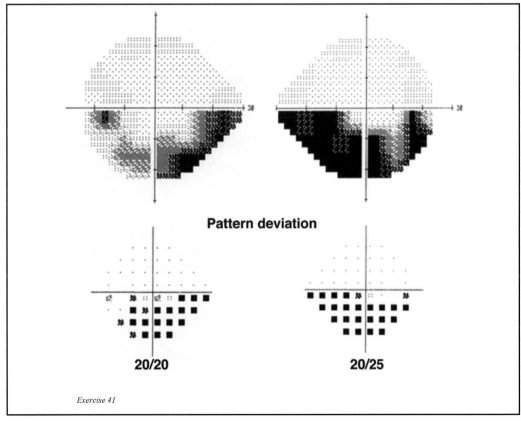

Pattern deviation

20/20   20/25

Exercise 41

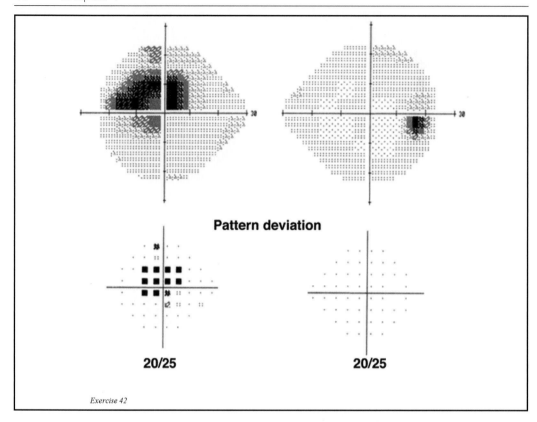

Pattern deviation

20/25   20/25

Exercise 42

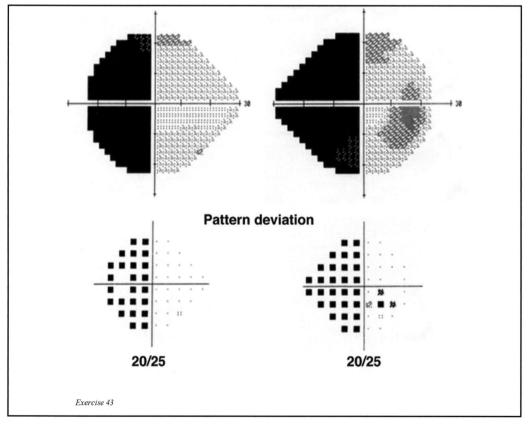

Pattern deviation

20/25   20/25

Exercise 43

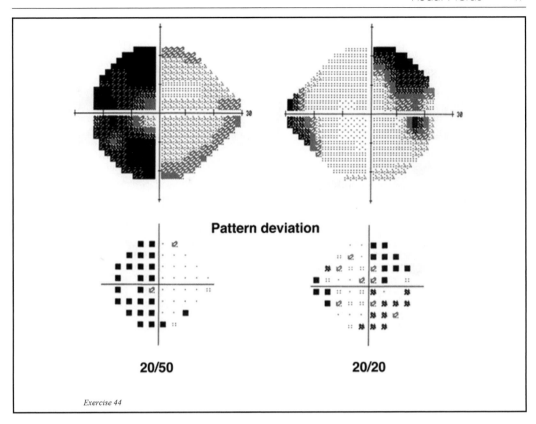

Pattern deviation

20/50   20/20

Exercise 44

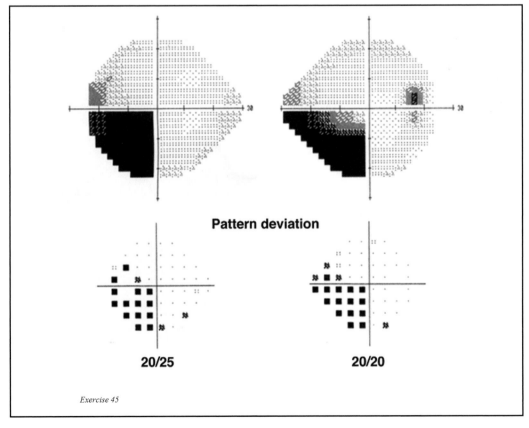

Pattern deviation

20/25   20/20

Exercise 45

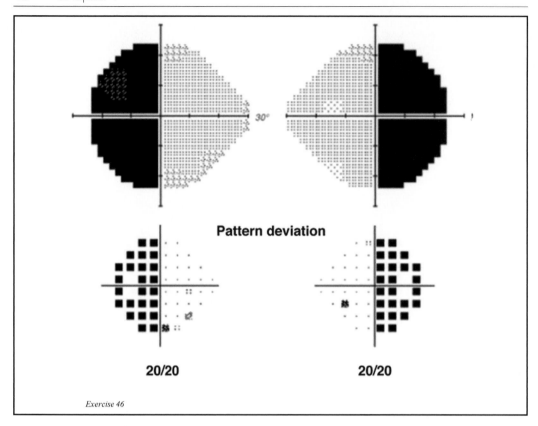

Pattern deviation

20/20   20/20

Exercise 46

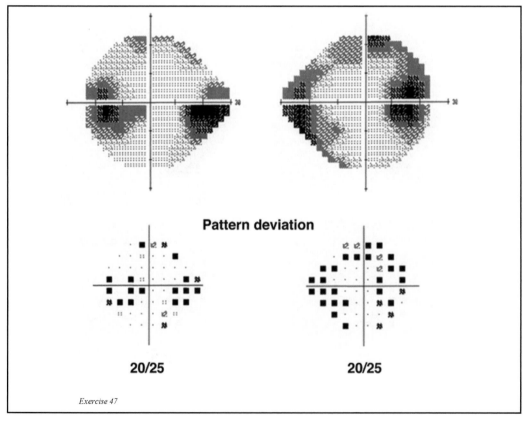

Pattern deviation

20/25   20/25

Exercise 47

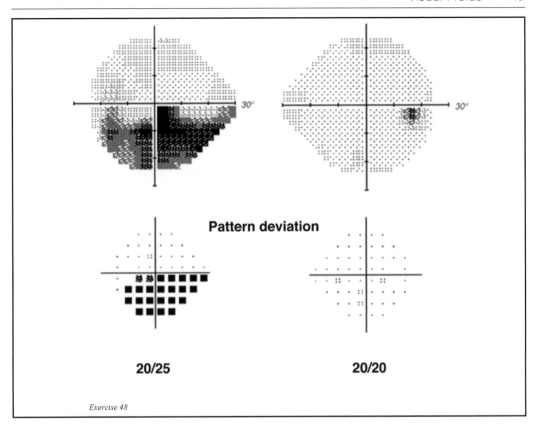

Exercise 48

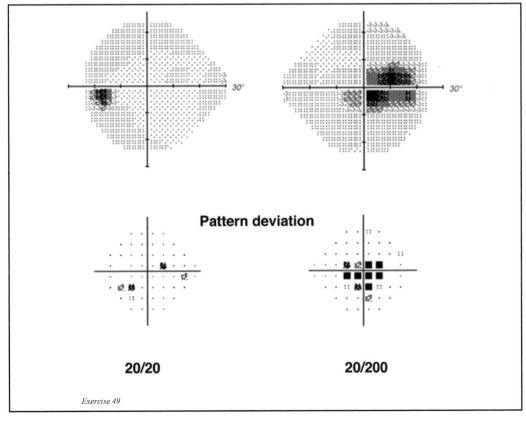

Exercise 49

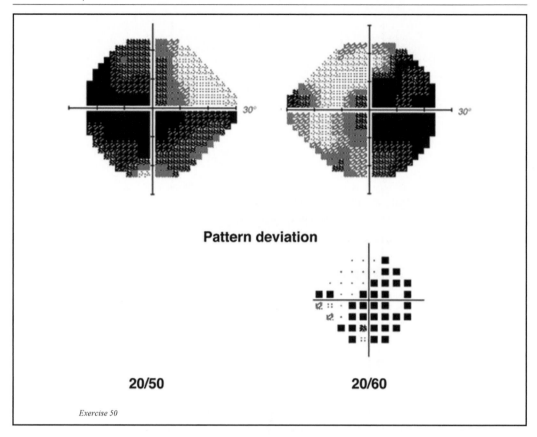

Pattern deviation

20/50   20/60

Exercise 50

PLAUSIBLE INTERPRETATIONS OF THE MYSTERY VISUAL FIELD DEFECTS

E1.   R homonymous hemianopia, incongruous, denser above but extending to fixation and into the inferior quadrants. L temporal lobe lesion extending to the L parietal lobe.

E2.   R homonymous hemianopia, central (macular), congruous. L occipital tip.

E3.   L homonymous hemianopia, denser above, markedly incongruous. Marked incongruity suggests possibility of R optic tract lesion, but greater density above suggests possibility of R temporal lobe lesion, which would also be 10 times more likely statistically.

E4.   R central scotoma; L temporal hemianopia; R optic nerve lesion at the junction of nerve and chiasm.

E5.   Bilateral ring scotomas with preservation of central 10 to 20 degrees with vision of 20/25 OU. Retinitis pigmentosa versus advanced glaucoma.

E6.   R homonymous superior quadrantanopia; congruous. L parietal versus occipital lesion. The congruity gives the edge to occipital localization.

E7.   Bilateral incomplete homonymous hemianopia, congruous. Bilateral occipital lesions.

E8.   Blind OD with temporal hemianopia OS. R optic nerve lesion extending into the chiasm.

E9.   Superior and inferior arcuate defects OS, creating a "ring" scotoma. OD: inferior arcuate scotoma and larger, superior arcuate scotoma breaking through nasally to create a nasal step. Glaucoma.

E10. L homonymous inferior quadrantanopia, congruous, with sparing of temporal crescent OS, and bilateral macular sparing. R occipital lesion, upper bank of the calcarine fissure.

E11. R superior NFL defect (Seidel scotoma). Glaucoma. Expect to see inferior elongation of the right cup.

E12. L homonymous hemianopia, complete (cannot make statement about congruity). R optic tract, parietal, or occipital lesion. OKN asymmetry would identify the parietal cases.

E13. Bilateral cecocentral scotomas. Bilateral optic neuropathy.

E14. Inferior nasal island remaining OD. Temporal hemianopia with involvement of central field OS. Extensive chiasmal lesion.

E15. Inferior NFB defect OS. OD normal. OS optic nerve lesion: glaucoma versus ischemic optic neuropathy (ION).

E16. Inferior NFB (altitudinal) defect OS with involvement of central field. Superior temporal cut OD. Lesion at junction of L optic nerve and chiasm (junctional scotoma).

E17. Inferior NFB (altitudinal) defect OS with involvement of the central field. Enlarged blind spot OD. Intracranial left optic nerve lesion. Be suspicious that the lesion is intracranial because the right optic disc appears to be edematous, probably due to increased intracranial pressure caused by the left optic nerve tumor (meningioma). Expect to see the disc changes associated with Foster Kennedy syndrome (optic atrophy OS and disc edema OD).

E18. R homonymous hemianopia, complete, with macular sparing. L occipital cortex.

E19. Inferior arcuate scotoma (NFB defect) OS. OD normal. Look for disc changes. Superior elongation of the cup (glaucoma). Lumpy disc (drusen).

E20. Tubular fields with discrepancy of size of remaining fields when comparing perimeter (20-A) and tangent screen (20-B) fields. "Tunnel" vision. Nonorganic field defects.

E21. Bitemporal hemianopia with central scotoma OS, junctional scotoma with lesion of the chiasm.

E22. Multiple central and paracentral defects OD. OS normal. Retinal lesions (chorioretinitis).

E23. R homonymous superior quadrantanopia, congruous, central, involving macular field. L occipital tip, inferior calcarine cortex.

E24. Bitemporal hemianopia. Chiasmatic lesion with some involvement of macular fibers, causing slightly decreased acuities.

E25. R homonymous hemianopia, markedly incongruous. L parietal lobe versus L optic tract.

E26. L homonymous superior quadrantanopia incongruous. "Pie in the sky" defects. R temporal lobe (Meyer loop) lesion.

E27. Temporal islands remaining OU. End-stage glaucoma.

E28. R homonymous hemianopia, incongruous, with central scotoma OS. L optic tract lesion at junction of tract and chiasm, affecting some of the crossing macular fibers of the left eye, causing decreased acuity in that eye.

E29. Bilateral inferior nasal contraction. Optic nerve or retinal lesions (optic disc drusen, glaucoma, retinoschisis).

E30. Bitemporal hemianopia, central (macular). Chiasm.

E31. Enlarged blind spots OU, causing pseudobitemporal (central) hemianopia: papilledema.

E32. Inferior-temporal wedge-shaped field defect OS. OD normal. A NFB defect affecting the superior-nasal bundle of nerve fibers (see Figures 1-8 and 1-10). An uncommon but well-documented glaucomatous field defect. May also represent the residual of optic neuropathy.

E33. Congruous horizontal wedge-shaped left homonymous, horizontal sectoranopia. A rare field defect due to a lesion of right LGN.

E34. Bilateral central scotomas. Bilateral maculopathy from hydroxychloroquine toxicity.

E35. R homonymous hemianopia, congruous, with slight macula sparing. L posterior cerebral artery (PCA) infarction.

E36. Bilateral homonymous hemianopia, congruous, checkerboard field. Bilateral occipital lobe damage.

E37. R homonymous hemianopia, congruous, enlarged blind spot OS. L hemispheric meningioma with papilledema.

E38. L homonymous hemianopia, incongruous. Demyelinating right optic tract lesion.

E39. Cecocentral scotoma OU. Bilateral optic neuropathy from Leber hereditary optic neuropathy (LHON).

E40. R inferior altitudinal defect OD, normal field OS. Nonarteritic anterior ION OD.

E41. Inferior arcuate defects OU. Optic nerve drusen OU.

E42. Superior defect nearly respecting the horizontal meridian OS, normal field OD. Retinal scar inferiorly OS.

E43. L homonymous hemianopia, congruous. Right PCA infarction.

E44. Superior temporal depression OD and a dense temporal defect with central involvement (decreased visual acuity) OS. Chiasmal syndrome.

E45. L homonymous inferior quadrantanopia, relatively congruous. R parietal tumor.

E46. Dense bitemporal hemianopia. Large sellar/suprasellar pituitary adenoma.

E47. Enlarged blind spot with nasal depression OU. Papilledema.

E48. L inferior altitudinal defect, normal field OD. Nonarteritic anterior ION OS.

E49. Cecocentral scotoma OD, normal field OS. Neuroretinitis OD.

E50. Constricted field more temporally with central and nasal involvement OD and a defect more temporally and inferiorly OS. Bilateral optic neuritis.

REFERENCES

1. Horton JC. Wilbrand's knee of the primate chiasm is an artifact of monocular enucleation. *Trans Am Ophthalmol Soc*. 1997;95:579-609.

2. Karanjia N, Jacobson DM. Compression of the prechiasmatic optic nerve produces a junctional scotoma. *Am J Ophthalmol*. 1999;128:256-258.

BIBLIOGRAPHY

Anderson DR. *Perimetry: With and Without Automation*. 2nd ed. St. Louis, MO: CV Mosby; 1987.

Barton JJS, Hefter R, Chang B, et al. The field defects of anterior temporal lobectomy: a quantitative reassessment of Meyer's loop. *Brain*. 2005;128:2123-2133.

Bundez PL. *Atlas of Visual Fields*. Philadelphia, PA: Lippincott-Raven; 1997.

Frisén L. Identification of functional visual field loss by automated static perimetry. *Acta Ophthalmol*. 2014;92:805-809.

Hershenfeld SA, Sharpe JA. Monocular temporal hemianopia. *Br J Ophthalmol*. 1993;77:424-427.

Horton JC, Hoyt WF. The representation of the visual field in human striate cortex. A revision of the classic Holmes map. *Arch Ophthalmol*. 1991;109:816-824.

Kedar S, Zhang X, Lynn MJ, Newman NJ, Biousse V. Congruency in homonymous hemianopia. *Am J Ophthalmol*. 2007;143:772-780.

Kerr NM, Chew SS, Eady EK, et al. Diagnostic accuracy of confrontation visual field tests. *Neurology*. 2010;74:1184-1190.

Lee JH, Tobias S, Kwon JT, Sade B, Kosmorsky G. Wilbrand's knee: does it exist? *Surg Neurol*. 2006;66:11-17.

Liu GT, Volpe NJ, Galetta SL. Visual loss: overview, visual field testing, and topical diagnosis. In: *Neuro-Ophthalmology: Diagnosis and Management*. 2nd ed. New York, NY: Saunders Elsevier; 2010:39-52.

Marsiglia M, Odel JG, Rudich DS, et al. Photopsia and a temporal visual field defect. *Surv Ophthalmol*. 2016;61:363-367.

Pandit RJ, Gales K, Griffiths PG. Effectiveness of testing visual fields by confrontation. *Lancet*. 2001;358:1339-1340.

Pasu S, Ridha BH, Wagh V, et al. Homonymous sectoranopia: asymptomatic presentation of a lateral geniculate nucleus lesion. *Neuroophthalmology*. 2015;39:289-294.

Sadun AA, Agarwal MR. Topical diagnosis of acquired optic nerve disorders. In: Miller NR, Newman NJ, eds. *Walsh and Hoyt's Clinical Neuro-Ophthalmology*. 6th ed. Vol 1. Philadelphia, PA: Lippincott Williams & Wilkins; 2005:197-236.

Walsh TJ, ed. *Visual Fields: Examination and Interpretation. Ophthalmology Monographs Volume 3*. San Francisco, CA: American Academy of Ophthalmology; 1996.

Wang AMF, Sharpe JA. Representation of the visual field in the human occipital cortex. A magnetic resonance imaging and perimetric correlation. *Arch Ophthalmol*. 1999;117:208-217.

Zhang X, Kedar S, Lynn MJ, et al. Homonymous hemianopias: clinical-anatomic correlations in 904 cases. *Neurology*. 2006;66:906-910.

CHAPTER 2

Supranuclear and Internuclear Gaze Pathways

MARK F. WALKER, MD

I. **SIX TYPES OF EYE MOVEMENTS, 5 CONJUGATE AND 1 DISCONJUGATE, AND THE FIXATION SYSTEM CONTROL THE POSITION OF THE FOVEA (TABLE 2-1)**

    A. Saccades and quick phases direct the fovea to a new location in the visual scene

    B. Pursuit, optokinetic slow phases, and vestibular slow phases stabilize images on the fovea

    C. Vergence moves the eyes in opposite directions to realign the 2 foveas

II. **FUNCTIONAL CLASSIFICATION OF EYE MOVEMENTS**

    A. Saccades

        1. Purpose: to shift gaze (the fovea) to a new location in the visual scene

        2. Stimuli

            a. Sudden appearance of a new stimulus (visual, auditory, somatosensory): reflexive saccade (look toward a possible threat)

            b. Voluntary change in gaze direction to another point in an already visible scene: voluntary saccade (eg, visual scanning)

        3. Saccades are very fast, and the speed of the saccade depends on its size (bigger saccades are faster)

        4. Visual "suppression" during saccades: even though the visual world is sweeping rapidly across the retina, there is no sense of a blurred image

        5. Saccades are assessed by asking the patient to look back and forth between 2 targets, observing accuracy (are corrections required because the eyes do not land on target?), speed (the eyes should jump quickly from one target to the next), and latency (how long does it take for the eyes to move?)

    B. Quick phases

        1. Purpose: to reset the position of the eyes during nystagmus so they do not reach an extreme orbital position

        2. Quick phases are very similar to saccades, for which they are the phylogenetic forerunner

        3. Quick phases can be examined during optokinetic stimulation (see page 56, II, D) or during prolonged rotation (eg, on a swivel chair)

Foroozan R, Vaphiades MS. *Kline's Neuro-Ophthalmology Review Manual, Eighth Edition (pp 55-81).* © 2018 SLACK Incorporated.

Table 2-1

CLASSIFICATION OF EYE MOVEMENTS

Type	Function
Conjugate Eye Movements	
Saccades	Redirect the fovea
Quick phases of nystagmus	Reset eye position toward the oncoming visual scene
Pursuit	Tracks a moving object
Vestibular slow phases	Keep image on the fovea when the head is moving
Optokinetic slow phases	Track full-field visual motion
Disconjugate Eye Movements	
Vergence	Aligns both foveas on the same object in the visual scene

C. Pursuit
   1. Purpose: to allow the fovea to maintain fixation of a moving target
   2. Stimuli
      a. Motion of the image of a target across the foveal and parafoveal retina (retinal slip)
      b. Nonvisual stimuli, such as proprioception, can also evoke pursuit (eg, following one's own fingers in darkness)
   3. When a target starts moving, the eyes first accelerate (over about 100 ms) to the target speed, then track it by matching eye speed to target speed
   4. Pursuit gain is defined as the ratio of eye speed to target speed
   5. If the eyes cannot keep up with the target (either because the target is moving too fast or because pursuit is deficient), then catch-up saccades bring the foveas back on target, leading to jerky-appearing saccadic pursuit
   6. Pursuit is examined by having the patient track a slow- and smooth-moving target (eg, a pen or light); both horizontal and vertical pursuit should be assessed as they can be differentially impaired
D. Optokinetic responses
   1. Purpose: to stabilize the visual image on the retina when the whole visual scene is moving
   2. Stimulus: motion of the entire visual scene across the retina due to prolonged self-motion (eg, looking out of the window while riding on a train)
   3. The optokinetic system supplements vestibular responses during prolonged motion
   4. OKN can be elicited with a striped tape or drum: observe both slow and quick phases
E. Vestibulo-ocular reflex (VOR)
   1. Purpose: the VOR generates an eye movement in the direction opposite to that of the head motion in order to keep the stationary visual image stable on the retina, maintaining clear vision when the head moves
   2. Stimuli: the vestibular system is activated by 2 types of head motion—rotations and translations (linear motion)

3. Head motion is sensed by the vestibular labyrinth of the inner ear
    a. The 3 semicircular canals (horizontal or lateral, anterior or superior, posterior) sense head rotations
    b. The 2 otolith organs (utricle and saccule) sense head translations
4. The compensatory eye movement of the VOR is called a "slow phase," although it can be fast (> 200 degrees/second) if the head is rotating quickly
5. Failure of the VOR leads to oscillopsia (the illusion that the world is moving) during head motion
6. The VOR is tested with the head impulse maneuver (see page 69, V, E, 1, b)

F. Vergence
1. Purpose: vergence eye movements realign the foveas on a new object at a different depth (viewing distance)
2. Stimuli:
    a. Different positions of the image of an object on the retinas of the 2 eyes (retinal disparity). This leads to fusional vergence
    b. Loss of focus of images on the retina (retinal blur). This leads to accommodative vergence
3. Vergence movements are disconjugate: they rotate the eyes in opposite directions
4. Vergence eye movements can be horizontal (convergence, divergence), vertical, or torsional (excyclovergence, incyclovergence)
5. To test convergence, ask the patient to fixate a target and move the target slowly toward the head; observe adduction of both eyes

G. Fixation
1. Purpose: the fixation system is an additional system that keeps the eyes still in the orbits to maintain gaze when neither the head nor the object is moving
2. To examine fixation, instruct the patient to maintain steady gaze of a fixed target; fixation may be interrupted by nystagmus or saccadic intrusions (see Chapter 3)

III. NEURAL PATHWAYS FOR EYE MOVEMENTS (FIGURE 2-1)
A. Saccade pathways
1. Mediated by parallel pathways (Figure 2-2)
    a. Frontal cortex—frontal eye field (FEF), supplementary eye field, dorsolateral prefrontal cortex (to the superior colliculus [SC] and directly to the brainstem saccade generators [BSGs])
    b. Posterior parietal cortex (PPC) to the SC
2. The frontocollicular pathway generates voluntary saccades, and the parietocollicular pathway generates reflexive saccades to novel targets
3. Horizontal saccades
    a. Originate in the FEF and PPC, contralateral to the saccade direction (eg, the right FEF and PPC generate leftward saccades)
    b. Cortical saccade neurons project to the SC on the same side. The FEF also projects to the BSG directly and through the basal ganglia. This allows for saccades to be preserved if the SC is lesioned
    c. Natural or electrical stimulation of the SC elicits a contraversive saccade. The SC has a topographic map; each position corresponds to a saccade of a particular size and direction
    d. The SC projects to the BSG on the opposite side
    e. The BSG converts the spatial code of the SC signal (specifying the saccade vector) to a rate code (the innervation signal for the ocular motor neurons)

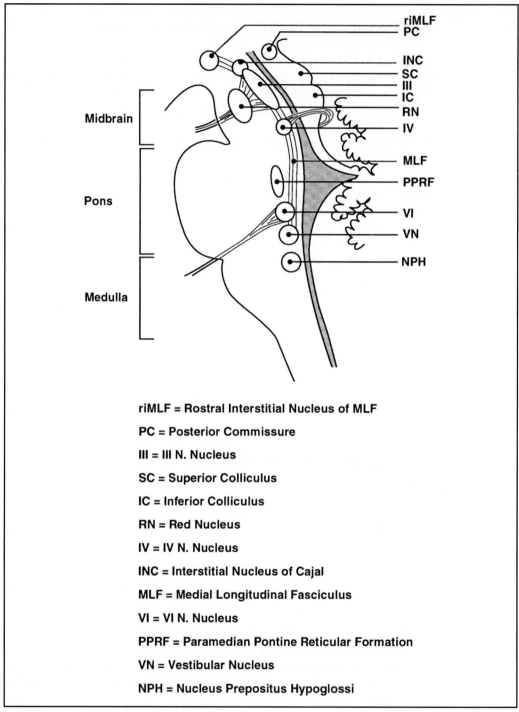

Figure 2-1. Sagittal view of the brainstem showing structures important for the generation of horizontal and vertical gaze.

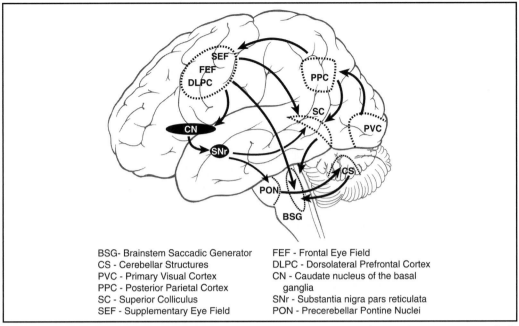

BSG- Brainstem Saccadic Generator
CS - Cerebellar Structures
PVC - Primary Visual Cortex
PPC - Posterior Parietal Cortex
SC - Superior Colliculus
SEF - Supplementary Eye Field

FEF - Frontal Eye Field
DLPC - Dorsolateral Prefrontal Cortex
CN - Caudate nucleus of the basal
    ganglia
SNr - Substantia nigra pars reticulata
PON - Precerebellar Pontine Nuclei

Figure 2-2. Saccadic eye movement pathways. Cerebellar structures (CS) of particular importance include the vermis and fastigial nucleus.

    f.   The saccade signal consists of 2 elements (Figure 2-3)
        i.   A high-frequency burst (the pulse) immediately preceding the saccade overcomes orbital viscosity to move the eye quickly to its new position. The pulse is generated by the burst neurons. Without a pulse, the eyes move very slowly
        ii. A new tonic signal (the step) provides the appropriate innervation to hold the eyes at the new position against elastic restoring forces. The step is generated by integrating the pulse (the neural integrator). Without a step, the eye drifts back to the center of the orbit
    g.   There are separate saccade generators for horizontal and vertical saccades (Table 2-2)
    h.   Excitatory burst neurons are tonically inhibited by omnipause neurons in the raphe interpositus to prevent unwanted saccades. This inhibition must be released for a saccade to occur
    i.   The cerebellar vermis, through the fastigial nucleus, adjusts innervation to maintain saccade accuracy and adapt to changes (eg, extraocular muscle weakness)

  4. Vertical saccades
    a.   Cortical pathways descend to the rostral interstitial nucleus of the medial longitudinal fasciculus (riMLF) in the midbrain just rostral to the oculomotor (III cranial nerve) nucleus at the junction of the midbrain and thalamus
    b.   Bilateral FEF or SC stimulation is required to elicit purely vertical saccades
    c.   There are different pathways for upward and downward saccades: upward burst neurons in the riMLF project bilaterally, whereas downward burst neurons project only ipsilaterally (Figure 2-4)

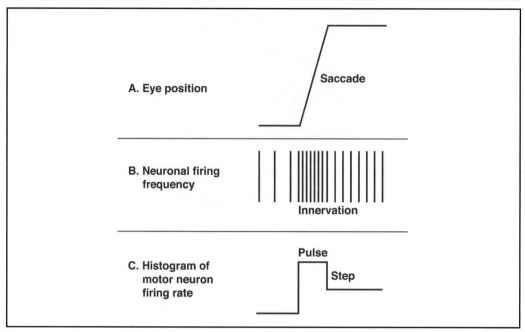

Figure 2-3. Pulse-step change of innervation that produces saccades and quick phases of nystagmus. Ocular motor neurons generate a high frequency discharge (pulse) that moves the eye at high velocity, followed by a tonic discharge (step) that maintains the desired eye position.

Table 2-2		
BRAINSTEM SACCADE GENERATORS		
	Horizontal Saccades	**Vertical Saccades**
Burst neurons	Paramedian pontine reticular formation (PPRF)	riMLF
Integrator	Nucleus prepositus hypoglossi (NPH) and medial vestibular nucleus (MVN)	Interstitial nucleus of Cajal (INC)

    B.   Pursuit pathways
        1.   Although classically viewed as distinct, data are suggesting that there is substantial overlap between the brain areas controlling pursuit and saccades
        2.   Several cortical areas are involved in pursuit (Figure 2-5)
            a.   Medial temporal (MT) and medial superior temporal (MST) cortex: these areas at the parieto-temporal-occipital junction process visual motion signals that drive pursuit
            b.   FEF: lesions dramatically reduce pursuit gain
            c.   PPC

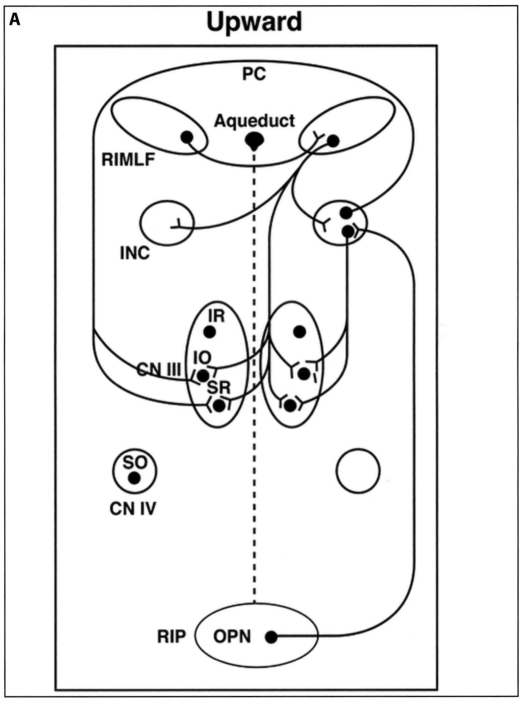

Figure 2-4. Brainstem pathways for vertical saccades. (A) Upward: The riMLF contains saccadic excitatory burst neurons (EBN) and receives an inhibitory input from omnipause neurons (OPN) of the nucleus raphe interpositus (RIP). Upward EBNs project bilaterally to the INC and to the motoneurons of both SR and IO muscles. The INC integrates the pulse of the EBNs to a tonic signal for upward gaze that is delivered to the ipsilateral III cranial nerve and, via the posterior commissure (PC), to the contralateral III cranial nerve. (Adapted from Leigh RJ, Zee DS. *The Neurology of Eye Movements*. 5th ed. New York, NY: Oxford University Press; 2015:396.)[1] *(continued)*

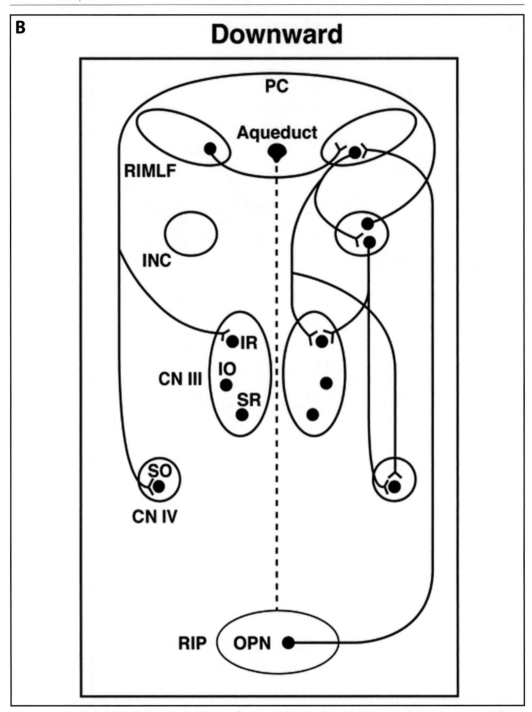

Figure 2-4 (continued). Brainstem pathways for vertical saccades. (B) Downward: EBNs project unilaterally to the INC and to the motoneurons of the ipsilateral IR and contralateral SO (remember that trochlear nerve axons cross the midline before exiting the brainstem). As for upward saccades, INC neurons carry the tonic signal bilaterally to the III and IV cranial nerves. (Adapted from Leigh RJ, Zee DS. *The Neurology of Eye Movements*. 5th ed. New York, NY: Oxford University Press; 2015:396.)[1]

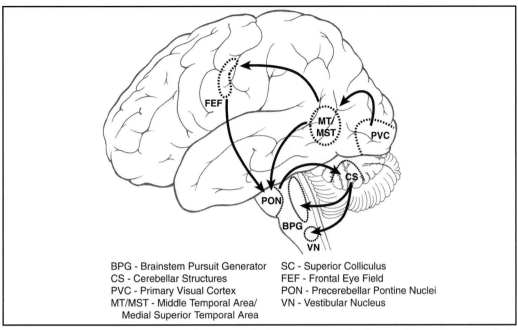

BPG - Brainstem Pursuit Generator
CS - Cerebellar Structures
PVC - Primary Visual Cortex
MT/MST - Middle Temporal Area/
　　　　Medial Superior Temporal Area

SC - Superior Colliculus
FEF - Frontal Eye Field
PON - Precerebellar Pontine Nuclei
VN - Vestibular Nucleus

Figure 2-5. Pursuit eye movement pathways. Cerebellar structures (CS) of particular importance include vermis, flocculus, and paraflocculus.

d. The cerebral cortex primarily controls ipsiversive pursuit (opposite to saccades). Hemispheric lesions generally impair pursuit toward the side of the lesion

e. Pure occipital lesions cause homonymous hemianopia, but patients can generally pursue in either direction as long as the target is in the intact visual hemifield

f. Parietal lesions may also cause akinetopsia (impaired motion perception)

g. Because several cerebellar structures are important for pursuit (see Figure 2-5), diffuse cerebellar disease severely impairs pursuit

C. Optokinetic slow-phases

1. In afoveates, optokinetic responses are elicited via the accessory optic system through retinal projections to the nucleus of the optic tract in the pretectum

2. In humans, responses to full-field visual motion likely involve both cortical and subcortical mechanisms

D. Vergence

1. Visual signals from occipital cortex project to vergence premotor neurons in the midbrain reticular formation (MRF)

2. Three types of premotor neurons in the MRF:

a. Vergence tonic cells: discharge in relation to vergence angle

b. Vergence burst cells: discharge in relation to vergence velocity

c. Vergence burst-tonic cells: combine position and velocity signals

3. Premotor neurons project to the oculomotor (III cranial nerve) nuclear complex to elicit the near triad: convergence, accommodation, miosis

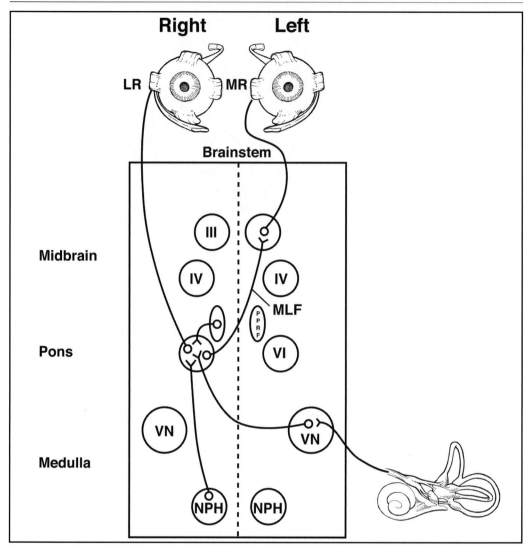

Right   Left

LR   MR

Brainstem

Midbrain

III

IV   IV

MLF

P
P
R
F

Pons

VI

Medulla

VN   VN

NPH   NPH

Figure 2-6. Brainstem pathways for horizontal gaze. Axons from cell bodies in the PPRF travel to ipsilateral VI where they synapse with abducens motoneurons, axons of which travel to ipsilateral lateral rectus (LR). Abducens internuclear neurons have axons that cross the midline and travel in the MLF to contact medial rectus (MR) motoneurons in contralateral III. Eye position information (neural integrator) reaches VI from neurons within the NPH and VN. (Adapted from Leigh RJ, Zee DS. *The Neurology of Eye Movements*. 4th ed. New York, NY: Oxford University Press; 2006:263.)[2]

IV. Binocular Coordination

A. Most eye movements (except for vergence) are conjugate—the eyes move together in the same direction by roughly the same amount. To accomplish this, the brain must coordinate the movements of the 2 eyes

B. Horizontal eye movements are coordinated through the projection of abducens interneurons via the MLF to contralateral medial rectus (MR) motoneurons (Figure 2-6)

1. Premotor commands for horizontal saccades (in the PPRF) and horizontal pursuit (from the VN) are sent to the adjacent abducens nucleus, to both abducens motoneurons and abducens interneurons

2. Abducens motoneurons innervate the ipsilateral lateral rectus, leading to abduction

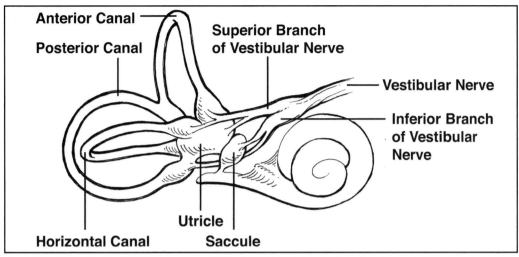

Figure 2-7. Membranous labyrinth of inner ear. Superior branch of vestibular nerve innervates anterior canal, horizontal canal, and utricle. Inferior branch innervates posterior canal and saccule.

3. Abducens interneurons send their axons across the midline to the contralateral MLF, where they ascend to the oculomotor nucleus (III cranial nerve), synapsing on MR motoneurons

4. Thus, there is a coordinated abduction of one eye and adduction of the other

C. Vertical eye movements are coordinated in the midbrain

1. Burst neurons (riMLF) and tonic neurons (INC) project directly to motoneurons of yoked muscles (eg, right SR and left IO). This differs from the horizontal system, where the eyes are yoked by abducens interneurons

2. The SR and SO muscles have crossed innervation (eg, the left trochlear nucleus innervates the right SO muscle). This facilitates binocular coordination because cell bodies innervating yoked muscles (eg, right SO and left IR muscles) are on the same side of the brainstem (left)

V. **VESTIBULO-OCULAR REFLEX**

A. The VOR generates an eye movement in the opposite direction as the head movement and of the appropriate speed to keep the visual image of the external world still on the retina as the head moves

B. Head motion is sensed by the vestibular labyrinth (Figure 2-7)

1. The 3 semicircular canals (horizontal or lateral, anterior or superior, posterior) sense head rotations

2. The 2 otolith organs (utricle, saccule) sense head orientation relative to gravity and linear motion of the head

3. "Labyrinth-within-a-labyrinth": The membranous labyrinth (filled with potassium-rich endolymph) sits within the bony labyrinth (filled with cerebrospinal fluid [CSF]-like perilymph) in the petrous portion of the temporal bone

C. Each semicircular canal has a particular orientation that determines the direction of the rotations that stimulate it. The 3 canals are roughly orthogonal to each other (Figure 2-8)

1. The horizontal canals (HCs) are located in a plane that is tilted about 30 degrees up from the earth-horizontal plane. Each HC is excited by a rotation toward it and inhibited by a rotation away from it (eg, rightward rotation excites the right HC and inhibits the left HC)

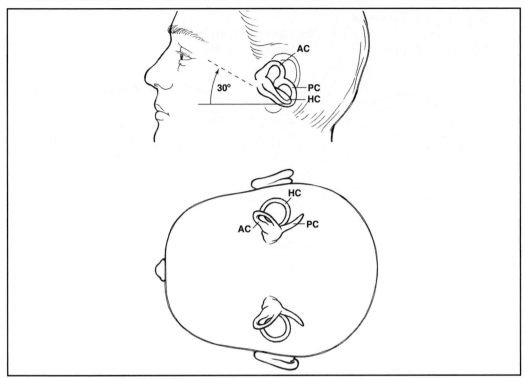

Figure 2-8. Orientation of semicircular canals on sagittal (top) and axial (bottom) projections. AC = anterior canal, HC = horizontal canal, PC = posterior canal.

2. The anterior (AC) and posterior canals (PC) are each oriented about midway between the sagittal and coronal planes

3. The canals are arranged in 3 pairs (RHC-LHC, RAC-LPC, LAC-RPC), each of which is roughly in a common plane. These canals operate in a "push-pull" fashion: a given rotation excites one canal in the pair and inhibits the other

4. Each canal pair is associated with a pair of extraocular muscles that lies roughly in the same plane (Figure 2-9; Table 2-3)

5. The basic pathway of the VOR is a "3-neuron arc": primary vestibular afferent, secondary vestibular neuron, extraocular motoneuron (see Figure 2-9)

6. When the head rotates, inertia of the endolymph causes it to lag behind, resulting in a relative motion of endolymph within the membranous canal (eg, rightward rotation leads to leftward endolymph motion)

7. At one end of each canal is a membrane called the *cupula*. Endolymph motion bows the cupula, causing deflection of hair cell stereocilia

8. Bending of the stereocilia affects the opening of ion channels, controlling hair cell potential

9. A change in hair cell potential is transmitted to the vestibular afferent, which changes its firing rate up or down, depending on whether the rotation is in the excitatory or inhibitory direction

10. The vestibular afferent projects to secondary vestibular neurons in the VN

11. Secondary neurons project to the ocular motor nuclei (eg, abducens for the horizontal VOR)

12. Binocular gaze pathways ensure that movements of the 2 eyes are coordinated

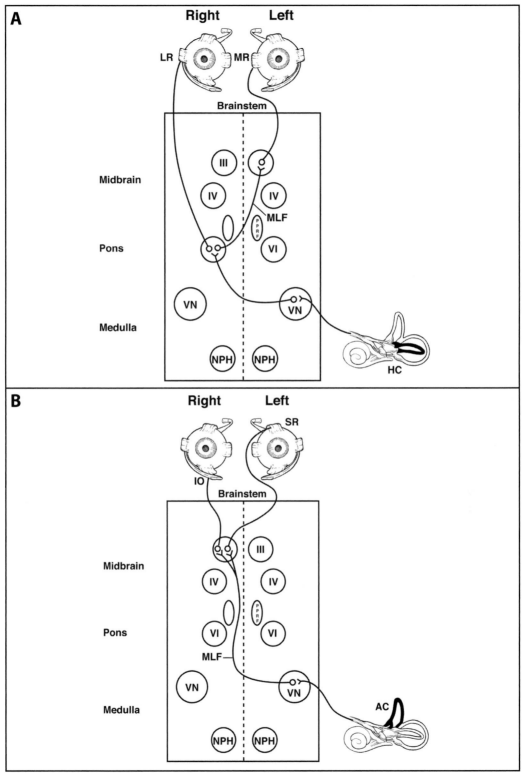

Figure 2-9. (A) Excitatory connections between horizontal semicircular canal and yoked extraocular muscles. (B) Excitatory connections between anterior semicircular canal and yoked extraocular muscles. *(continued)*

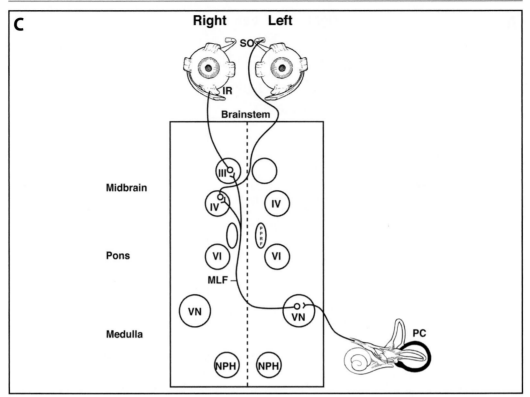

Figure 2-9 (continued). (C) Excitatory connections between posterior semicircular canal and yoked extraocular muscles.

Table 2-3

SEMICIRCULAR CANAL PAIRS AND ACTIVATED EYE MUSCLES				
Head Motion	**Excited Canal**	**Inhibited Canal**	**Right Eye**	**Left Eye**
Rightward	Right horizontal	Left horizontal	Medial rectus	Lateral rectus
Leftward	Left horizontal	Right horizontal	Lateral rectus	Medial rectus
Down/right	Right anterior	Left posterior	Superior rectus	Inferior oblique
Up/left	Left posterior	Right anterior	Inferior rectus	Superior oblique
Up/right	Right posterior	Left anterior	Superior oblique	Inferior rectus
Down/left	Left anterior	Right posterior	Inferior oblique	Superior rectus

D. Vestibular imbalance produces nystagmus
1. Each vestibular nerve has a resting discharge rate (~100 spikes/sec)
2. When the head is not moving, both vestibular nerves are discharging at the same rate (balanced)
3. When the head rotates, the discharge rate increases on one side and decreases on the other (eg, rightward rotation leads to an increased firing rate of the right vestibular nerve and a decreased rate of the left vestibular nerve)

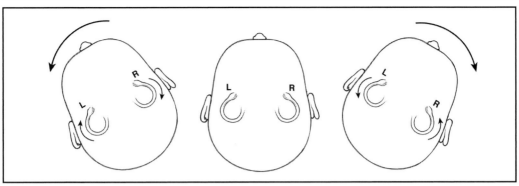

Figure 2-10. Doll's eye testing. When the head is rotated to the left, the endolymph moves toward the left ampulla and away from the right ampulla. When the head is rotated to the right, the endolymph moves toward the right ampulla and away from the left ampulla.

    4.   The imbalance in vestibular nerve inputs tells the brain that the head is moving

    5.   The VOR generates a compensatory eye movement (the slow phase) in the direction opposite to that of head rotation

    6.   Quick phases reset the position of the eyes and keep them from reaching extreme positions in the orbits

    7.   The combination of slow and quick phases is nystagmus

    8.   Nystagmus is often described by the direction of its quick phases, even though the slow phases are what really indicate what is happening in the vestibular system (eg, rightward rotation elicits leftward slow phases and a right-beating nystagmus)

  E.   Clinical testing of vestibular function

    1.   Head rotation

        a.   The "doll's eye" maneuver (Figure 2-10): the examiner moves the head back and forth slowly while the subject maintains visual fixation (eg, of the examiner's nose)

        b.   The head impulse test (Figure 2-11): the head is moved quickly but not far

           i.   A catch-up saccade at the end of the head rotation indicates a poor VOR

          ii.   The head impulse test has 2 advantages over slow ("doll's eye") rotations: it can test any single canal in isolation and it is less likely to be confounded by pursuit. The head impulse test is the best bedside test for impaired peripheral vestibular function

        c.   Head rotation testing is helpful in assessing the range of eye movements in infants (Figure 2-12)

    2.   Caloric testing

        a.   Test of HC function

        b.   Uses a combination of gravity and a thermal gradient across the labyrinth to cause cupular deflection

        c.   The subject is positioned so that the HCs are oriented vertically, to maximize the effect of gravity on the endolymph (about 30 degrees up from the supine position; Figure 2-13A)

        d.   The external auditory canal (EAC) is irrigated with warm (44°C) or cool (30°C) water (Figures 2-13B and C)

        e.   Warm water is excitatory and cool water is inhibitory, eliciting a corresponding nystagmus

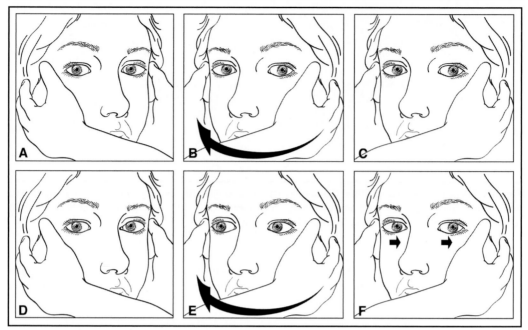

Figure 2-11. Head impulse test. Testing of the right HC is illustrated (A through C: normal response; D through F: patient with vestibular hypofunction). The examiner begins with the patient's head turned slightly to the left (A, D). While the patient attempts to maintain fixation of a target, the head is turned quickly to the right. When vestibular function is intact, the eyes will rotate to the left in the orbits as the head turns, so that they are still looking at the target at the end of the head movement (B). No corrective saccade is needed (C). When right HC function is impaired, the eyes do not counter-rotate, but move with the head, taking fixation off the target (E). A leftward corrective saccade is made to refixate the target (F). This corrective saccade is the "head impulse sign" that indicates right vestibular hypofunction.

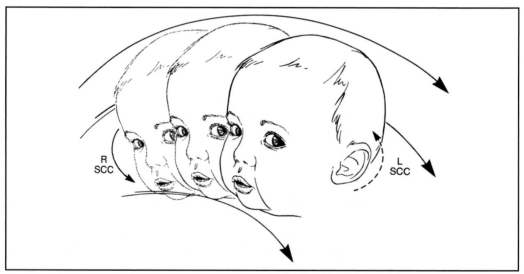

Figure 2-12. Rotational testing for eye movement function in infants. As the infant is turned toward his or her left (toward the examiner's right), the eye will tonically deviate in the direction of the movement with jerk phase of nystagmus toward the opposite side. This leads to stimulation of the right semicircular canals (SCC) and inhibition of the left SCC.

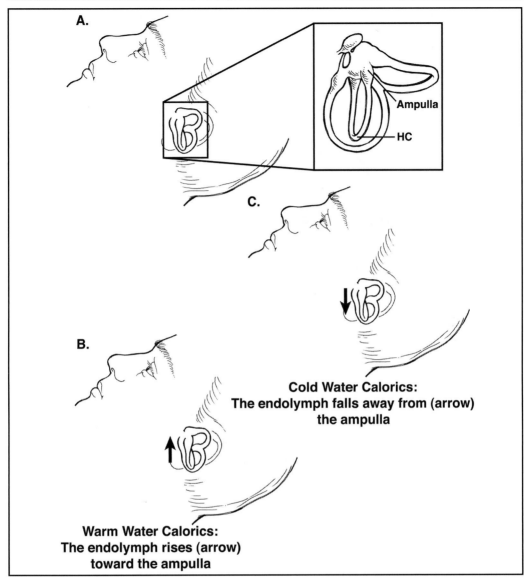

A.

Ampulla

HC

C.

Cold Water Calorics:
The endolymph falls away from (arrow)
the ampulla

B.

Warm Water Calorics:
The endolymph rises (arrow)
toward the ampulla

Figure 2-13. With head elevated 30 degrees, HC is oriented in vertical direction, allowing for maximal effect with caloric testing.

    f.   Example: warm water in the right EAC excites the right HC, eliciting leftward slow phases and a right-beating nystagmus (Figures 2-14 and 2-15)

    g.   Cool water inhibits the right HC and causes a left-beating nystagmus (Figure 2-16)

    h.   A lesion of one labyrinth will result in a reduced nystagmus response from irrigation of that side

3.   Comatose patients

    a.   Caloric irrigation is used to test whether the lower brainstem is intact in comatose patients

    b.   To maximize the stimulus, ice water is used

    c.   Comatose patients do not have quick phases, so there is no nystagmus, only a tonic drift of the eyes toward the irrigated (inhibited) ear

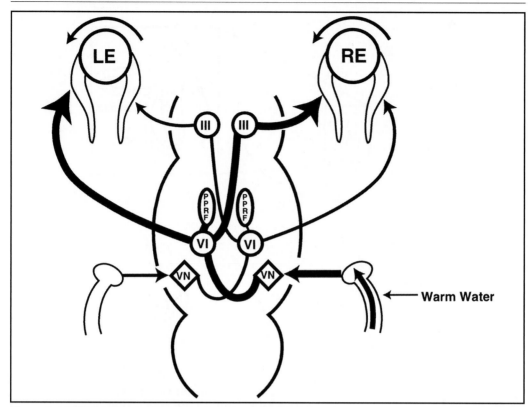

Figure 2-14. Warm water in the right ear causes shift of endolymph toward the ampulla, thereby increasing the vestibular tone and resulting in a slow movement of the eyes to the left side. The compensatory fast phase will be directed back to the right side.

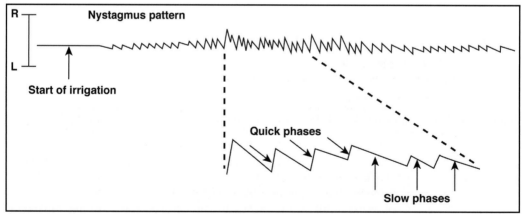

Figure 2-15. Caloric nystagmus. Horizontal eye position as a function of time in response to irrigation of the right EAC with warm (44°C) water. The temperature gradient set up across the horizontal semicircular canal in the presence of gravity leads to a convection current that causes a deflection of the cupula in the excitatory direction. The resulting nystagmus has leftward slow phases and rightward quick phases. Nystagmus intensity increases as the temperature gradient builds up and then dissipates. The maximum slow-phase velocity for each irrigation is recorded and the responses between the 2 ears are compared for symmetry.

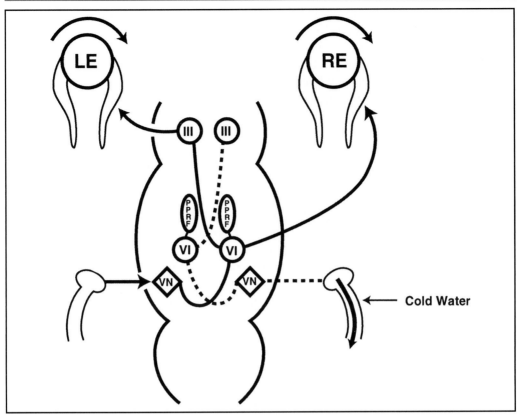

Figure 2-16. Cold water in the right ear causes shift of endolymph away from the ampulla, thereby decreasing the vestibular tone and allowing the vestibular tone from the left side to be dominant. This results in a slow movement of the eyes to the right. The compensatory fast phase will therefore be directed to the left side.

VI. DISORDERS OF HORIZONTAL GAZE

    A. Cerebral cortical lesions

        1. Acute cerebral hemisphere infarcts may cause conjugate eye deviation toward the side of the lesion

            a. Frontal and/or parietal ocular motor areas may be involved

            b. Gaze deviation results from unopposed activity of the normal contralateral hemisphere and, with right hemisphere lesions, spatial neglect

            c. Vestibular reflexes (VOR, calorics) remain intact and can still drive the eyes toward the contralateral side

            d. Acute FEF lesions transiently impair contraversive saccades

            e. Lesions of prefrontal cortex impair suppression of unwanted reflexive saccades

        2. Congenital ocular motor apraxia

            a. Impairment of voluntary horizontal eye movements

            b. Reflexive saccades and combined eye-head saccades (shifts of gaze with the head unrestrained) may be relatively spared

            c. The VOR is normal

            d. In more severe cases, quick phases may also be impaired

e. "Head thrusts" may be used to redirect gaze when head-free saccades and vestibular quick phases are impaired
  i. The head is rotated toward the target
  ii. Without quick phases, the intact VOR moves the eyes to an extreme orbital position
  iii. Further head rotation "drags" the eyes in the direction of the target
  iv. Once the target is foveated, the head is rotated back, but gaze direction does not change because the VOR is again active
f. Associated with ataxia-telangiectasia (A-T); ataxia with ocular motor apraxia, types 1 and 2; Joubert syndrome; Niemann-Pick disease, type C; Gaucher disease

3. Balint syndrome
  a. A form of acquired ocular motor apraxia due to bilateral posterior parietal lesions
  b. Inability to shift gaze or attention to another location in the visual field
  c. Simultanagnosia: inability to perceive more than one object at a time
  d. The VOR is intact
  e. Optic ataxia: impaired visually guided reaching

B. Pontine lesions
  1. Pontine conjugate gaze palsy
    a. A lesion of the PPRF eliminates all ipsiversive saccades due to loss of horizontal saccade burst neurons
    b. If the abducens (VI cranial nerve) nucleus is involved, there will be a complete conjugate gaze palsy, affecting horizontal saccades, pursuit, optokinetic, and vestibular eye movements. The effect is conjugate because both abducens motoneurons and interneurons are lost
    c. This gaze palsy distinguishes an abducens nucleus lesion from one affecting the abducens nerve, which only affects abduction of the ipsilateral eye
    d. If only the PPRF (and not the abducens nucleus) is affected, the VOR is preserved

  2. Internuclear ophthalmoplegia (INO)
    a. A lesion of the MLF affects axons of contralateral abducens neurons that project to MR motoneurons of the ipsilateral oculomotor nucleus ("internuclear" = between nuclei VI and III)
    b. Impaired adduction of the eye ipsilateral to the MLF lesion during attempted conjugate gaze away from the lesion (Figure 2-17)
    c. There may be nystagmus of the abducting eye when looking away from the lesion
    d. A complete INO eliminates adduction past the midline for all conjugate eye movements
    e. A partial INO may only slow the adducting eye during contraversive saccades without affecting the overall range of adduction (brought out clinically by asking the patient to initiate a horizontal saccade)
    f. The INO is named for the side of the lesion (a right INO impairs right eye adduction)
    g. Usually, adduction during convergence is relatively spared (Cogan posterior INO)
    h. INO caused by a midbrain lesion may also affect convergence and is usually bilateral (Cogan anterior INO)

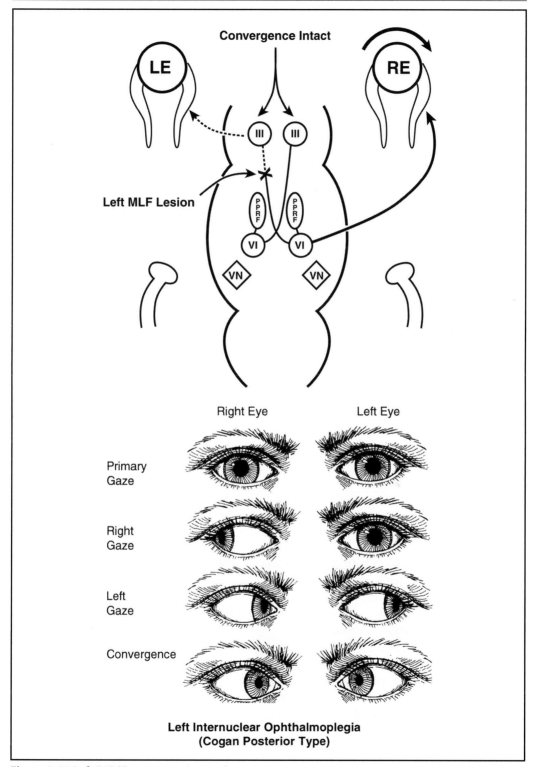

Figure 2-17. Left INO (Cogan posterior type).

        i.   INO (unilateral or bilateral) in a young adult is most commonly due to multiple sclerosis; in adults over age 50 years, ischemia is the most common cause

        j.   WEBINO (wall-eyed bilateral INO) refers to exotropia with bilateral INOs. It is impossible to exclude involvement of the MR subnuclei along with both MLFs, unless convergence is spared

        k.   INO may be accompanied by the following:

            i.   Skew deviation (hypertropia [HT] of the ipsilateral eye)/ocular tilt reaction (OTR)

            ii.   Disjunctive vertical-torsional nystagmus

            iii.   Impaired VOR in response to head impulses exciting the contralateral PC

    3.   One-and-a-half syndrome (Figure 2-18)

        a.   Caused by a unilateral pontine lesion that affects both the PPRF/abducens nucleus and the MLF

        b.   Conjugate ipsiversive gaze palsy ("one")

        c.   INO leading to impaired adduction of the ipsilateral eye during contraversive gaze (the "half")

        d.   For example, with a right one-and-a-half syndrome, neither eye can make rightward saccades, and only the left eye can make leftward saccades

        e.   For the first few days, there may be an exotropia due to tonic abduction of the contralateral eye (paralytic pontine exotropia)

VII. DISORDERS OF VERTICAL GAZE

    A.   Downgaze palsy: due to midbrain disease (stroke, tumor) with lesions involving the riMLF just rostral to the oculomotor (III cranial nerve) nucleus and dorsomedial to the red nucleus. A unilateral riMLF lesion impairs downward (but not upward) saccades and ipsilesional torsional quick phases. The latter can be tested with head roll

    B.   Upgaze palsy: associated with lesions located more dorsally, including the posterior commissure

    C.   Vertical gaze palsies are occasionally monocular

    D.   riMLF control of upward saccades is bilateral while riMLF control of downward saccades is unilateral at the oculomotor nucleus level. Each riMLF projects to the neurons innervating the ipsilateral inferior rectus and contralateral superior oblique. Thus, a unilateral riMLF lesion impairs downward (but not upward) saccades. Bilateral riMLF lesions may impair both downward and upward saccades

    E.   The riMLF also generates torsional components of saccades and quick phases. A unilateral riMLF lesion impairs ipsilesional torsional quick phases (eg, a right riMLF lesion affects clockwise—from the patient's perspective—quick phases)

    F.   Dorsal midbrain syndrome

        1.   Also known as *pretectal syndrome*, *Sylvian aqueduct syndrome*, and *Parinaud syndrome*

        2.   Supranuclear paresis of vertical gaze, especially upward, reflecting involvement of the INC and its projections through the posterior commissure

        3.   Other associated eye signs:

            a.   Light-near dissociation of the pupils—pupils constrict with near viewing but not to light

            b.   Convergence-retraction nystagmus

            c.   Lid retraction (Collier sign)

            d.   Convergence spasm or paresis

            e.   Accommodative spasm or paresis

            f.   Skew deviation (see page 79, IX)

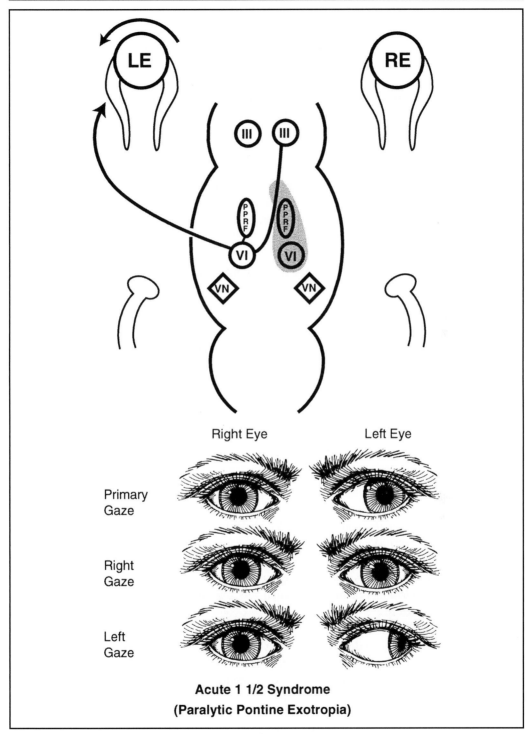

Figure 2-18. Acute one-and-a-half syndrome (paralytic pontine exotropia).

G. Progressive supranuclear palsy (PSP)

1. Supranuclear impairment of voluntary and reflexive saccades

2. Vertical saccades are affected first, but horizontal saccades also become involved as the disease progresses

3. First, saccade velocities are reduced, but eventually all gaze movements are lost

4. Neck rigidity makes it difficult for patients to use head movements to shift gaze

5. The VOR remains intact until very late in the disease course (there is preservation of oculocephalic reflex with fixation of gaze and examiner-led head motion)

6. Other features:

   a. Strabismus

      i. Particularly convergence insufficiency

   b. Reduced blinking, leading to corneal drying

   c. Apraxia of eyelid opening (slowed eye opening after eye closure)

   d. Gaze-evoked nystagmus

   e. Square-wave jerks (horizontal saccadic intrusions)

   f. Patients cannot look down nor move their neck well and thus cannot see objects unless brought up to eye level. They also often fall backward

   g. Hummingbird sign, also known as the *penguin silhouette sign*, refers to the midsagittal magnetic resonance imaging (MRI) appearance of the brainstem

7. Similar syndromes can occur due to central nervous system (CNS) ischemia and after cardiac surgery

H. Oculogyric crisis

1. Tonic, involuntary deviation of the eyes, usually upward, sometimes horizontal

2. Associated with neuroleptics and other drugs, encephalitis lethargica (post-encephalitic parkinsonism)

VIII. **DISORDERS OF VERGENCE**

A. Spasm of the near reflex

1. Triad of convergence, accommodation, miosis

2. May simulate unilateral or bilateral abducens palsies

3. Usually nonorganic with a variable esotropia

4. Rarely due to organic disease: head trauma, dorsal midbrain syndrome, intoxication, Wernicke syndrome

B. Convergence paresis/paralysis

1. Characterized by the following:

   a. Orthophoria or subtle ocular misalignment at distance

   b. Exotropia at near

   c. Full extraocular movements

2. Patients report diplopia at near or easy fatigability when reading

3. Usual causes: aging, lack of effort

4. Rarely due to organic cause: dorsal midbrain syndrome, PSP, multiple sclerosis, encephalitis, diphtheria, botulism

C. Divergence paresis/paralysis

1. Characterized by the following:

   a. Orthophoria or subtle ocular misalignment at near

   b. Comitant esotropia at distance

   c. Full extraocular movements

2. May present in isolation in adults without other neurologic findings

3. Must exclude the following:
    a. Decompensated esophoria
    b. Subtle bilateral abducens palsies
4. Causes: head trauma, PSP, brainstem stroke, cerebellar lesions including Arnold-Chiari I malformation
5. Esotropia when looking at distance is a characteristic finding in cerebellar disease (most likely due to involvement of the vermis)

D. Horizontal ocular misalignments should be measured at a distance and near to avoid overlooking a vergence disorder

IX. **SKEW DEVIATION**

A. Vertical/torsional strabismus from a supranuclear lesion
B. Must be distinguished from a cyclovertical extraocular muscle palsy (eg, superior oblique palsy; see Chapter 6)
C. Reduction of HT when supine supports a skew deviation rather than a superior oblique palsy
D. Usually due to lesion in central otolith pathways or INC. May be part of a full OTR (see section X next) or may occur in isolation
E. May be comitant or incomitant
F. Sometimes associated with INO (MLF lesion) or vertical/torsional nystagmus
G. With lower brainstem lesions, the ipsilateral eye is usually hypotropic; with pontine and midbrain lesions, the ipsilateral eye is usually hypertropic
H. An alternating skew deviation is a characteristic finding in cerebellar degeneration; usually the abducting eye is higher

X. **OCULAR TILT REACTION**

A. Physiologic OTR (Figure 2-19A)
    1. Normally, the utricle is excited by ipsilateral head tilt and inhibited by contralateral head tilt
    2. The normal response to head tilt is to move the head back toward upright, to counterroll the eyes, and (in lateral-eyed animals) to produce a vertical vergence movement to realign both eyes with the horizontal
B. Pathologic OTR (Figure 2-19C)
    1. Caused by a lesion in the peripheral or central otolith pathways that carry signals from the utricle
    2. If one utricle is lesioned, the tonic signal from the other side is unopposed, leading to an input imbalance, as if the head were tilted toward the good side
    3. Head tilt toward the lesioned ear (because the brain thinks the head is tilted toward the good side and wants to restore it to upright)
    4. Ocular rotation (torsion), with the upper poles of the eyes moving toward the lesioned side (the appropriate ocular counterroll if the head were tilted toward the good side, as the brain thinks)
    5. Skew deviation: disconjugate vertical deviation with the eye on the lesioned side lower (the appropriate response in a lateral-eyed animal, if the head were tilted toward the good side)
    6. Differentiate from a IV cranial nerve palsy where there is higher eye excyclotorsion; in OTR, there is higher eye incyclotorsion
C. Utricular afferents synapse in the VN, whose neurons project across the midline into the contralateral MLF. Thus, an MLF lesion produces a contraversive OTR (the head tilts and the eyes rotate away from the side of the MLF lesion and the ipsilateral eye is higher)

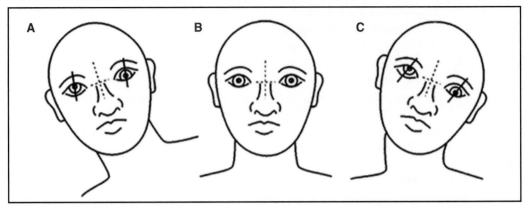

Figure 2-19. Figure showing physiologic and pathologic skew deviation. (A) In the physiologic OTR, a rightward body tilt activates right utricular and inhibits left utricular pathways subserving graviceptive tone in the roll plane, resulting in vertical divergence with conjugate torsion of the eyes and head tilt toward the lowermost eye and thus the compensatory head tilt predominates, with only a small skew deviation or static ocular counterroll. (B) Normal eye position with head upright. (C) In the pathologic OTR, all 3 components of the OTR are present (head tilt toward the lesioned ear, ocular torsion with the upper poles of the eyes moving toward the lesioned side, skew deviation with the eye on the lesioned side lower). (Reprinted from *Surv Ophthalmol*, vol 51, Brodsky MC, Donahue SP, Vaphiades M, Brandt T, Skew deviation revisited, pp 105-128, Copyright 2006, with permission from Elsevier.)[3]

XI. WERNICKE ENCEPHALOPATHY

A. Critical to recognize because it must be treated promptly

B. Triad: ophthalmoplegia, mental confusion, gait ataxia

C. Caused by thiamine deficiency (alcoholism, malnutrition, gastric bypass surgery)

D. Ocular motor findings include the following:
1. Impaired abduction
2. Partial or complete ophthalmoplegia
3. Vertical nystagmus, usually upbeat, that may change direction with convergence or with orbital position
4. Vestibular hypofunction
5. Gaze-evoked nystagmus
6. INO

E. Lesions occur throughout the brainstem, thalamus, hypothalamus, cerebellum

F. Treated emergently with intravenous thiamine

G. Magnesium deficiency must be tested for and treated if present

H. If untreated, may progress to Korsakoff syndrome with permanent memory loss and persistent eye movement abnormalities

REFERENCES

1. Leigh RJ, Zee DS. *The Neurology of Eye Movements.* 5th ed. New York, NY: Oxford University Press; 2015.

2. Leigh RJ, Zee DS. *The Neurology of Eye Movements.* 4th ed. New York, NY: Oxford University Press; 2006:263.

3. Brodsky MC, Donahue SP, Vaphiades M, Brandt T. Skew deviation revisited. *Surv Ophthalmol.* 2006;51:105-128.

BIBLIOGRAPHY

Brodsky MC. Dissociated vertical divergence: a righting reflex gone wrong. *Arch Ophthalmol.* 1999;117:1216-1222.

Buttner–Ennever JA, ed. *Neuroanatomy of the Oculomotor System, Volume 151 (Progress in Brain Research).* New York, NY: Elsevier; 2006.

Chen AL, Riley DE, King SA, et al. The disturbance of gaze in progressive supranuclear palsy: implications for pathogenesis. *Front Neurol.* 2010;1:147.

Donahue SP, Lavin PJ, Hamed LM. Tonic ocular tilt reaction simulating a superior oblique palsy. Diagnostic confusion with the three-step test. *Arch Ophthalmol.* 1999;117:347-352.

Graber JI, Staudinger R. Teaching NeuroImages: "penguin" or "hummingbird" sign and midbrain atrophy in progressive supranuclear palsy. *Neurology.* 2009;72:e81.

Kheradmand A, Zee DS. Cerebellum and ocular motor control. *Front Neurol.* 2011;2:53.

Krauzlis RJ. Recasting the smooth pursuit eye movement system. *J Neurophysiol.* 2004;91:591-603.

Lavin PJM. Eye movement disorders: ocular motor system. In: Daroff RB, Jankovic J, Mazziotta JC, Pomeroy SL, eds. *Neurology in Clinical Practice.* 7th ed. Boston, MA: Butterworth-Heineman; 2016:528-572.

Liu GT, Volpe NJ, Galetta SL. Eye movement disorders: conjugate gaze abnormalities. In: *Neuro-Ophthalmology: Diagnosis and Management.* 2nd ed. New York, NY: Saunders Elsevier; 2010:551-586.

Ramat S, Leigh RJ, Zee DS, Optican LM. What clinical disorders tell us about the neural control of saccadic eye movements. *Brain.* 2007;130:10-35.

Sander T, Sprenger A, Neumann G, et al. Vergence deficits in patients with cerebellar lesions. *Brain.* 2009;132:103-115.

Sechi GP, Serra A. Wernicke's encephalopathy: new clinical settings and recent advances in diagnosis and management. *Lancet Neurol.* 2007;6:442-455.

Sharpe J, Wong AMF. Anatomy and physiology of ocular motor systems. In: Miller NR, Newman NJ, eds. *Walsh and Hoyt's Clinical Neuro-Ophthalmology.* 6th ed. Vol 1. Philadelphia, PA: Lippincott Williams & Wilkins; 2005:809-885.

Solomon D, Ramat S, Tomsak RL, et al. Saccadic palsy after cardiac surgery: characteristics and pathogenesis. *Ann Neurol.* 2008;63:355-365.

Versino M, Zee DS. Disorders of binocular control of eye movements in patients with cerebellar dysfunction. *Brain.* 1996;119:1933-1950.

Wong AM, Colpa L, Chandrakumar M. Ability of an upright-supine test to differentiate skew deviation from other vertical strabismus causes. *Arch Ophthalmol.* 2011;129:1570-1575.

Zee DS, Newman-Toker DE. Supranuclear and internuclear ocular motility disorders. In: Miller NR, Newman NJ, eds. *Walsh and Hoyt's Clinical Neuro-Ophthalmology.* 6th ed. Vol 1. Philadelphia, PA: Lippincott Williams & Wilkins; 2005:907-967.

CHAPTER 3

Nystagmus and Related Ocular Oscillations

MARK F. WALKER, MD

I. **NYSTAGMUS IS A RHYTHMIC, INVOLUNTARY, BACK-AND-FORTH OSCILLATION OF THE EYES**
   A. Nystagmus is categorized by its waveform (Figure 3-1)
      1. Jerk (most common): slow drift (slow phase) followed by quick reset (quick phase). Slow phase waveform can be:
         a. Increasing velocity exponential (eg, integrator instability, congenital)
         b. Decreasing velocity exponential (eg, gaze-evoked)
         c. Constant (linear) velocity (eg, vestibular)
      2. Pendular: sinusoidal oscillation (like a pendulum), phases have equal speed
   B. Trajectory: nystagmus can be horizontal, vertical, torsional, or a combination of the 3
      1. Combined horizontal and vertical pendular nystagmus can be diagonal or elliptical, depending on the difference in phase between the 2 components
      2. Seesaw nystagmus: alternating upward/incyclotorsional movement of one eye with downward/excyclotorsional movement of the other eye (hemi-seesaw: one direction is a quick phase)
   C. The direction of jerk nystagmus is usually defined by its quick phases ("right-beating nystagmus": eyes drift left and beat right)
   D. Conjugacy: nystagmus can be conjugate (both eyes move in the same direction) or disconjugate (the eyes move in different directions, also called *disjunctive*)
   E. Dissociated: the 2 eyes move in the same direction but by different amounts
   F. Alexander law: jerk nystagmus usually increases in intensity when looking in the direction of the quick phase
   G. Null zone: the field of gaze where nystagmus intensity is minimal
II. **PHYSIOLOGIC NYSTAGMUS (NOT ALL NYSTAGMUS IS PATHOLOGICAL)**
   A. End-position nystagmus: a few beats of horizontal nystagmus when the eyes are first moved to extreme horizontal positions in the orbit
   B. Vestibular nystagmus (see Chapter 2)
      1. Caloric nystagmus
         a. Irrigation with warm water (in the head-up supine position) causes endolymph in the HC to move toward the ampulla, exciting the hair cells and driving a slow phase eye movement away from the irrigated side

Foroozan R, Vaphiades MS. *Kline's Neuro-Ophthalmology Review Manual, Eighth Edition (pp 83-90).* © 2018 SLACK Incorporated.

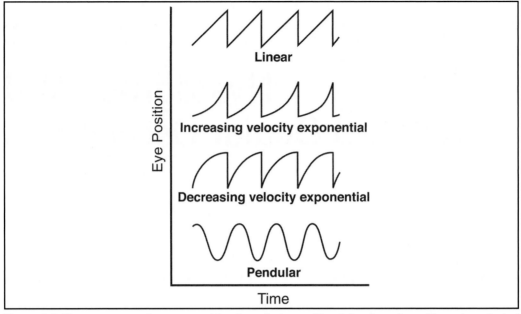

Figure 3-1. Nystagmus waveforms named for the velocity profile of the slow phase. Linear is typical of vestibular nystagmus; increasing velocity exponential of congenital nystagmus, decreasing velocity exponential of gaze-evoked nystagmus, and pendular may be seen with congenital or acquired nystagmus.

  b. Irrigation with cold water inhibits the HC and produces a slow phase toward the irrigated side

 2. Rotational nystagmus (VOR)

  a. Prolonged head rotation produces a slow phase in the direction opposite to head movement interrupted by quick phases in the same direction as head movement

  b. This serves to stabilize the retinal image as the head moves

C. OKN

 1. Driven by prolonged full-field visual motion

 2. In natural circumstances, most often occurs during sustained self-rotation in the light

 3. Supplements the VOR to stabilize vision

III. PATHOLOGIC NYSTAGMUS

A. Congenital nystagmus (infantile nystagmus syndrome)

 1. May be present at birth but more commonly appears later in infancy

 2. May be sporadic or genetic

  a. Autosomal dominant (6p12), autosomal recessive, and X-linked recessive patterns seen

  b. Associated with oculocutaneous albinism

 3. Commonly accentuated by attempted fixation and anxiety

 4. Typically damped by eye closure and convergence

 5. May or may not be accompanied by abnormalities of the visual system

 6. Does not cause oscillopsia

 7. Distinct waveforms

  a. Usually conjugate horizontal-torsional pendular and/or jerk nystagmus

  b. Similar amplitude in both eyes

       c. Jerk nystagmus has increasing velocity slow phases

       d. Foveation periods: brief cessation of eye motion, often following quick phases, during which clear vision is possible (if there are no afferent visual abnormalities)

  8. There is often an orbital position (null point) where nystagmus is minimal and vision is best

  9. May be associated with other abnormalities: strabismus, latent nystagmus, head oscillations

B. Latent nystagmus (fusional maldevelopment nystagmus syndrome)

  1. Seen only when one eye is covered

  2. Binocular jerk nystagmus with slow phases directed toward the covered eye

  3. Linear or exponentially decreasing slow phase velocity profile

  4. Retinal slip from nystagmus causes visual acuity to be diminished during monocular viewing

  5. Binocular viewing suppresses nystagmus and improves visual acuity

  6. May occur in association with congenital pendular or jerk nystagmus

  7. May be associated with dissociated vertical deviation and strabismus (usually esotropia)

C. Manifest latent nystagmus

  1. Similar to latent nystagmus but present with both eyes uncovered

  2. Suppression of vision in one eye (eg, due to strabismus and amblyopia) is the functional equivalent of covering one eye

  3. Slow phases directed away from the viewing eye (as in latent nystagmus)

  4. Vision may be improved when the eyes are moved eccentrically in the orbits in the direction of the slow phase

D. Spasmus nutans

  1. Triad of head turn, head nodding, and nystagmus

  2. Typically develops during the first year of life

  3. Resolves by age 10 years

  4. Horizontal or vertical pendular nystagmus with low amplitude and high frequency

  5. May be monocular or of different amplitude and/or phase in each eye

  6. Optic pathway glioma can cause acquired monocular nystagmus and should be ruled out by MRI

E. Seesaw nystagmus

  1. A disconjugate vertical-torsional nystagmus

  2. The torsional component has the same direction in both eyes, but the vertical movement is in the opposite direction

  3. During each half cycle, one eye moves upward and intorts and the other eye moves downward and extorts

  4. May be pendular (seesaw nystagmus) or jerk (hemi-seesaw nystagmus)

  5. Associated with the following:

      a. Midbrain stroke

      b. Medial medullary stroke

      c. Multiple sclerosis

      d. Chiari malformation

      e. Head trauma

      f. Visual loss

      g. Parasellar masses

      h. Congenital

F. Convergence-retraction nystagmus
1. Convergence and/or retraction of the eyes elicited by attempted upward saccades or quick phases
2. Best seen during stimulation with a downward-moving OKN stimulus
3. Part of the dorsal midbrain (Parinaud) syndrome
    a. Impaired vertical gaze (particularly upward)
    b. Light-near dissociation of the pupillary responses
    c. Lid retraction (Collier sign)
    d. Convergence-retraction nystagmus
    e. Spasm or paresis of convergence
    f. Spasm or paresis of accommodation
    g. Skew deviation
4. Due to lesions affecting the area of the posterior commissure
    a. Tumors (eg, pineal)
    b. Hydrocephalus (eg, aqueductal stenosis)
    c. Hemorrhage or infarction (midbrain, thalamus)
    d. Multiple sclerosis and other inflammatory lesions

G. Downbeat nystagmus
1. Spontaneous upward drift of the eyes
2. Characteristic sign of a lesion of the vestibulocerebellum or its pathways in the brainstem (cerebellar degeneration, multiple sclerosis, stroke, Chiari malformation)
3. Other important causes include drug toxicity (lithium, anticonvulsants), Wernicke encephalopathy
4. Often occurs in the context of a more general cerebellar syndrome but may present in isolation and be nonprogressive
5. Slow phase waveform may have constant, decreasing, or increasing velocity
6. Commonly enhanced by down and lateral gaze
7. May be affected by vergence state, position of the head relative to gravity (eg, prone versus supine positioning)

H. Upbeat nystagmus
1. Spontaneous nystagmus with downward slow phases in primary position
2. Different from upbeat nystagmus that may be a part of gaze-evoked nystagmus and is only present when looking up (not in primary position) and also from the transient upbeat-torsional nystagmus seen in benign paroxysmal positioning vertigo (BPPV; see page 88, III, L, 4)
3. Etiologies:
    a. Focal lesions (infarction, tumor, demyelinating) of the medulla or cerebellum
    b. Cerebellar degeneration
    c. Wernicke encephalopathy
4. Downbeat nystagmus may convert to upbeat nystagmus with convergence (or vice versa)

I. Gaze-evoked and rebound nystagmus
1. Loss of eccentric gaze holding, in which the eyes tend to drift back to the center of the orbit
2. A weak neural integrator does not produce a sufficiently strong tonic innervation to hold the eyes against elastic forces
3. Etiologies
    a. Vestibulocerebellar lesions (eg, cerebellar degenerations)

        b.   Functional neural integrator impairment due to drugs (sedatives, anticonvulsants), metabolic derangements

    4.   The direction of nystagmus depends on gaze direction: the eyes drift toward the center and quick phases beat back in the direction of attempted gaze

    5.   Typically horizontal: right-beating nystagmus with right gaze and left-beating nystagmus with left gaze

    6.   May also include upbeat nystagmus with upgaze

    7.   With sustained gaze, the nystagmus will often diminish

    8.   Upon return to center position, there may be a brief oppositely directed nystagmus (rebound nystagmus)

    9.   Gaze-evoked and downbeat nystagmus often occur together in patients with cerebellar degeneration

J.   Pendular nystagmus

    1.   Sinusoidal oscillation (no quick phases)

    2.   May have a complex waveform that includes horizontal, vertical, and torsional components

    3.   Elliptical nystagmus: horizontal and vertical components out of phase

    4.   May be congenital (see pages 84-85, III, A) or acquired

    5.   Etiologies of acquired pendular nystagmus

        a.   Multiple sclerosis

        b.   Oculopalatal tremor syndrome

            i.   Usually vertical pendular nystagmus with variable horizontal and torsional components

            ii.   Synchronous contraction of face, palate, pharynx, diaphragm, extremities

            iii.   Persists during sleep

            iv.   Delayed effect of lesion in the central tegmental tract connecting the deep cerebellar nuclei to the inferior olive

            v.   Seen with hypertrophy of inferior olive (latency from acute infarction: 2 to 49 months); not a manifestation of an acute lesion

        c.   Whipple disease

        d.   Pelizaeus-Merzbacher disease

        e.   Toluene toxicity

        f.   Severe visual loss

    6.   May respond to gabapentin or memantine

K.   Periodic alternating nystagmus (PAN)

    1.   Horizontal jerk nystagmus that changes direction every 2 minutes

    2.   Present in the primary position, unlike gaze-evoked nystagmus

    3.   May be accompanied by periodic head deviations that reduce the nystagmus by moving the eyes into a relative null position

    4.   Results from lesions to the nodulus/uvula combined with either flocculus/paraflocculus lesions or visual loss

    5.   Baclofen abolishes nystagmus

    6.   In cases where visual loss contributes, improvement of vision (eg, vitrectomy, cataract extraction) may eliminate nystagmus

    7.   Congenital PAN is less regularly periodic than acquired PAN and does not respond as well to baclofen

    8.   In comatose patients with no quick phases, PAN may be seen as a periodic alternating gaze deviation

L. Peripheral vestibular nystagmus
    1. Jerk nystagmus due to imbalance of vestibular inputs (see Chapter 2)
    2. Unilateral vestibular hypofunction
        a. An acute lesion to one labyrinth or vestibular nerve (eg, vestibular neuritis) results in a spontaneous horizontal/torsional nystagmus because the tonic input from the intact side is suddenly unopposed
        b. The eyes drift (slow phase) toward the lesioned side and quick phases beat toward the intact side
        c. The intensity is usually greatest when looking toward the intact side (Alexander law), but the direction does not change with gaze, unlike gaze-evoked nystagmus
        d. May be partially or fully suppressed by vision and is best seen when fixation is removed
            i.   Frenzel goggles
            ii. When looking at one optic nerve with a direct ophthalmoscope, cover the fellow eye
        e. Slowly growing tumors (eg, vestibular schwannomas) do not usually produce much nystagmus because the vestibular imbalance is compensated centrally as it develops (may see Bruns nystagmus—see section 3 next)
        f. Bilateral vestibular lesions do not cause nystagmus because the lesion is symmetric and there is no imbalance
    3. Bruns nystagmus
        a. May be seen with large tumors in the cerebellopontine angle
        b. Two components:
            i.   Horizontal nystagmus beating away from the lesion when looking away from the lesion (vestibular nystagmus—accentuated by Alexander law) due to vestibular nerve involvement
            ii. Horizontal nystagmus beating toward the lesion when looking toward the lesion (unilateral gaze-evoked nystagmus) due to compression of the adjacent brainstem and cerebellar flocculus
    4. BPPV
        a. Brief (<1 min) nystagmus provoked by changes in head position relative to gravity (lying down, looking up, rolling over in bed)
        b. Caused by free-moving otoconia that have become lodged in a semicircular canal
        c. Usually affects the PC: slow phases are directed downward with a torsional component in which the upper poles of the eyes rotate away from the affected ear (upbeating-torsional nystagmus)
        d. Diagnosed by the Dix-Hallpike maneuver
        e. Treated by repositioning maneuvers (eg, Epley, Semont) that move the otoconia out of the affected canal
    5. Sound- (Tullio phenomenon) and pressure-induced nystagmus
        a. Loud noise, Valsalva, or pressure in the external ear causes endolymph motion when the pressure change is transmitted to the inner ear through a fistula
        b. Usually caused by superior semicircular canal dehiscence (defect in the bony roof of the superior canal leading to a communication between the labyrinth and the middle cranial fossa)
        c. If severe, treated surgically by closing the fistula

IV. **SACCADIC INTRUSIONS AND OSCILLATIONS**

A. Saccadic intrusions are undesired, involuntary saccades that interfere with visual fixation

B. Repeated saccadic intrusions result in saccadic oscillations

C. Saccadic oscillations differ from nystagmus in that they are made up only of saccades; there are no slow phases

D. Saccadic oscillations are defined by their amplitude, frequency, and direction and whether they have a normal intersaccadic interval

E. Square-wave jerks and square-wave oscillations
   1. A square-wave jerk consists of an involuntary saccade (amplitude 0.5 to 3 degrees) followed by a second saccade after a normal interval (about 200 msec) that brings the eyes back to the point of fixation
   2. Square-wave jerks may be seen in normal individuals but are enhanced in neurological diseases such as cerebellar lesions and PSP
   3. Named for their rectangular appearance on eye movement recordings
   4. Macro–square-wave jerks are larger (> 5 degrees) and have a shorter intersaccadic interval
   5. Macrosaccadic oscillations are repeated saccades with a normal intersaccadic interval that are related to saccadic hypermetria and usually seen with lesions of the cerebellar vermis

F. Ocular flutter and opsoclonus
   1. Continuous back-to-back saccades without an intersaccadic interval
   2. Symptoms are blurred vision and oscillopsia
   3. May be associated with limb and body myoclonus
   4. Ocular flutter is a one-dimensional (usually horizontal) saccadic oscillation; opsoclonus has horizontal, vertical, and torsional components
   5. Causes:
      a. Parainfectious encephalitis of the brainstem
      b. Paraneoplastic syndrome
      c. Toxic-metabolic
      d. Idiopathic
   6. The opsoclonus-myoclonus syndrome in children is characteristic of a neuroblastoma
   7. In adults, other tumors (breast, small-cell lung, ovary) are associated with paraneoplastic flutter and opsoclonus
   8. Treatment includes removing the tumor, if present. Immune therapies such as intravenous immunoglobulin may help

G. Microsaccadic oscillations (microflutter)
   1. Very small amplitude flutter
   2. Usually requires an ophthalmoscope to visualize
   3. May be isolated and benign, but evaluation for an occult malignancy should be performed
   4. Can be multidirectional: microsaccadic opsoclonus

H. Voluntary flutter (voluntary "nystagmus")
   1. Saccadic oscillation (not true nystagmus) that can be induced, often by vergence effort
   2. Unlike involuntary flutter and opsoclonus, it is not sustained
   3. May produce oscillopsia when present

V. OCULAR BOBBING VARIANTS AND PING-PONG GAZE

A. Ocular bobbing and its variants are vertical nystagmoid movements that occur in comatose patients

B. Ocular bobbing is typically seen with pontine lesions (eg, hemorrhage or compression) but may occur with toxic-metabolic insults; the other variants are less well localized

C. Ocular bobbing variants are distinguished by the pattern of slow and fast eye motion

1. Ocular bobbing: rapid downward movement followed by slow upward drift back to the center of the orbit

2. Reverse ocular bobbing: rapid upward movement followed by slow downward drift to center position

3. Ocular dipping (inverse ocular bobbing): slow downward drift with rapid upward return to center position

4. Reverse ocular dipping (converse ocular bobbing): slow upward drift followed by rapid downward return to center position

D. Ping-pong gaze is an alternating horizontal gaze deviation (changes every few seconds) that is seen in comatose patients

BIBLIOGRAPHY

Brodsky MC, Dell'Osso LF. A unifying neurologic mechanism for infantile nystagmus. *JAMA Ophthalmol*. 2014;132:761-768.

Burde RM, Savino PJ, Trobe JD. Ocular oscillations. In: *Clinical Decisions in Neuro-Ophthalmology*. 3rd ed. St Louis, MO: CV Mosby; 2002:220-245.

Gottlob I, Wizov SS, Reinecke RD, et al. Spasmus nutans. A long term follow-up. *Invest Ophthalmol Vis Sci*. 1995;36:2768-2771.

Lavin PJM. Eye movement disorders: ocular motor system. In: Daroff RB, Jankovic J, Mazziotta JC, Pomeroy SL, eds. *Neurology in Clinical Practice*. 7th ed. Boston, MA: Butterworth-Heineman; 2016:528-572.

Leigh RJ, Rucker JC. Nystagmus and related motility disorders. In: Miller NR, Newman NJ, eds. *Walsh and Hoyt's Clinical Neuro-Ophthalmology*. 6th ed. Vol 1. Philadelphia, PA: Lippincott Williams & Wilkins; 2005:1133-1173.

Leigh RJ, Zee DS. *The Neurology of Eye Movements*. 5th ed. New York, NY: Oxford University Press; 2015.

Liu GT, Volpe NJ, Galetta SL. Eye movement disorders: nystagmus and nystagmoid eye movements. In: *Neuro-Ophthalmology: Diagnosis and Management*. 2nd ed. New York, NY: Saunders Elsevier; 2010:587-610.

McLean R, Proudlock F, Thomas S, Degg C, Gottlob I. Congenital nystagmus: randomized, controlled, double-masked trial of memantine/gabapentin. *Ann Neurol*. 2007;61:130-138.

Ramat S, Leigh RJ, Zee DS, Optican LM. What clinical disorders tell us about the neural control of saccadic eye movements. *Brain*. 2007;130:10-35.

Self J, Lotery A. The molecular genetics of congenital idiopathic nystagmus. *Semin Ophthalmol*. 2006;21:87-90.

Shaikh AG, Hong S, Liao K, et al. Oculopalatal tremor explained by a model of inferior olivary hypertrophy and cerebellar plasticity. *Brain*. 2010;133:923-940.

Straube A. Therapeutic considerations for eye movement disorders. *Dev Ophthalmol*. 2007;40:175-192.

Strupp M, Thrutell MJ, Shaikh AG, Brandt T, Zee DS, Leigh RJ. Pharmacotherapy of vestibular and ocular motor disorders, including nystagmus. *J Neurol*. 2011;258:1207-1222.

Thurtell MJ, Joshi AC, Leone AC, et al. Crossover trial of gabapentin and memantine as treatment for acquired nystagmus. *Ann Neurol*. 2010;67:676-680.

Wagner JN, Glaser M, Brandt T, Strupp M. Downbeat nystagmus: etiology and comorbidity in 117 patients. *J Neurol Neruosurg Psychistry*. 2008;79:672-677.

CHAPTER 4

The Six Syndromes of the VI Nerve (Abducens)

MICHAEL S. VAPHIADES, DO

I. **ANATOMICAL CONSIDERATIONS**
   A. Figure 4-1 identifies the structures in the posterior fossa, base of the skull, and middle cranial fossa that serve as landmarks in the study of the VI nerve
   B. Figure 4-2 is a schematic representation of these structures and includes a sagittal section of the brainstem
   C. Figure 4-3 is a schematic representation of these structures when viewed from an occipital view
   D. Figure 4-4 illustrates the S-shaped course of the VI nerve and shows its relationship to the VII and VIII cranial nerves and the internal carotid artery
   E. Figure 4-5 adds the III, IV, and V cranial nerves
   F. Figure 4-6 shows the composite diagram and the division of the course of the VI nerve into 5 portions, each associated with a different syndrome:
      1. VI_1: the brainstem syndrome
      2. VI_2: the subarachnoid space syndrome
      3. VI_3: the petrous apex syndrome
      4. VI_4: the cavernous sinus syndrome
      5. VI_5: the orbital syndrome

II. **THE BRAINSTEM SYNDROME (VI_1)**
   A. Figure 4-6 reminds us that a brainstem lesion of the VI nerve may also affect the V, VII, and VIII nerves and the cerebellum
   B. The VI nerve nucleus contains motoneurons that supply the lateral rectus muscle and abducens internuclear neurons that project via the MLF to the medial rectus subdivision of the contralateral oculomotor nucleus. Thus, a nuclear VI nerve palsy causes an ipsilateral conjugate horizontal gaze palsy
   C. Figure 4-7 illustrates the structures within the substance of the lower pons that may be affected by a lesion affecting the VI nerve
      1. Oculosympathetic central neuron: ipsilateral Horner syndrome
      2. PPRF: ipsilateral horizontal conjugate gaze palsy
      3. MLF: ipsilateral INO
      4. Pyramidal tract: contralateral hemiparesis

Foroozan R, Vaphiades MS. *Kline's Neuro-Ophthalmology Review Manual, Eighth Edition (pp 91-100).*
© 2018 SLACK Incorporated.

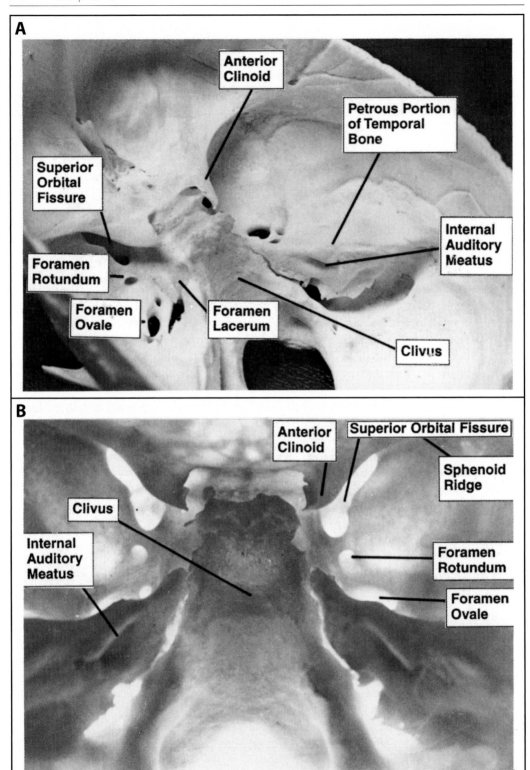

Figure 4-1. Human skull. Anatomical landmarks in the study of the VI nerve. Occipital view, retroilluminated skull.

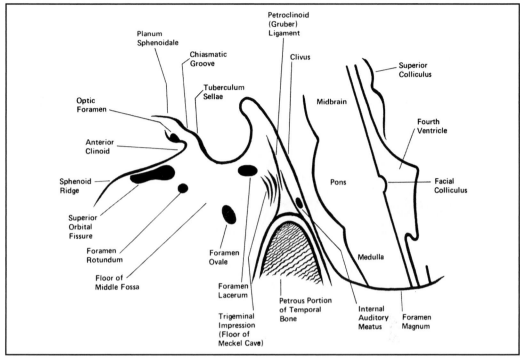

Figure 4-2. Schematic representation of the anatomical landmarks, temporal view.

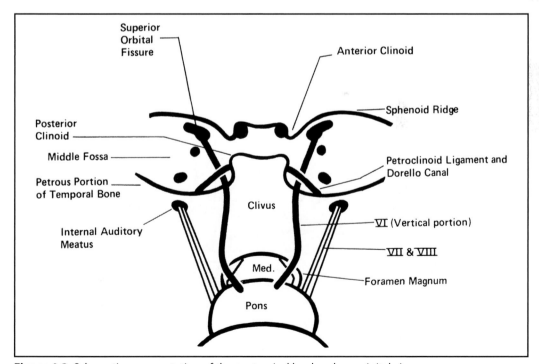

Figure 4-3. Schematic representation of the anatomical landmarks, occipital view.

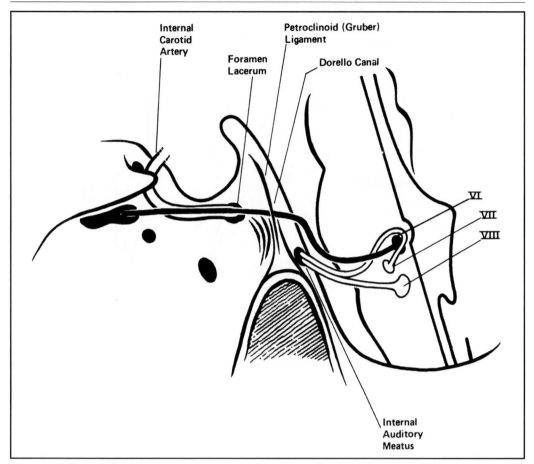

Figure 4-4. Course of the VI nerve (highlighted in black) from the pons to the superior orbital tissue.

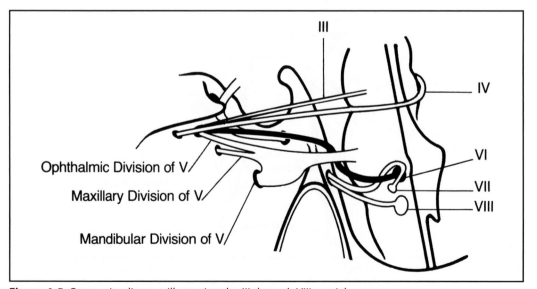

Figure 4-5. Composite diagram illustrating the III through VIII cranial nerves.

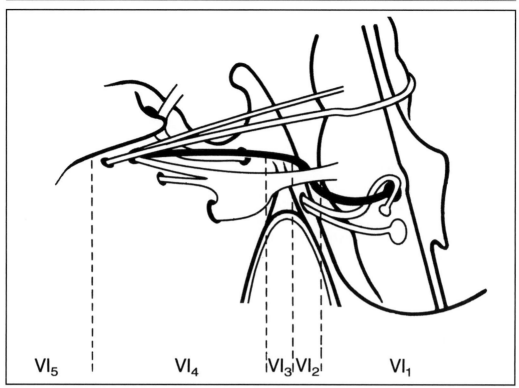

Figure 4-6. Composite diagram divided into 5 sections, corresponding to the first 5 syndromes of the VI nerve (VI_1 to VI_5).

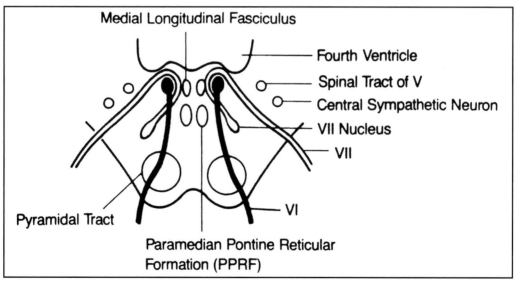

Figure 4-7. Diagram of cross-section of the lower pons through the VI nucleus and fascicle (highlighted in black).

    D. The brainstem syndrome may consist of any combination of the deficits listed previously; the following are frequently encountered syndromes:

1. Millard-Gubler syndrome
   a. VI nerve paresis
   b. Ipsilateral VII nerve paresis
   c. Contralateral hemiparesis
2. Raymond syndrome
   a. VI nerve paresis
   b. Contralateral hemiparesis
3. Foville syndrome
   a. Horizontal conjugate gaze palsy
   b. Ipsilateral V, VII, VIII cranial nerve palsies
   c. Ipsilateral Horner syndrome

III. THE SUBARACHNOID SPACE SYNDROME (VI$_2$)

    A. Elevated intracranial pressure may result in downward displacement of the brainstem, with stretching of the VI nerve, which is tethered at its exit from the pons and in the Dorello canal

1. Gives rise to "nonlocalizing" VI nerve palsies of raised intracranial pressure
2. Approximately 30% of patients with pseudotumor cerebri have VI nerve paresis

    B. Other disturbances in the subarachnoid space causing VI nerve palsies include hemorrhage, meningeal or parameningeal infection (eg, viral, bacterial, fungal), inflammation (eg, sarcoidosis), or infiltration (eg, lymphoma, leukemia, carcinoma)

    C. Low intracranial pressure (intracranial hypotension) may also result in downward displacement of the brain with damage to the VI nerve. May see descent of the brain and cerebellar tonsillar ectopia

1. Causes:
   a. Trauma
   b. Iatrogenic (post–lumbar puncture [LP] or after epidural)
   c. Idiopathic
2. LP frequently shows low opening pressure but may be normal
3. Treatment includes blood patch and surgery to correct tear in the involved dura

IV. THE PETROUS APEX SYNDROME (VI$_3$)

    A. Contact with the tip of the petrous pyramid makes the portion of the VI nerve within the Dorello canal susceptible to pathologic processes affecting the petrous bone

    B. Gradenigo syndrome

1. Clinical findings:
   a. VI nerve palsy
   b. Ipsilateral decreased hearing
   c. Ipsilateral facial pain in the distribution of the V nerve
   d. Ipsilateral facial paralysis
2. Due to localized inflammation or extradural abscess of petrous apex following complicated otitis media

    C. Petrous bone fracture

1. Basal skull fracture following head trauma
2. Potential cranial nerve involvement: V, VI, VII, VIII
3. Associated findings: hemotympanum, Battle sign, mastoid ecchymosis, CSF otorrhea

    D.   Pseudo-Gradenigo syndrome

        1.   Nasopharyngeal carcinoma: may cause serous otitis media due to obstruction of the eustachian tube and the carcinoma may subsequently invade the cavernous sinus, causing VI nerve paresis

        2.   Cerebellopontine angle tumor: may cause VI nerve paresis and other clinical findings, including the following:

            a.   Decreased hearing

            b.   VII nerve palsy

            c.   V nerve paralysis

            d.   Ataxia

            e.   Papilledema

V. THE CAVERNOUS SINUS SYNDROME (VI_4)

    A.   Lesions in cavernous sinus rarely produce isolated VI nerve palsy; associated involvement of the following:

        1.   III, IV, and ophthalmic (V_1) nerves

        2.   Carotid oculosympathetic plexus (Horner syndrome)

        3.   Optic nerve and chiasm

        4.   Pituitary gland (pituitary apoplexy, radiation-induced abducens nerve palsy in patients with pituitary tumor)

    B.   Differential diagnosis of cavernous sinus disease includes the following:

        1.   Trauma

        2.   Vascular

        3.   Neoplastic

        4.   Inflammatory

    C.   See Chapter 7

VI. THE ORBITAL SYNDROME (VI_5)

    A.   Proptosis is an early sign and may be accompanied by congestion of the conjunctival vessels and chemosis

    B.   The optic nerve may appear normal or demonstrate atrophy or edema

    C.   Trigeminal signs are limited to the ophthalmic division

    D.   It is frequently difficult to distinguish between cranial nerve (III, IV, VI) pareses and mechanical restriction of the globe

    E.   Etiologies

        1.   Tumor (local, metastatic)

        2.   Trauma

        3.   Nonspecific orbital inflammation (orbital pseudotumor)

        4.   Cellulitis

        5.   Allergic fungal rhinosinusitis

VII. ISOLATED VI NERVE PALSY (VI_6)

    A.   The sixth syndrome of the VI nerve

        1.   No signs of the first 5 syndromes

        2.   As a general rule:

            a.   Ocular motor cranial nerve palsy in young patient—greater likelihood of neoplasm; aggressive evaluation

            b.   Ocular motor cranial nerve palsy in older patient—greater likelihood of ischemic mononeuropathy; less aggressive evaluation

            c.   Ischemic mononeuropathy often preceded or accompanied by pain, which usually resolves within 2 to 4 weeks

Table 4-1

ETIOLOGIES OF ACQUIRED VI NERVE PALSY

	Rucker[1]	Schrader & Schlezinger[2]	Rucker[3]	Johnston[4]	Robertson et al[5] (children)	Rush & Younge[6]	Kodsi & Younge[7] (children)	Richards et al[8]	Park et al[9]
Total Patients	**545**	**104**	**607**	**158**	**133**	**419**	**88**	**575**	**108**
Etiologies (%)									
Neoplasm	21	7	33	13	39	15	21	20	6
Trauma	16	3	12	32	20	17	42	20	19
Aneurysm	6	0	3	1	3	3	0	3	5
Ischemic	11	36	8	16	0	18	0	10	28
Misc	16	30	24	30	29	18	22	23	19
Undetermined	30	24	20	8	9	29	15	23	23

3. Note in series by Robertson et al[5] and Kodsi and Younge[7] (Table 4-1) that if cases due to trauma are excluded, a child with a VI nerve palsy has a 50-50 chance of harboring a neoplasm, usually a brainstem glioma
4. In pediatric patients, the syndrome of benign, postviral VI nerve palsy may occur
    a. Acute onset
    b. Usually complete absence of abduction
    c. Antecedent febrile viral illness or after vaccination
    d. Absence of other cranial nerve dysfunction
    e. No signs of increased intracranial pressure
    f. Complete resolution within 3 months
    g. May be recurrent
    h. Careful follow-up mandatory

B. Initial evaluation
    1. Blood pressure determination
    2. Blood tests
        a. Complete blood count (CBC) with differential
        b. Basic metabolic panel (BMP)
        c. Sedimentation rate; C-reactive protein
        d. VDRL (Venereal Disease Research Laboratory) and if positive, FTA-ABS (fluorescent treponemal antibody absorbed; or TPHA [*Treponema pallidum haemagglutination*])
        e. Myasthenia gravis panel (acetylcholine receptor and striated muscle antibodies) and thyroid stimulating hormone (TSH), consider anti-GQ1b antibody
    3. Neuroimaging studies
        a. Consider neuroimaging in patients under age 50 years
        b. In patients over age 50 years, the most likely cause is an ischemic mononeuropathy. If the VI nerve palsy has not resolved in 3 months, or if other cranial nerve involvement occurs, then comprehensive evaluation is recommended
            i.   Medical and neurologic examinations
            ii. MRI brain and orbits with contrast and fat suppression

        iii. LP

        iv. If a vascular cause is suspected consider magnetic resonance angiography (MRA), computed tomographic angiography (CTA), and cerebral angiography

        v. If signs of elevated intracranial pressure (IIH), magnetic resonance venography (MRV) and LP

VIII. **TABLE 4-1 CONTAINS A SUMMARY OF 9 RETROSPECTIVE STUDIES OF PATIENTS WITH PARESIS OF THE VI NERVE**

    A. Eight percent to 30%, etiology undetermined, reflecting the vulnerability of the nerve to influences that are transient, benign, and unrecognizable

    B. Sixteen percent to 30% attributed to a miscellaneous group of causes that includes leukemia, migraine, idiopathic intracranial hypertension, and multiple sclerosis. The miscellaneous group of etiologies reflects the poor localizing value of paresis of the VI nerve

IX. **SEVEN IMPOSTERS OF THE VI NERVE**

    A. Thyroid eye disease

    B. Neuromuscular junction disorders (Myasthenia gravis and botulism)

    C. Duane syndrome

    D. Spasm of the near reflex

    E. Medial wall orbital blowout fracture with restrictive myopathy

    F. Break in fusion of a congenital esophoria

    G. Miller Fisher syndrome (see Chapter 7)

REFERENCES

1. Rucker CW. Paralysis of the third, fourth, and sixth cranial nerves. *Am J Ophthalmol*. 1958;46:787-794.

2. Schrader EC, Schlezinger NS. Neuroophthalmic evaluation of abducens nerve paralysis. *Arch Ophthalmol*. 1960;63:1184-1191.

3. Rucker CW. The causes of paralysis of the third, fourth, and sixth cranial nerves. *Am J Ophthalmol*. 1966;61:1293-1298.

4. Johnston AC. Etiology and treatments of abducens palsy. *Trans Pac Coast Oto-ophthalmol Soc*. 1968;49:259-277.

5. Robertson DM, Hines JD, Rucker CW. Acquired sixth nerve paresis in children. *Arch Ophthalmol*. 1970;83:574-579.

6. Rush JA, Younge BR. Paralysis of cranial nerves III, IV and VI. Cause and prognosis in 1,000 cases. *Arch Ophthalmol*. 1981;99:76-79.

7. Kodsi SR, Younge BR. Acquired oculomotor, trochlear, abducent cranial nerve palsies in pediatric patients. *Am J Ophthalmol*. 1992;114:568-574.

8. Richards BW, Jones FR, Young BR. Causes and prognosis in 4278 cases of paralysis of the oculomotor, trochlear, and abducens cranial nerves. *Am J Ophthalmol*. 1992;113:489-496.

9. Park UC, Kim SJ, Hwang JM, Yu YS. Clinical features and natural history of acquired third, fourth, and sixth cranial nerve palsy. *Eye*. 2008;22:691-696.

BIBLIOGRAPHY

Illing EA, Dunlap Q, Woodworth BA. Outcomes of pressure-induced cranial neuropathies from allergic fungal rhinosinusitis. *Otolaryngol Head Neck Surg*. 2015;152:541-545.

Kayayurt K, Gündogdu ÖL, Yavaşi Ö, Metin Y, Ugras E. Isolated abducens nerve palsy due to pituitary apoplexy after mild head trauma. *Am J Emerg Med*. 2015;33:1539.e3-e4.

Kontzialis M, Choudhri AF, Patel VR, et al. High-resolution 3D magnetic resonance imaging of the sixth cranial nerve: anatomic and pathologic considerations by segment. *J Neuroophthalmol*. 2015;35:412-425.

Leigh RJ, Zee DS. *The Neurology of Eye Movements*. 5th ed. New York, NY: Oxford University Press; 2015.

Liu GT, Volpe NJ, Galetta SL. Eye movement disorders: third, fourth, and sixth nerve palsies and other causes of diplopia and ocular misalignments. In: *Neuro-Ophthalmology: Diagnosis and Management*. 2nd ed. New York, NY: Saunders Elsevier; 2010:491-550.

Lyons CJ, Godoy F, ALQahtani E. Cranial nerve palsies in childhood. *Eye (Lond)*. 2015;29:246-251.

Mokri B. Spontaneous low pressure, low CSF volume headaches: spontaneous CSF leaks. *Headache*. 2013;53:1034-1053.

Sargent JC. Nuclear and infranuclear ocular motility disorders. In: Miller NR, Newman NJ, eds. *Walsh and Hoyt's Clinical Neuro-Ophthalmology*. 6th ed. Vol 1. Philadelphia, PA: Lippincott Williams & Wilkins; 2005:969-1040.

Vaphiades MS, Spencer SA, Riley K, Francis C, Deitz L, Kline LB. Radiation-induced ocular motor cranial nerve palsies in patients with pituitary tumor. *J Neuroophthalmol*. 2011;31:210-213.

Wilker SC, Rucker JC, Newman NJ, Biousse V, Tomsak RL. Pain in ischemic ocular motor cranial nerve palsies. *Br J Ophthalmol*. 2009;93:1657-1659.

CHAPTER 5

The Seven Syndromes of the III Nerve (Oculomotor)

MICHAEL S. VAPHIADES, DO

I. **ANATOMICAL CONSIDERATIONS**
   A. Figure 5-1 represents a cross-section through the rostral midbrain at the level of the SC
   B. Figure 5-2 is a copy of Figure 5-1 with superimposition of sites 1 through 6, representing 6 sites in which the III cranial nerve may be affected and present with distinct ocular manifestations, or in the company of different neurologic signs and symptoms, or as a result of specific disease processes. The seventh syndrome is the isolated III nerve palsy
   C. Figure 5-3 illustrates the relationship of the III nerve (highlighted in black) to other cranial nerves

II. **THE 7 SYNDROMES OF THE III NERVE**
   A. Nuclear III nerve paresis (see Figure 5-2, site 1)
      1. Least common of all the sites, yet not rare
      2. The arrangement of the III nerve subnuclei places strict prerequisites on the diagnosis of a nuclear III nerve palsy
         a. Each superior rectus is innervated by the contralateral III nerve nucleus; therefore, a nuclear III nerve palsy on one side causes paresis of the contralateral superior rectus
         b. Both levators are innervated by one subnuclear structure—the central caudal nucleus; therefore, a nuclear III nerve palsy causes bilateral ptosis
      3. Some cases of skew deviation may actually represent instances of one or more III nerve subnuclei (subserving the vertical recti or the inferior oblique) being affected (see Chapter 2)
   B. III nerve fascicle syndrome (see Figure 5-2, site 2)
      1. Topical diagnosis depends upon the coexistence of other neurologic signs
      2. Fascicles have already left the III nerve nucleus so that the ocular manifestations are present only on one side (no longer subject to the rules governing nuclear III nerve paresis)
      3. Nothnagel syndrome
         a. Lesion in the area of the superior cerebellar peduncle
         b. Ipsilateral III nerve paresis and cerebellar ataxia

Foroozan R, Vaphiades MS. *Kline's Neuro-Ophthalmology Review Manual, Eighth Edition (pp 101-110).* © 2018 SLACK Incorporated.

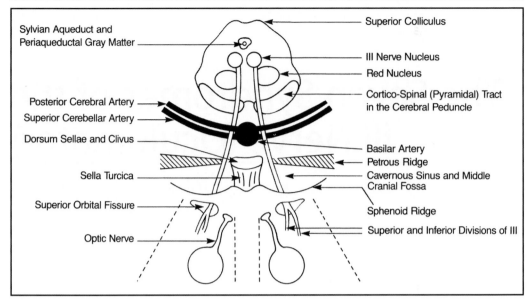

Figure 5-1. Cross-section through the rostral midbrain at the level of the SC.

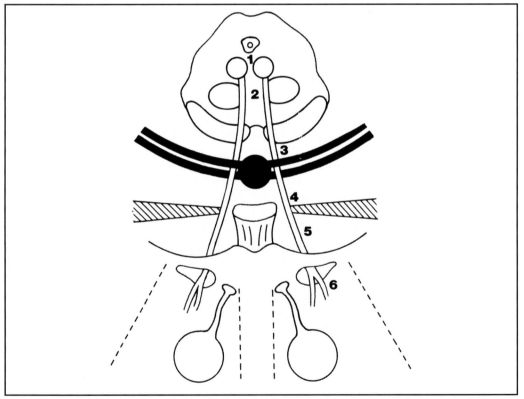

Figure 5-2. Superimposition on the rostral midbrain (see Figure 5-1) of sites 1 through 6, representing 6 sites in which the III cranial nerve may be affected.

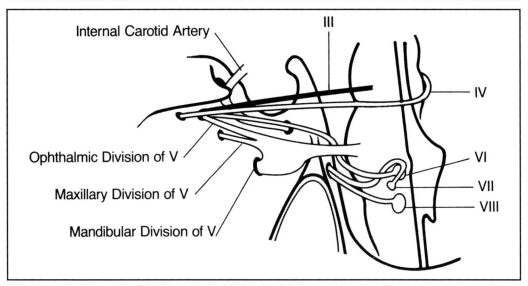

Figure 5-3. Relationship of the III nerve (highlighted in black) to other cranial nerves.

4. Benedikt syndrome
   a. Lesion in the region of the red nucleus
   b. Ipsilateral III nerve paresis with contralateral hemitremor
5. Weber syndrome
   a. Involvement of the III nerve in the neighborhood of the cerebral peduncle
   b. Ipsilateral III nerve paresis with contralateral hemiparesis
6. Claude syndrome
   a. Features of both Benedikt and Nothnagel syndromes
7. Fascicular lesions are virtually always ischemic, infiltrative (tumor), or rarely inflammatory
8. Fascicular lesion may cause partial III nerve palsy due to topographic anatomy (Figure 5-4)

C. Uncal herniation syndrome (see Figure 5-2, site 3)
   1. In its course toward the cavernous sinus, the III nerve rests on the edge of the tentorium cerebelli
   2. The portion of the brain overlying the III nerve, at the tentorial edge, is the uncal portion of the undersurface of the temporal lobe
   3. A supratentorial space-occupying mass, located anywhere in or above this cerebral hemisphere, may cause a downward displacement and herniation of the uncus across the tentorial edge, thereby compressing the III nerve (Figure 5-5)
   4. A dilated and fixed pupil (Hutchinson pupil) may be the first indication that altered consciousness is due to a space-occupying intracranial lesion

D. Posterior communicating artery aneurysm (see Figure 5-2, site 4)
   1. In its course toward the cavernous sinus, the III nerve travels alongside (lateral to) the posterior communicating artery
   2. The most common cause of nontraumatic isolated III nerve paresis with pupillary involvement is an aneurysm at the junction of the posterior communicating artery and the internal carotid artery (Figure 5-6)
   3. Hemorrhage suddenly enlarges the aneurysmal sac to which the III nerve is adherent or there is actual hemorrhage into the substance of the nerve

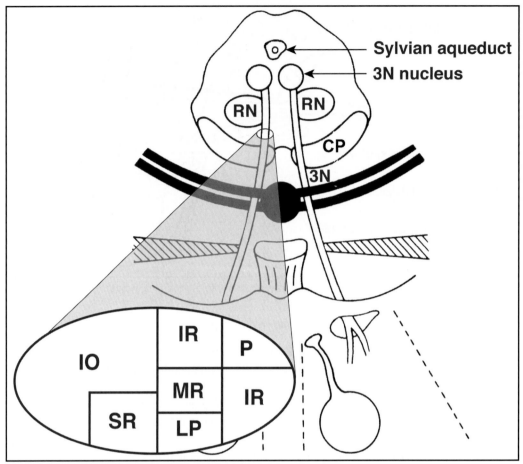

Figure 5-4. Topographic anatomy of right III nerve fascicle at level of rostral midbrain. CP = corticospinal tract, IO = inferior oblique, IR = inferior rectus, LP = levator palpebrae, MR = medial rectus, P = pupillary fibers, RN = red nucleus, SR = superior rectus. (Adapted from Purvin V. Isolated fascicular third nerve palsy. *J Neuroophthalmol.* 2010;30:263-265.)[1]

    4.   On occasion, the pupil is spared early in the course of aneurysmal compression of the III nerve. The patient must be followed carefully during the initial 5 to 7 days to be certain of the status of the pupil

  E. Cavernous sinus syndrome (see Figure 5-2, site 5)

    1.   III nerve paresis is usually seen in association with other cranial nerve involvement: IV, V, VI, and oculosympathetic paralysis

    2.   III nerve paresis due to cavernous sinus lesion tends to be partial (ie, all muscles innervated by the III nerve are not equally involved)

    3.   Pupillary fibers are frequently "spared," such that the pupil may be normal or minimally involved

    4.   Cavernous sinus lesions may lead to primary aberrant regeneration of the III nerve (see page 108, IV)

    5.   Isolated oculomotor nerve palsy occasionally occurs in patients with cavernous sinus invasion from pituitary adenoma with or without pituitary apoplexy

    6.   Radiation-induced oculomotor cranial nerve palsy in patients with pituitary tumor or sellar-based lesions

    7.   See Chapter 7

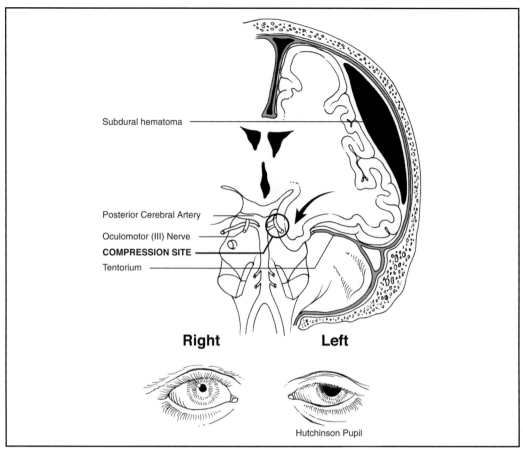

Figure 5-5. Transtentorial herniation of the uncus of the temporal lobe with III nerve compression.

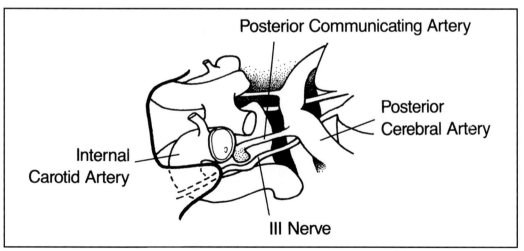

Figure 5-6. Compression of the left III nerve due to aneurysm at the junction of the posterior communicating and internal carotid arteries.

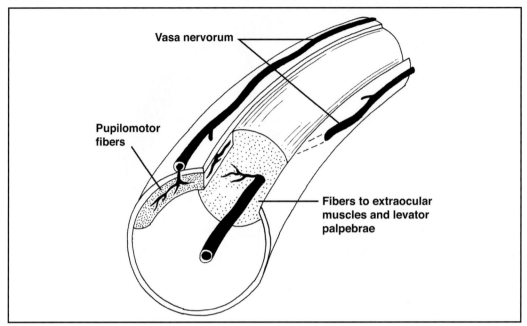

Figure 5-7. Blood supply to portions of III nerve supplying the pupil and extraocular muscles.

    F.   Orbital syndrome (see Figure 5-2, site 6)
        1.   See the orbital syndrome of the VI nerve (see Chapter 4)
        2.   Just before entering the superior orbital fissure, the III nerve splits into 2 divisions
        3.   The superior division innervates the following:
            a.   Superior rectus
            b.   Levator palpebrae
        4.   The inferior division innervates the following:
            a.   Inferior rectus
            b.   Medial rectus
            c.   Inferior oblique
            d.   Iris sphincter muscle (pupil)
            e.   Ciliary muscle (accommodation)
        5.   Orbital involvement of the III nerve may result in selective paresis of structures innervated by only one of the divisions
    G.   Pupil-sparing isolated III nerve paresis (the seventh syndrome of the III nerve)
        1.   The pupillomotor fibers of the III nerve travel in the outer layers of the nerve and are therefore closer to the nutrient blood supply enveloping the nerve (Figure 5-7)
        2.   This may explain why the pupillomotor fibers are spared in 80% of ischemic III nerve paresis but are affected in 95% of cases of compressive (trauma, tumor, aneurysm) III nerve paresis
        3.   Patients with pupil-sparing isolated III nerve palsies are evaluated and managed in a similar manner to patients with isolated IV and VI nerve paresis
            a.   Laboratory evaluation, including for presumed ischemic cranial nerve palsy
                i.   Blood pressure determination
                ii.   CBC
                iii.   Sedimentation rate and C-reactive protein

          iv.   Glucose tolerance test (GTT); hemoglobin A1C

          v.   Fasting lipid panel

          vi.   VDRL, if positive, FTA-ABS or TPHA

          vii. Antinuclear antibody (ANA)

    b.   Follow the patient

          i.   The III nerve paresis is truly isolated

          ii.   The patient is over 50 years of age

          iii. The patient has a history of vasculopathic risk factors such as diabetes and hypertension

    c.   Most patients with ischemic III nerve paresis demonstrate improvement of the motility measurements within 1 month and complete recovery by 3 months

    d.   Recommend additional testing, which may include MRI, MRA, CTA, possibly LP, and 4-vessel cerebral angiography if:

          i.   The pupil becomes dilated in the initial 5 to 7 days after onset

          ii.   No significant improvement in 3 months

          iii. The patient develops signs of aberrant regeneration of the III nerve

          iv.   Other neurologic findings develop

    e.   **Caution:** ocular myasthenia can mimic a pupil-sparing III nerve palsy so consider ice/rest test, myasthenia panel (acetylcholine receptor and striated muscle antibodies)

H.   Diagnostic guidelines for patient with isolated III nerve palsy

    1.   While the size and reactivity of the pupil are major determinants in patient evaluation, other important considerations include the following:

      a.   Age of patient (see page 108, III, C)

      b.   Degree of somatic (motility, lid) involvement

      c.   Some pupillary involvement (<2 mm anisocoria) is found in up to one-third of patients with ischemic (eg, diabetic) III nerve palsies

      d.   Pupillary involvement may develop during the initial 5 to 7 days of a compressive III nerve palsy

      e.   Periorbital pain does not reliably distinguish between compressive versus vasculopathic etiology

      f.   Remember: "pupil-sparing" III nerve palsy designates complete involvement of the levator palpebrae and extraocular muscles innervated by the III nerve without anisocoria

    2.   Guidelines:

      a.   All children less than age 10 years (no matter the pupillary findings) should undergo MRI, MRA, and CTA. If normal, consider cerebral angiography (occult aneurysm). If a normal pupil, consider acetylcholine antibodies and an ice/rest test (myasthenia gravis), LP (infectious, neoplastic etiology), anti-GQ1b antibody (Miller Fisher syndrome)

      b.   All patients older than 10 years with pupil-involving III nerve palsy should undergo MRI, MRA, and CTA. Depending on results, may need cerebral angiography

      c.   All patients age 10 to 50 years with pupil-sparing III nerve palsy should undergo MRI and MRA. If normal:

          i.   Medical evaluation—diabetes mellitus, hypertension

          ii.   Observe for pupillary involvement

          iii. Follow for development of other neurologic abnormalities

	Rucker[2]	Goldstein & Cogan[3] (isolated III)	Green et al[4]	Rucker[5]	Rush & Younge[6]	Kodsi & Younge[7] (children)	Richards et al[8]	Schumacher-Feero et al[9] (children)	Park et al[10]	Fang et al[11]
Total Patients	**335**	**61**	**130**	**274**	**290**	**35**	**244**	**49**	**48**	**145**
Etiologies (%)										
Neoplasm	11	10	4	18	12	14	10	12	7	11
Trauma	15	8	11	13	16	40	14	31	18	12
Aneurysm	19	18	30	18	14	0	12	8	10	6
Ischemic*	19	47	19	17	21	0	23	0	35	42
Misc	8	6	13	12	14	29	18	47	11	10
Undetermined	28	11	23	20	23	17	23	2	19	19

Table 5-1

ETIOLOGIES OF ACQUIRED III NERVE PALSY

*Including diabetes mellitus.

    d.   All patients age 50 years and older with pupil-sparing III nerve palsy with total somatic involvement
       i.   Observation versus neuroimaging (MRI/MRA or CT/CTA)
       ii.   Consider laboratory evaluation (see page 106, II, G, 3, a)
    e.   All patients age 50 years and older with partial pupillary involvement (anisocoria >2 mm but pupil not fixed and dilated) should undergo neuroimaging (may include MRI, MRA, and CTA). If results are normal, strongly consider cerebral angiography, which may be necessary for interventions including coiling, clipping, or flow-diversion

III. INCIDENCE OF VARIOUS CAUSES OF III NERVE PALSIES
    A.   Table 5-1 summarizes 10 major published series of patients with paresis of the oculomotor nerve
    B.   Although neoplasm, aneurysm, and ischemia are the most common etiologies, approximately 10% to 25% of cases of III nerve palsies have an undetermined cause
    C.   Approximately one-half of III nerve palsies in children are congenital, and a high percentage have signs of aberrant regeneration. However, approximately 10% to 20% are due to aneurysm or neoplasm; therefore, all children should undergo neuroimaging (see Chapter 20)

IV. ABERRANT REGENERATION (MISDIRECTION) OF THE III NERVE
    A.   Regeneration of the disrupted III nerve fibers may result in fibers of one structure being hooked up ("axon sprouting") to fibers that terminate in another structure
    B.   Clinical phenomena may be classified as the following:
       1.   Lid-gaze dyskinesis
         a.   Some of the inferior rectus fibers may end up innervating the levator so that the lid retracts when the patient looks down: pseudo-Graefe sign

        b.   Some of the medial rectus fibers may end up supplying some of the innervation to the levator so that the lid retracts when the patient adducts his or her eye: inverse Duane syndrome

    2.   Pupil-gaze dyskinesis

        a.   Some of the medial rectus fibers may end up innervating the pupillary sphincter muscle so that there is more pupil constriction during convergence than as a response to light: pseudo-Argyll Robertson pupil

        b.   Some of the fibers destined to innervate the inferior rectus may end up innervating the pupillary sphincter so that on attempted downgaze, the pupil constricts

  C. Two forms of aberrant regeneration

    1.   Primary aberrant regeneration

        a.   No preceding acute III nerve palsy

        b.   Insidious development of III nerve palsy with accompanying signs of misdirection

        c.   Sign of an intracavernous lesion: meningioma, aneurysm, neurinoma

    2.   Secondary aberrant regeneration

        a.   Observe weeks to months during recovery from a III nerve palsy

        b.   Seen after trauma and tumor compression of the III nerve, but never after ischemic III nerve paresis. If you are following a patient with a presumed diagnosis of ischemic III nerve palsy and he or she develops signs of aberrant regeneration, then neuroimaging is indicated

V.   RARE CAUSES OF III NERVE PALSY

  A. Minor head trauma

    1.   In general, head trauma causing III nerve palsy is severe enough to cause loss of consciousness and often other neurologic deficits

    2.   Rarely, a patient may harbor a basal intracranial tumor and, with only minor head trauma, develop a III nerve palsy

    3.   Minimal head injury resulting in a III nerve palsy is an indication for neuroimaging

  B. Ophthalmoplegic migraine (see Chapter 15, VII, I on page 217)

    1.   Onset almost always in childhood

    2.   Usually a family history of migraine

    3.   III nerve palsy may occur at any time in relation to headache but usually appears as the headache phase abates

    4.   As a rule, III nerve palsy clears completely within 1 month, but occasionally permanent oculomotor paresis occurs

    5.   MRI may demonstrate thickening and enhancement of the cisternal (site 3) portion of III nerve

    6.   Pathophysiology uncertain: ischemia, inflammation, demyelination

    7.   Disorder may be mimicked by mass lesion (schwannoma, angioma) of III nerve

  C. Cyclic oculomotor palsy

    1.   Disorder usually present at birth or in early childhood

    2.   Occurs in the setting of a total III nerve palsy

    3.   Spastic movements of the muscles innervated by the III nerve results in lid elevation, adduction, miosis, and increased accommodation

    4.   These movements occur at regular intervals, lasting 10 to 30 seconds

    5.   Etiology unknown

References

1. Purvin V. Isolated fascicular third nerve palsy. *J Neuroophthalmol*. 2010;30:263-265.
2. Rucker CW. Paralysis of the third, fourth, and sixth cranial nerves. *Am J Ophthalmol*. 1958;46:787-794.
3. Goldstein JE, Cogan DG. Diabetic ophthalmoplegia with special reference to the pupil. *Arch Ophthalmol*. 1960;64:592-600.
4. Green WR, Hackett ER, Schlezinger NS. Neuro-ophthalmic evaluation of oculomotor nerve paralysis. *Arch Ophthalmol*. 1964;72:154-167.
5. Rucker CW. The causes of paralysis of the third, fourth, and sixth cranial nerves. *Am J Ophthalmol*. 1966;61:1293-1298.
6. Rush JA, Younge BR. Paralysis of cranial nerves III, IV, and VI. Cause and prognosis in 1,000 cases. *Arch Ophthalmol*. 1981;99:76-79.
7. Kodsi SR, Younge BR. Acquired oculomotor, trochlear and abducent cranial nerve palsies in pediatric patients. *Am J Ophthalmol*. 1992;114:568-574.
8. Richards BW, Jones FR, Younge BR. Causes and prognosis in 4278 cases of paralysis of the oculomotor, trochlear and abducens cranial nerves. *Am J Ophthalmol*. 1992;113:489-496.
9. Schumacher-Feero LA, Yoo KW, Solari FM, et al. Third cranial nerve palsy in children. *Am J Ophthalmol*. 1999;128:216-221.
10. Park UC, Kim SJ, Hwang JM, Yu YS. Clinical features and natural history of acquired third, fourth, and sixth cranial nerve palsy. *Eye*. 2008;22:691-696.
11. Fang C, Leavitt JA, Hodge DO, Holmes JM, Mohney BG, Chen JJ. Incidence and etiologies of acquired third nerve palsy using a population-based method. *JAMA Ophthalmol*. 2017;135:23-28.

Bibliography

Chen PK, Wang SJ. Ophthalmoplegic migraine: migraine variant or cranial neuralgia? *Cephalalgia*. 2012;32:515-517.

Jacobson DM. Pupil involvement in patients with diabetes-associated oculomotor nerve palsy. *Arch Ophthalmol*. 1998;116:723-727.

Jacobson DM, Broste SK. Early progression of ophthalmoplegia in patients with ischemic oculomotor nerve palsies. *Arch Ophthalmol*. 1995;113:1525-1537.

Kissel JT, Burde RM, Klingele TG, et al. Pupil-sparing oculomotor palsies with internal carotid-posterior communicating artery aneurysms. *Ann Neurol*. 1983;13:149-154.

Kobayashi H, Kawabori M, Terasaka S, Murata J, Houkin K. A possible mechanism of isolated oculomotor nerve palsy by apoplexy of pituitary adenoma without cavernous sinus invasion: a report of two cases. *Acta Neurochir (Wien)*. 2011;153:2453-2456.

Lepore FE, Glaser JS. Misdirection revisited: a critical appraisal of acquired oculomotor nerve synkinesis. *Arch Ophthalmol*. 1980;98:2206-2209.

Murchison AP, Gilbert ME, Savino PJ. Neuroimaging and acute ocular motor mononeuropathies. *Arch Ophthalmol*. 2011;129:301-305.

Tamhankar MA, Volpe NJ. Management of acute cranial nerve 3, 4 and 6 palsies: role of neuroimaging. *Curr Opin Ophthalmol*. 2015;26:464-468.

Vaphiades MS, Spencer SA, Riley K, Francis C, Deitz L, Kline LB. Radiation-induced ocular motor cranial nerve palsies in patients with pituitary tumor. *J Neuroophthalmol*. 2011;31:210-213.

Volpe NJ, Lee AG. Do patients with neurologically isolated ocular motor cranial nerve palsies require prompt neuroimaging? *J Neuroophthalmol*. 2014;34:301-305.

Wilker SC, Rucker JC, Newman NJ, Biousse V, Tomsak RL. Pain in ischemic ocular motor cranial nerve palsies. *Br J Ophthalmol*. 2009;93:1657-1659.

CHAPTER 6

The Five Syndromes of the IV Nerve (Trochlear)

Michael S. Vaphiades, DO

I. **ANATOMICAL CONSIDERATIONS**

    A. Figure 6-1 is a diagram of a cross-section of the lower midbrain at the level of the inferior colliculi

    B. The IV nerve

        1. The only cranial nerve that exits at the dorsal aspect of the brainstem (Figure 6-2)

        2. The cranial nerve with the longest intracranial course (75 mm)

    C. The IV nerve fascicles cross in the anterior medullary velum (roof of the Sylvian aqueduct) prior to exiting dorsally and coursing anteriorly around the midbrain to travel forward between the superior cerebellar and posterior cerebral arteries (just as, but laterally separated from, the III cranial nerve)

    D. Therefore, the left IV nerve fascicle becomes the right IV nerve and innervates the right superior oblique muscle; and the right IV nerve fascicle becomes the left IV nerve and innervates the left superior oblique muscle

II. **CLINICAL SYNDROMES OF THE IV NERVE (FIGURE 6-3): NUCLEAR-FASCICULAR SYNDROME, SUBARACHNOID SPACE SYNDROME, CAVERNOUS SINUS SYNDROME, ORBITAL SYNDROME, ISOLATED IV NERVE PALSY (CONGENITAL OR ACQUIRED)**

    A. Nuclear-fascicular syndrome (see Figure 6-3, site 1)

        1. Distinguishing nuclear from fascicular lesions is virtually impossible due to the short course of the fascicles within the midbrain, thus the lack of associated neurologic signs

        2. Frequent etiologies include hemorrhage, infarction, demyelination, trauma (including neurosurgical)

        3. Fascicular lesion may be seen with contralateral Horner syndrome since the sympathetic pathways descend through the dorsolateral tegmentum of the midbrain adjacent to the trochlear fascicles

    B. Subarachnoid space syndrome (see Figure 6-3, site 2)

        1. IV nerve particularly susceptible to injury as it emerges from the dorsal surface of the brainstem

        2. When bilateral IV nerve palsies occur, the site of injury is likely in the anterior medullary velum. Contrecoup forces transmitted to the brainstem by the free tentorial edge may injure the nerves at this site

        3. Less frequent causes include tumor (eg, pinealoma, tentorial meningioma), meningitis, neurosurgical trauma

Foroozan R, Vaphiades MS. *Kline's Neuro-Ophthalmology Review Manual, Eighth Edition (pp 111-121).* © 2018 SLACK Incorporated.

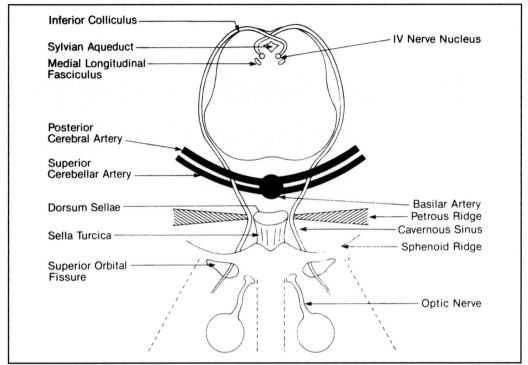

Figure 6-1. Diagram of a cross-section of the lower midbrain at the level of the inferior colliculi showing the petrous ridge (hatched) and the posterior cerebral artery and superior cerebellar artery (highlighted in black) and their relationship to the IV nerve.

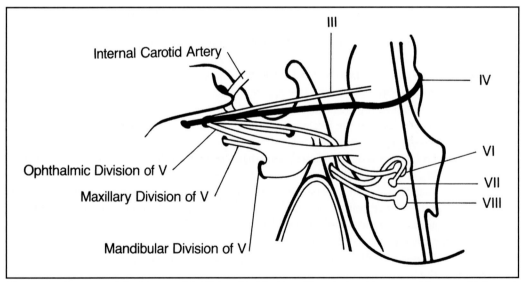

Figure 6-2. Diagram of the IV nerve (highlighted in black) and its relationship to cranial nerves III through VIII.

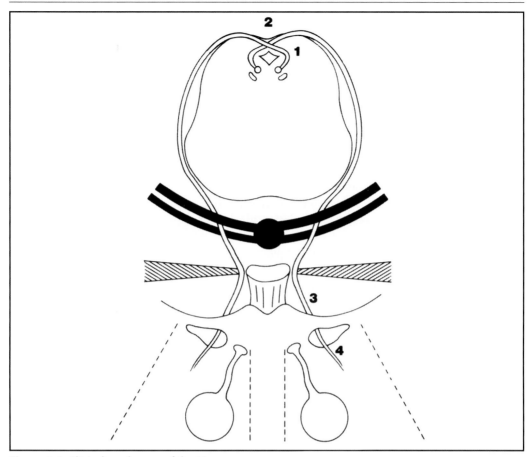

Figure 6-3. Clinical syndromes of the IV nerve.

    C.   Cavernous sinus syndrome (see Figure 6-3, site 3)
        1.   Seen in association with other cranial nerve palsies: III, V, VI, and oculosympathetic paralysis
        2.   Checking IV nerve function in the setting of a III nerve paresis
            a.   Since the involved eye cannot be adducted well, the vertical actions of the superior oblique muscle cannot be tested
            b.   Therefore, the eye is moved into abduction and then the patient is instructed to look down; the ability of the eye to intort is examined as a measure of IV nerve function
            c.   If a limbal or conjunctival landmark (eg, pterygium or blood vessel) is noted to intort, then the IV nerve is presumed intact
        3.   See Chapter 7
    D.   Orbital syndrome (see Figure 6-3, site 4)
        1.   Usually seen in association with III, IV, and VI cranial nerve palsies: orbital signs including proptosis, chemosis, conjunctival injection
        2.   Most common etiologies include trauma, inflammation, tumor

E.   Isolated IV nerve palsy (the fifth syndrome of the IV nerve)

1.   Congenital

a.   See page 119, VI for incidence of this condition

b.   Most often seen in pediatric population and late in life (fifth to seventh decades) as patient's IV nerve palsy may decompensate

c.   Diagnostic keys

i.   Large vertical fusion amplitude (10 to 15 prism diopters)

ii. Family album tomography (FAT) scan: look at old photographs (including on social media) to detect long-standing head-tilt, suggestive of congenital etiology

iii. Look for facial asymmetry

d.   Some cases might be a cranial dysinnervation disorder as MRI may show superior oblique hypoplasia with absence of the IV nerve

2.   Acquired

a.   Acute onset of vertical diplopia, usually with torsional component

b.   Characteristic head position

i.   Tilt to opposite shoulder

ii. Head turned downward with chin depressed, eyes up

iii. Face turned to opposite side

c.   Perform Parks-Bielschowsky 3-step test (see section III next) to confirm diagnosis

d.   Initial evaluation (always ask about head trauma)

i.   Blood pressure determination

ii. CBC, BMP including glucose, lipids, hemoglobin A1C, VDRL, if positive, FTA-ABS or TPHA, ANA

iii. Sedimentation rate; C-reactive protein (in patients with suspected of giant cell arteritis)

iv. Myasthenia gravis panel (acetylcholine receptor and striated muscle antibodies) if atypical features

e.   As with other isolated ocular motor neuropathies, if the IV nerve palsy has not improved or resolved within 3 months, or if other neurologic signs develop, further evaluation is indicated

i.   Medical and neurologic examinations

ii. MRI of the brain and orbits with and without fat suppression and contrast

iii. Cerebrovascular studies: MRA, CTA, cerebral angiography if an aneurysm is suspected (very unusual cause of an isolated IV nerve palsy)

iv. LP if infection, demyelinating disease or neoplasm suspected

III. **Diagnosis of recently acquired IV nerve palsy**

A.   If a patient has vertical misalignment (HT) due to recently acquired weakness of a single vertically acting muscle, then determine the weak muscle by performing the Parks-Bielschowsky 3-step test (Figures 6-4 and 6-5)

1.   The medial and lateral rectus muscles do not have primarily vertical actions

2.   Therefore, HT of paretic etiology is caused by weakness of one or more of the following 8 vertically acting muscles:

a.   Right inferior oblique (RIO); left inferior oblique (LIO)

b.   Right superior oblique (RSO); left superior oblique (LSO)

c.   Right inferior rectus (RIR); left inferior rectus (LIR)

d.   Right superior rectus (RSR); left superior rectus (LSR)

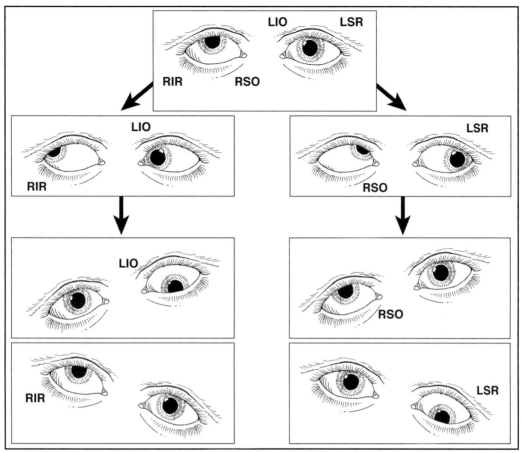

Figure 6-4. Parks-Bielschowsky 3-step test in a patient with a right HT. Potential paretic muscle. LIO = left inferior oblique, LSR = left superior rectus, RIR = right inferior rectus, RSO = right superior oblique.

3. If the HT is due to weakness of only 1 of these 8 muscles, the paretic muscle is identified by answering the 3 questions asked in the Parks-Bielschowsky 3-step test

4. Each step cuts the possible number of muscles in half
    a. After the first step, there are 4 possible muscles remaining
    b. After the second step, there are 2 remaining
    c. After the third step, only one muscle remains

5. Parks-Bielschowsky first step: which is the higher eye?
    a. If the patient has an RHT, then the weak muscle is either a depressor of the right eye (RIR, RSO) or an elevator of the left eye (LSR, LIO; see Figure 6-4)
    b. If the patient has an LHT, then the weak muscle is either an elevator of the right eye (RSR, RIO) or a depressor of the left eye (LIR, LSO; see Figure 6-5)
    c. Therefore, by determining if the patient has an RHT or a LHT, you have narrowed down the number of suspected muscles from 8 to 4

6. Parks-Bielschowsky second step: HT worse on gaze right or left?
    a. The vertical rectus muscles (superior and inferior recti) have their greatest vertical action (and least torsional action) when the eye is abducted
    b. Therefore, LHT due to paresis of LIR will be worse on gaze left (since OS is abducted on gaze left); LHT due to paresis of RSR will be worse on gaze right (since OD is abducted on right gaze)

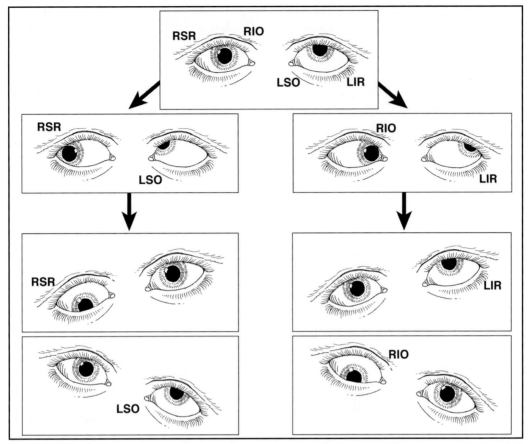

Figure 6-5. Parks-Bielschowsky 3-step test in a patient with a left HT. Potential paretic muscle. LIR = left inferior rectus, LSO = left superior oblique, RIO = right inferior oblique, RSR = right superior rectus.

   c.   The oblique muscles (superior and inferior obliques) have their greatest vertical action (and least torsional action) when the eye is adducted

   d.   Therefore, LHT due to paresis of LSO will be worse on gaze right; LHT due to paresis of RIO will be worse on gaze left

   e.   LHT worse on gaze right is due to weakness of either LSO or RSR

   f.   LHT worse on gaze left is due to weakness of either LIR or RIO

   g.   Thus, in the case of LHT, by answering the question, "Is LHT worse on gaze right or left?" you have narrowed the possible muscles from 4 (LSO, RSR, LIR, RIO) to 2 (either LSO/RSR or LIR/RIO)

   h.   Similarly, the possible causes of RHT are narrowed down from 4 (RIR, LIO, LSR, RSO) to 2 (RIR/LIO if RHT worse on gaze right; RSO/LSR if RHT worse on gaze left). **Note:** in each case:

      i.   RHT worse on gaze right (RIR or LIO)

      ii.   RHT worse on gaze left (RSO or LSR)

      iii.   LHT worse on gaze right (LSO or RSR)

      iv.   LHT worse on gaze left (LIR or RIO)

      You are left with either 2 superior or 2 inferior muscles; 1 will be a rectus and 1 an oblique, and 1 will be of the right eye and 1 of the left. If this is not the case (eg, if you have narrowed it down after the second step to "RIR versus LSR" or "LSO versus LIO"), then you have made a mistake and need to retrace your steps

      7. Parks-Bielschowsky third step: is the HT worse on head-tilt right (head tilted so that the right ear is near the right shoulder) or head-tilt left (head tilted so that the left ear is near the left shoulder)?

         a. The superior muscles (SR and SO) intort the eyes; the inferior muscles (IR and IO) extort the eye

         b. When the head is tilted downward to the right shoulder, the eyes undergo corrective torsion (ie, OD intorted and OS extorted)

         c. Therefore, when the head is tilted to the right, OD will be intorted by contraction of RSR and RSO; these 2 muscles work together in affecting the intorsion and neutralize each other's vertical action (RSR is an elevator and RSO a depressor)

         d. If one of these muscles is the paretic muscle responsible for the HT, then the vertical action will not be neutralized and the HT will be worse on tilting the head to the right shoulder

         e. Therefore, the mnemonic for the third step is as follows:

            i. If you are left with 2 superior muscles, then the paretic muscle is the one on the same side as the shoulder toward which the head-tilt makes the HT worse (eg, if it is narrowed down to "RSO versus LSR," then the paretic muscle is "RSO if RHT worse on tilt to right" and "LSR if RHT is worse to tilt left")

            ii. If you are left with 2 inferior muscles, then the paretic muscle is the one on the side opposite the shoulder toward which the head-tilt makes the HT worse (eg, if it is narrowed down to "RIO versus LIR," then the paretic muscle is "RIO if LHT worse on tilt left" and "LIR if LHT worse on tilt right")

    8. Not all IV nerve palsies (30% in one series) will conform to the expected pattern of the Parks-Bielschowsky 3-step test. There may be spread of comitance, particularly with long-standing deficits

    9. Orbital MRI may show atrophy of the involved superior oblique muscle

B. Do not forget Bielschowsky's "missing step": is the HT worse on gaze up or gaze down?

    1. This step confirms step 3

    2. Note again that after step 2, we are down to either 2 superior or 2 inferior muscles

         a. RSR versus LSO

         b. RSO versus LSR

         c. RIR versus LIO

         d. RIO versus LIR

    3. Note also that in each case, one muscle is an elevator and the other a depressor

    4. Therefore, we can confirm the paretic muscle identified by step 3 by noting if the HT is worse on gaze up (RSR, LSR, LIO, RIO) or gaze down (LSO, RSO, RIR, LIR)

    5. In patients with IV nerve palsy, HT that is equal or greater in gaze up compared to gaze down is suggestive of a long-standing deficit

    6. A mnemonic for a unilateral IV nerve palsy is **GOTS-D**, meaning the HT (side of the IV) increased in vertical prism diopters if the patients "**g**aze" in the "**o**pposite" direction and "**t**ilts" to the "**s**ame" side, and it also increases in "**d**owngaze"

IV. **MEASURING THE TORSIONAL COMPONENT OF IV NERVE PALSY**

A. Double Maddox rod test to quantitate torsional component of diplopia

B. The patient will report intorsion of image seen by eye with IV nerve palsy. Actually, this indicates extorsion of the patient's eye caused by action of the antagonist inferior oblique muscle (Figure 6-6)

C. Greater than 10 degrees of torsion is suggestive of bilateral IV nerve palsies

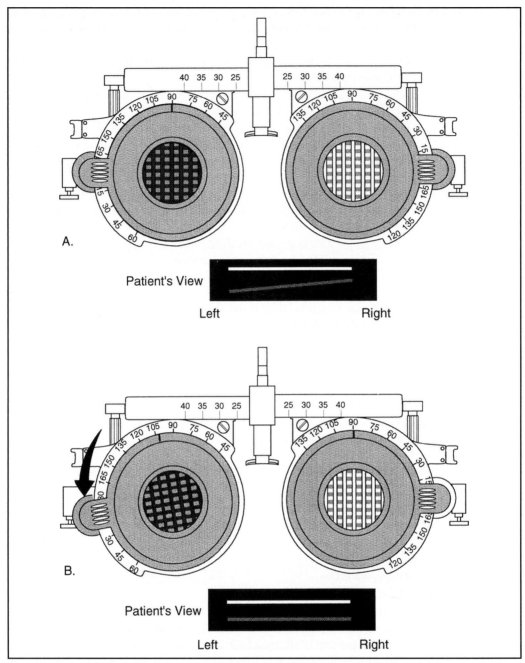

Figure 6-6. Double Maddox rod test for cyclodeviation in a patient with a right IV nerve palsy. Red and white Maddox rods are inserted into a trial frame, with the red lens before the eye with a suspected cyclodeviation. Special care must be taken to align the direction of the glass rods with the 90-degree mark of the trial frame. The trial frame must be adjusted carefully to a more exact horizontal position. (Adapted from Van Noorden GK. *Atlas of Strabismus.* 4th ed. St Louis, MO: CV Mosby; 1983:52-53.)[1]

V. Bilateral IV nerve palsies

A. Usually due to severe head trauma with contusion of the anterior medullary velum where the IV nerve fascicles cross

	Rucker[2]	Rucker[3]	Khawam et al[4]	Burger et al[5]	Younge & Sutula[6]	Rush & Younge[7]	Kodsi & Younge[8] (children)	Richards et al[9]	Park et al[10]
Total Patients	**67**	**84**	**40**	**33**	**36**	**172**	**19**	**248**	**46**
Etiologies (%)									
Neoplasm	4	8	2.5	21	0	4	5	4	0
Trauma	36	27	67.5	39	44	32	37	26	31
Aneurysm	0	0	0	3	0	2	0	1	0
Ischemic	36	15	2.5	18	33	18	0	14	37
Misc	10	15	7.5	9	8	4	37	20	4
Undetermined	13	33	20	6	15	36	21	35	28

Table 6-1

ETIOLOGIES OF ACQUIRED IV NERVE PALSY

B. Parks-Bielschowsky 3-step test
 1. Either eye may be hypertropic in primary position or patient may be orthophoric
 2. RHT on gaze left; LHT on gaze right
 3. RHT on head-tilt right; LHT on head-tilt left
C. With double Maddox rods, measure greater than 10 degrees of torsion
D. There may be a V-pattern esotropia due to loss of the secondary function of abduction

VI. **INCIDENCE OF VARIOUS CAUSES OF IV NERVE PALSY**
 A. Table 6-1 summarizes 9 large series of patients with acquired paresis of the IV nerve
 B. Summary of cases of acquired, isolated IV paresis (10-20-30-40 rule)
 1. Ten percent: neoplasm-aneurysm
 2. Twenty percent: ischemic
 3. Thirty percent: undetermined or miscellaneous
 4. Forty percent: trauma
 C. In addition to acquired causes, a large proportion of IV nerve palsies are classified as congenital. In various series of patients, the frequency of congenital IV nerve palsies ranges from 29%[6] to 67%[11]
 D. The frequency of congenital IV nerve paresis cannot be overemphasized. Many adults presenting in the fifth and sixth decades of life may have decompensated, congenital IV nerve palsies

VII. **DIFFERENTIAL DIAGNOSIS OF VERTICAL DIPLOPIA**
 A. Ocular myasthenia
 B. Thyroid eye disease
 C. Orbital disease (tumor, trauma, inflammation, blowout fracture of the floor, silent sinus syndrome)
 D. III nerve paresis
 E. Brown syndrome
 F. Skew deviation
 G. Sagging eye syndrome
 H. Heavy eye syndrome

VIII.   OTHER SYNDROMES OF THE SUPERIOR OBLIQUE MUSCLE

    A.   Brown (sheath) syndrome

        1.   Limitation of elevation of the eye in adduction because movements of the superior oblique tendon in the trochlea are restricted; elevation in abduction normal or near normal

        2.   Affected eyes usually hypotropic, and the patient often develops abnormal head position (chin up) and face turn (away from the eye with Brown syndrome)

        3.   Forced ductions must be positive to establish diagnosis

        4.   Congenital etiology: superior oblique tendon is short and tethered

        5.   Acquired etiologies:

            a.   Tenosynovitis may prevent tendon from passing through the trochlear pulley

            b.   Orbital trauma to trochlear region

            c.   Superonasal orbital mass

    B.   Superior oblique myokymia

        1.   Episodic condition causing vertical diplopia or monocular blurred vision with tremulous sensations of the affected eye

        2.   Paroxysmal, rapid, vertical, and torsional movements of one eye that are usually small, necessitating slit-lamp examination or ophthalmoscopy

        3.   Precipitated by asking the patient to first look in the direction of action of the superior oblique muscle and then return to the primary position

        4.   Usually benign; occasionally seen with multiple sclerosis or posterior fossa tumor

        5.   Etiology: uncertain. Some cases may be due to neurovascular compression of IV nerve at root exit zone from the brainstem

        6.   Treatment:

            a.   Topical beta-blocker

            b.   Carbamazepine (Tegretol); propranolol (Inderal); gabapentin (Neurontin)

            c.   Superior oblique surgery

            d.   Neurosurgical decompression

REFERENCES

1. Van Noorden GK. *Atlas of Strabismus*. 4th ed. St Louis, MO: CV Mosby; 1983:52-53

2. Rucker CW. Paralysis of the third, fourth, and sixth cranial nerves. *Am J Ophthalmol*. 1958;46:787-794.

3. Rucker CW. The causes of paralysis of the third, fourth, and sixth cranial nerves. *Am J Ophthalmol*. 1966;61:1293-1298.

4. Khawam E, Scott AB, Jampolski A. Acquired superior oblique palsy. *Arch Ophthalmol*. 1967;77:761-768.

5. Burger LJ, Kalvin NH, Smith JL. Acquired lesions of the fourth cranial nerve. *Brain*. 1970;93:567-574.

6. Younge BR, Sutula F. Analysis of trochlear nerve palsies. *Mayo Clin Proc*. 1977;52:11-18.

7. Rush JA, Younge BR. Paralysis of cranial nerves III, IV, and VI. Cause and prognosis in 1,000 cases. *Arch Ophthalmol*. 1981;99:76-79.

8. Kodsi SR, Younge BR. Acquired oculomotor trochlear and abducent cranial nerve palsies in pediatric patients. *Am J Ophthalmol*. 1992;114:568-574.

9. Richards BW, Jones FR, Younge BR. Cause and prognoses of 4278 cases of paralysis of oculomotor, trochlear and abducens cranial nerves. *Am J Ophthalmol*. 1992;183:489-496.

10. Park UC, Kim SJ, Hwang JM, Yu YS. Clinical features and natural history of acquired third, fourth, and sixth cranial nerve palsy. *Eye*. 2008;22:691-696.

11. Harley RD. Paralytic strabismus in children: etiologic incidence and management of the third, fourth, and sixth nerve palsies. *Ophthalmology*. 1980;86:24-43.

BIBLIOGRAPHY

Chaudhuri Z, Demer JL. Sagging eye syndrome: connective tissue involution as a cause of horizontal and vertical strabismus in older patients. *JAMA Ophthalmol.* 2013;131:619-625.

Hashimoto M, Ohtsuka K, Suzuki Y, Minamida Y, Houkin K. Superior oblique myokymia caused by vascular compression. *J Neuroophthalmol.* 2004;24:237-239.

Jacobson DM, Warner JJ, Choucair AK, Ptacek LJ. Trochlear nerve palsy following minor head trauma. A sign of structural disorder. *J Clin Neuroophthalmol.* 1988;8:263-268.

Jeong SH, Kim SH, Lee SH, et al. Central trochlear palsy: report of two patients with ipsilesional palsy and review of the literature. *J Neuroophthalmol.* 2016;36:377-382.

Kaeser PF, Brodsky MC. Fourth cranial nerve palsy and Brown syndrome: two interrelated congenital cranial dysinnervation disorders? *Curr Neurol Neurosci Rep.* 2013;13:352.

Khaier A, Dawson E, Lee J. Clinical course and characteristics of acute presentation of fourth nerve paresis. *J Pediatr Ophthalmol Strabismus.* 2012;49:366-369.

Kim JH, Hwang JM. Absense of trochlear nerve in patients with superior oblique hypoplasia. *Ophthalmology.* 2010;117:2208-2213.

Manchandia AM, Demer JL. Sensitivity of the three-step test in diagnosis of superior oblique palsy. *J AAPOS.* 2014;18567-18571.

Muthusamy B, Irsch K, Peggy Chang HY, Guyton DL. The sensitivity of the Bielschowsky head-tilt test in diagnosing acquired bilateral superior oblique paresis. *Am J Ophthalmol.* 2014;157:901-907.

Shin SY, Demer JL. Superior oblique extraocular muscle shape in superior oblique palsy. *Am J Ophthalmol.* 2015;159:1169-1179.

Tamhankar MA, Kim JH, Ying GS, Volpe NJ. Adult hypertropia: a guide to diagnostic evaluation based on review of 300 patients. *Eye (Lond).* 2011;25:91-96.

Tan RJ, Demer JL. Heavy eye syndrome versus sagging eye syndrome in high myopia. *J AAPOS.* 2015;19:500-506.

Wilker SC, Rucker JC, Newman NJ, Biousse V, Tomsak RL. Pain in ischemic ocular motor cranial nerve palsies. *Br J Ophthalmol.* 2009;93:1657-1659.

CHAPTER 7

Cavernous Sinus Syndrome

MICHAEL S. VAPHIADES, DO

I. **GENERAL CONSIDERATIONS**
   A. The ocular motor cranial nerves lie in proximity within the cavernous sinus and superior orbital fissure
   B. Since the cavernous sinus contains structures that continue through the superior orbital fissure, it is often impossible to state whether a lesion is in the sinus or in the fissure. More general designation is parasellar syndrome
   C. Typically, patients present with periorbital or hemicranial pain, combined with ipsilateral ocular motor cranial nerve palsies, oculosympathetic paralysis, and sensory loss in the distribution of the ophthalmic (V^1) and occasionally maxillary (V^2) division of the trigeminal nerve. Clinically, various combinations of these cranial nerve palsies occur
   D. The "orbital apex syndrome" should be reserved for multiple ocular motor cranial nerve palsies plus optic nerve dysfunction

II. **ANATOMY (FIGURES 7-1 AND 7-2)**
   A. Traditionally, the cavernous sinus was thought to be an unbroken, trabeculated structure, but studies have demonstrated that it is a plexus of various-sized veins that divide and coalesce
   B. Major constituents:
      1. III nerve
      2. IV nerve
      3. VI nerve
      4. Ophthalmic nerve (V^1)
      5. Sympathetic carotid plexus
      6. Intracavernous carotid artery
   C. The III, IV, V^1 nerves all lie in a lateral wall of the cavernous sinus. The VI nerve lies freely within the sinus, just lateral to the intracavernous carotid

III. **CAUSES OF CAVERNOUS SINUS SYNDROME PRODUCING PAINFUL OPHTHALMOPLEGIA**
   A. Trauma
   B. Vascular
      1. Intracavernous carotid artery aneurysm
      2. Posterior cerebral artery aneurysm

Foroozan R, Vaphiades MS. *Kline's Neuro-Ophthalmology Review Manual, Eighth Edition (pp 123-127)*.
© 2018 SLACK Incorporated.

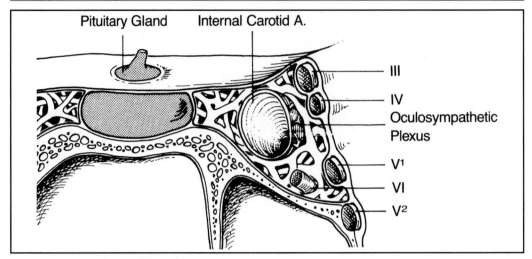

Figure 7-1. Coronal view of the left cavernous sinus and its contents.

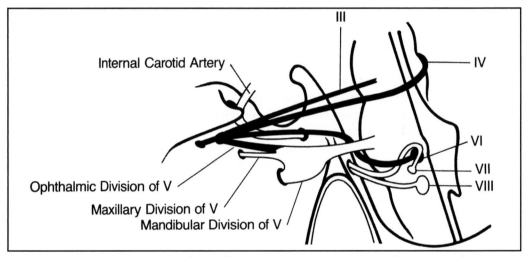

Figure 7-2. Lateral schematic view of the left cavernous sinus; cranial nerves that traverse the sinus are highlighted in black.

      3.   Carotid-cavernous fistula

      4.   Carotid-cavernous sinus thrombosis

   C. Neoplasm

      1.   Primary intracranial tumor

         a.   Pituitary adenoma

         b.   Meningioma

         c.   Craniopharyngioma

         d.   Sarcoma

         e.   Neurofibroma

         f.   Gasserian ganglion neuroma

         g.   Epidermoid

         h.   Hemangioma/hemangiopericytoma

         i.   Eosinophilic granuloma

         j.   Neuroblastoma

      2. Primary cranial tumor

         a. Chordoma

         b. Chondroma

         c. Giant cell tumor

      3. Local metastases

         a. Nasopharyngeal tumor

         b. Cylindroma

         c. Adamantinoma

         d. Squamous cell carcinoma

      4. Distant metastases

         a. Lymphoma

         b. Multiple myeloma

         c. Carcinomatous metastases

  D. Inflammation

      1. Bacterial: sinusitis, mucocele, periostitis

      2. Viral: herpes zoster

      3. Fungal: mucormycosis, aspergillosis

      4. Spirochetal: *T pallidum*

      5. Mycobacterial: *Mycobacterium tuberculosis*

      6. Unknown cause: sarcoidosis, granulomatosis with polyangiitis (Wegener granulomatosis), Tolosa-Hunt syndrome

IV. OF THE MORE COMMON CAUSES OF CAVERNOUS SINUS SYNDROME, THESE POINTS DESERVE EMPHASIS

  A. Intracavernous carotid artery aneurysm

      1. Typically produces slowly progressive, unilateral ophthalmoplegia

      2. May become painful

      3. Rarely rupture, but this occurrence produces a carotid-cavernous sinus fistula

      4. Neuroimaging: MRI, MRA, CTA

  B. Carotid-cavernous fistula

      1. Due to direct communication between intracavernous carotid artery and cavernous sinus

      2. High-flow, high-pressure fistula

      3. Most common cause is head trauma

      4. Clinical picture: chemosis, proptosis, ocular motor nerve palsies, bruit, retinopathy, increased intraocular pressure

  C. Dural-cavernous fistula

      1. Due to communication of dural branches of internal or external carotid arteries and cavernous sinus or vessels in the region of the cavernous sinus

      2. Low-flow, low-pressure fistula

      3. Most commonly occur spontaneously

      4. More subtle clinical picture: do not be fooled into treating these patients for "red eye"

      5. A minority of patients may develop cortical venous drainage of their fistula, with increased risk of intracerebral hemorrhage or cerebral venous infarction. Suggestive clinical signs are bilateral orbital congestion and postauricular bruit. Workup: MRI, MRA, MRV, cerebral angiography

      6. On occasion, fistula flow is directed posteriorly, causing chronic ocular motor cranial nerve palsies without orbital congestive signs ("white-eyed shunt"), may be painful and cranial CTA, MRA may be normal, a catheter angiogram may be the only way to diagnose this. Remember to ask about pulsatile tinnitus

D. Nasopharyngeal carcinoma
  1. Two to 3 times more common in males
  2. Predilection for Asian patients
  3. Varied clinical presentation
      a. Nasal obstruction
      b. Rhinorrhea
      c. Epistaxis
      d. Otitis media
      e. Proptosis
      f. Ipsilateral dry eye
  4. Ninety-five percent of patients with nasopharyngeal carcinoma have VI nerve paresis at some time during clinical course
  5. Neuroimaging: MRI with attention to subcranial soft tissue in region of nasopharynx
  6. Pharyngoscopy and biopsies of the nasopharynx if clinical suspicion high
E. Two aspects of neoplastic involvement of the parasellar region require particular attention
  1. Mode of onset and clinical course do not prognosticate the type of lesion (ie, neoplastic disease may have an acute clinical presentation as well as an expected insidious course)
  2. High-dose corticosteroid therapy may initially improve signs and symptoms due to neoplasm
F. Tolosa-Hunt syndrome
  1. Painful ophthalmoplegia due to granulomatous inflammation occurring in the cavernous sinus
  2. Spontaneous remissions may occur after days or weeks
  3. Recurring attacks may occur at intervals of months or years
  4. Systemic steroids usually lead to marked improvement of signs and symptoms within 48 hours
  5. Categorically, diagnosis of exclusion and patients with this diagnosis require careful follow-up
  6. Check an IgG-4 blood test for IgG4-related disease

V. **IMITATORS OF CAVERNOUS SINUS SYNDROME**
A. Myasthenia gravis (see Chapter 11)
B. Thyroid eye disease (see Chapter 11)
C. Orbital disease: inflammation, infection, neoplasm, trauma
D. Diabetic ophthalmoplegia
  1. Typically acute, often painful, mononeuropathy with full recovery within 3 months
  2. Less frequent occurrence of simultaneous paralysis of multiple ocular motor nerves. Often painful, recurrent, and not responsive to steroid therapy
E. Giant cell arteritis (see Chapter 9)
  1. Single or multiple ocular motor nerve palsies
  2. Produces ischemic necrosis of extraocular muscles
F. Botulism
  1. Occurs in 6 forms: food-borne, wound, infantile, infant, hidden, inadvertent
  2. Ophthalmologic findings include dilated, poorly reactive pupils, ptosis, and ophthalmoplegia
  3. Affected individuals have nausea; vomiting; facial, pharyngeal, and generalized proximal weakness; and no sensory deficits

    4. In its pure form, botulinum toxin is a potent poison

    5. Causes cholinergic blockage by preventing release of acetylcholine at neuromuscular junction

  G. Miller Fisher syndrome

    1. Bulbar variant of Guillain-Barré syndrome, characterized by triad of ataxia, areflexia, ophthalmoplegia

    2. In evolution, this cranial polyneuropathy may mimic unilateral or bilateral ocular motor cranial nerve palsies, but usually progresses to a virtually total ophthalmoplegia with involvement of pupils and accommodation

    3. Patients may also have facial diplegia, respiratory and swallowing difficulties, and confusion

    4. Often follows gastroenteritis from *Campylobacter jejuni* infection

    5. More than 90% of patients have antibodies to the ganglioside GQ1b, which cross-reacts with ganglioside structure in wall of *C jejuni*

    6. Anti-GQ1b antibodies have been shown to damage the motor nerve terminal by a complement-mediated mechanism, possibly targeting neuronal membrane of presynaptic Schwann cells

    7. Bickerstaff brainstem encephalitis is a closely related condition with alterations in consciousness and long tract signs seen in addition to ophthalmoplegia and ataxia

    8. Typically benign and self-limited

    9. If needed, treatment includes plasmapheresis and intravenous immunoglobulin

VI. OCULAR NEUROMYOTONIA

  A. Patient reports episodic diplopia or oscillopsia

  B. Failure of extraocular muscles to "relax" following sustained, eccentric gaze

  C. Previous history of invasive pituitary adenoma or other intracranial tumors treated with radiation therapy

  D. Due to episodic, involuntary discharge of ocular motor nerves producing sustained and inappropriate contraction of their respective ocular muscles

  E. Treatment: carbamazepine, gabapentin, phenytoin

BIBLIOGRAPHY

Aryasit O, Preechawai P, Aui-Aree N. Clinical presentation, aetiology and prognosis of orbital apex syndrome. *Orbit.* 2013;32:91-94.

Chua ML, Wee JT, Hui EP, Chan AT. Nasopharyngeal carcinoma. *Lancet.* 2016;387:1012-1024.

Curone M, Tullo V, Proietti-Cecchini A, Peccarisi C, Leone M, Bussone G. Painful ophthalmoplegia: a retrospective study of 23 cases. *Neurol Sci.* 2009;30 Suppl 1:S133-135.

Fernandez S, Godina O, Martinez-Yelamos S, et al. Cavernous sinus syndrome: a series of 126 patients. *Medicine.* 2009;86:278-281.

Kline LB, Hoyt WF. The Tolosa-Hunt syndrome. *J Neurol Neurosurg Psychiatry.* 2001;71:577-582.

Roper-Hall G, Chung SM, Cruz OA. Ocular neuromyotonia: differential diagnosis and treatment. *Strabismus.* 2013;21:131-136.

Spillane J, Beeson DJ, Kullmann DM. Myasthenia and related disorders of the neuromuscular junction. *J Neurol Neurosurg Psychiatry.* 2010;81:850-857.

Stiebel-Kalish H, Setton A, Berenstein A, et al. Bilateral orbital signs predict cortical venous drainage in cavernous sinus dural AVMs. *Neurology.* 2002;58:1521-1524.

Wakerley BR, Uncini A, Yuki N. Guillain-Barre and Miller Fisher syndromes--new diagnostic classification. *Nat Rev Neurol.* 2014;10:537-544.

Zanaty M, Chalouhi N, Tjoumakaris SI, Hasan D, Rosenwasser RH, Jabbour P. Endovascular treatment of carotid-cavernous fistulas. *Neurosurg Clin N Am.* 2014;25:551-563.

CHAPTER 8

The Pupil

MICHAEL S. VAPHIADES, DO

I. **ANATOMICAL CONSIDERATIONS**
   A. Sphincter muscle of the iris
      1. Innervated by parasympathetic fibers originating in the Edinger-Westphal (EW) nucleus, which forms part of the oculomotor nuclear complex in the midbrain
      2. Input that excites the EW nucleus
         a. Light reflex (Figure 8-1)
            i. Afferent neurons from retinal ganglion cells to the pretectal area; intercalated neurons from the pretectal complex to EW nuclei; parasympathetic outflow with the oculomotor nerve to the ciliary ganglion and then to the iris sphincter muscle
            ii. Monocular light information is carried by the optic nerve to the chiasm, where approximately half of the fibers decussate to the contralateral optic tract, and half of the fibers continue in the ipsilateral optic tract
            iii. Approximately two-thirds of the way along the optic tract, some of the axons leave the tract, enter the brachium of the SC, and synapse in the pretectal region
            iv. The information is then passed forward via the intercalated neurons to the EW nuclei bilaterally
            v. The pupillomotor information travels with the III nerve and through the superior orbital fissure with the inferior division
            vi. Thus, light information received by one eye is transmitted to both pupils equally
            vii. Intrinsically photosensitive retinal ganglion cells containing melanopsin also appear to play a role in pupillary light reflex (transient and sustained pupillary constriction)
         b. Near synkinesis (Figure 8-2)
            i. The peristriate cortex (area 19), at the upper end of the calcarine fissure, may be the origin of near synkinesis
            ii. Near synkinesis triad
               1. Convergence of eyes
               2. Accommodation of the lenses
               3. Miosis of the pupils

Foroozan R, Vaphiades MS. *Kline's Neuro-Ophthalmology Review Manual, Eighth Edition (pp 129-142).*
© 2018 SLACK Incorporated.

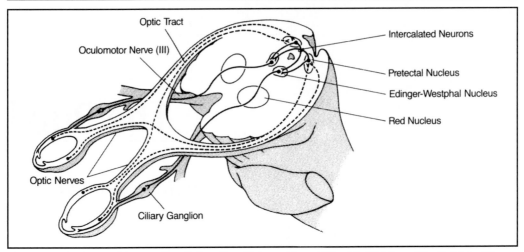

Figure 8-1. Pathway of the pupillary light reflex. (Adapted from Miller NR. *Walsh and Hoyt's Clinical Neuro-Ophthalmology.* 4th ed. Vol 2. Baltimore, MD: Williams & Wilkins; 1985:421.)[1]

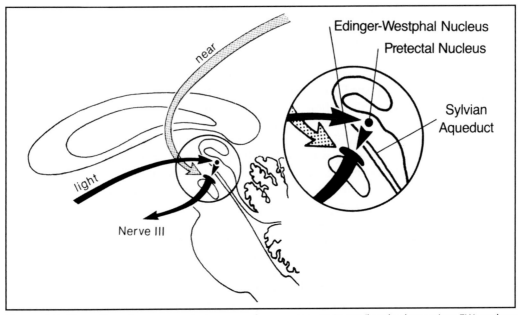

Figure 8-2. Illustration of a more ventral course of near response input (hatched arrow) to EW nucleus compared to light response input (solid arrow).

iii. The near synkinesis pathway is more ventrally located than the pretectal afferent limb of the light reflex. This separation of the "near" from "light" reflexes may be the anatomical basis for some instances of light-near dissociation of the pupils (eg, Argyll Robertson pupils, dorsal midbrain syndrome)

iv. The final pathway is the oculomotor nerve, ciliary ganglion, and the short posterior ciliary nerves. The ratio of ciliary ganglion cells that innervate the ciliary muscle versus cells related to iris sphincter is approximately 30:1

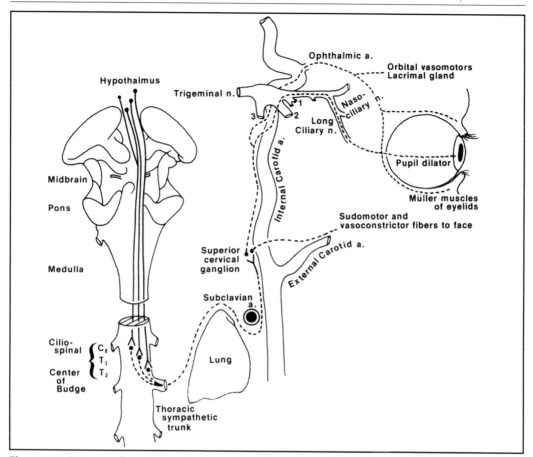

Figure 8-3. Diagram of oculosympathetic pathway. (Reprinted with permission from Slamovits TL, Glaser JS. The pupils and accommodation. In: Tasman W, Jaeger E, eds. *Duane's Clinical Ophthalmology*. Vol 2. Lippincott Williams & Wilkins; 1994.)[2]

      3.   Input that inhibits EW nucleus
         a. Cortical: dilated pupils during epileptic seizures
         b. Spinal-reticular: states of arousal, excitement
         c. Sleep, coma: inhibitory influences decline and pupils are miotic
   B. Dilator muscle of the iris
      1.   Innervated by sympathetic fibers
      2.   Three neuron pathways (Figure 8-3):
         a. First-order neuron originates in posterior hypothalamus and courses down through the brainstem to the C8-T2 level of the cord (ciliospinal center of Budge)
         b. Second-order (preganglionic) neurons leave the cord, enter the paravertebral sympathetic chain, and terminate in the superior cervical ganglion at the base of the skull
         c. Third-order (postganglionic) neuron fibers intended for the pupil and Müller muscle ascend the internal carotid artery to enter the skull, join the ophthalmic nerve in the cavernous sinus, and then to the orbit through the superior orbital fissure; the sudomotor and vasomotor fibers to the face travel with the external carotid artery

II. NORMAL PUPILLARY PHENOMENA

A. Physiologic anisocoria
1. Approximately 20% of the general population have clearly perceptible (generally <1 mm) anisocoria. The degree of anisocoria can vary from day to day and even switch sides

B. Pupillary unrest
1. During distance fixation and with constant, moderate, ambient illumination, the pupils will be noted to have bilaterally, symmetrically, nonrhythmical unrest or variation in size, usually less than 1 mm in amplitude of variation. This is termed *hippus*

C. Near synkinesis
1. With sufficient ambient illumination to allow visualization in the pupils, the patient is asked to shift fixation from the distant object to a near point, preferably the patient's own forefinger. Equal miosis of both pupils will be noted
2. After shifting fixation back to the distant object and maintaining the same ambient illumination, a bright light is placed before one or both eyes and the miosis of the light reflex is noted and compared to the "near" miosis. The "light" miosis will be equal to or greater than the "near" miosis
3. If a patient demonstrates normal reactions of the pupil to light, there is usually no clinical observation to be gained by testing the near response

D. Psychosensory reflex
1. While maintaining constant "near" and "light" stimuli, the examiner observes pupillary size with the use of a "startle" stimulus, such as a loud noise or pain
2. The pupils will dilate due to 2 neural mechanisms:
   a. Active sympathetic discharges (stimulate iris dilator muscle)
   b. Inhibition of ocular motor nuclei (relaxation of iris sphincter muscle)
3. The psychosensory reflex is helpful when demonstrating Horner syndrome

E. Direct pupillary light reflex
1. By having the subject fixate on a distant object (thereby obviating the miosis associated with accommodation) and the ambient illumination moderately subdued, the direct pupillary response is noted when a bright light is placed before one eye
2. The pupil constricts briskly, with a subsequent slow dilation to an intermediate size, followed by a state of pupillary unrest (hippus)
3. The normalcy of the briskness and the latency of the initial response can be evaluated by clinical experience but will be further evaluated by comparison with the fellow eye during the direct light reflex test as well as during the swinging flashlight test (see section G below and on page 133)
4. The amplitudes of the initial constriction and subsequent redilation (pupillary escape) depend on the ambient illumination and the relative brightness of the test light. These amplitudes are also subject to marked individual variation and are best evaluated by comparison with the fellow eye during the swinging flashlight test

F. Consensual pupillary reflex
1. Because of the equal distribution (to both III nerves) of the photic information provided by one eye, the fellow pupil will behave in the same manner described previously for the direct light reflex

G. Swinging flashlight test (Figure 8-4)
1. While maintaining the same test conditions described in testing the direct pupillary light reflex, the examiner projects the light on (for example) the right eye and

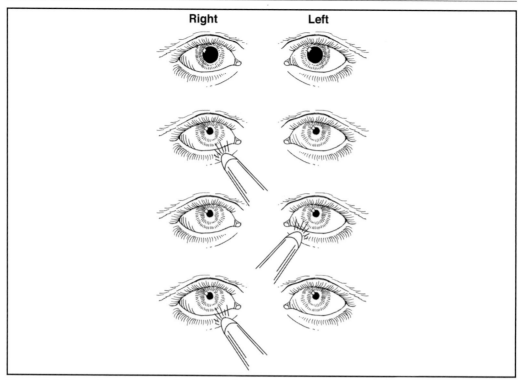

Figure 8-4. Normal response to swinging flashlight test with no change in size of pupils without an RAPD.

allows the right pupil to go through the phase of initial constriction to a minimum size and subsequent escape to an intermediate size

2. At this point, the examiner quickly swings the light to the left eye, which will begin at the intermediate size and go through the phase of initial constriction to a minimum size and subsequent escape to an intermediate size

3. As soon as the left pupil redilates to the intermediate size, the light is swung to the right eye and a mental note made of the intermediate (starting) size, the latency and briskness of the response, the minimum size, and the latency and briskness of the redilation of the intermediate size

4. These characteristics will be exactly the same in both eyes as the light is alternately swung to each eye

5. Key points in proper testing:
    a. A bright hand light in a darkened room is essential
    b. The patient should fixate on a distant object
    c. The light should cross from one eye to the other fairly rapidly (across the bridge of the nose) and remain 3 to 5 seconds on each eye to allow pupillary stabilization

III. ABNORMAL PUPILLARY STATES
A. RAPD (Figure 8-5)
1. During the swinging flashlight test, if the amount of light information transmitted from one eye is less than that carried from the fellow eye, the following phenomenon may be noted when the light is swung from the normal eye to the defective eye
    a. Immediate dilation of the pupil, instead of normal initial constriction (3+ to 4+ RAPD)

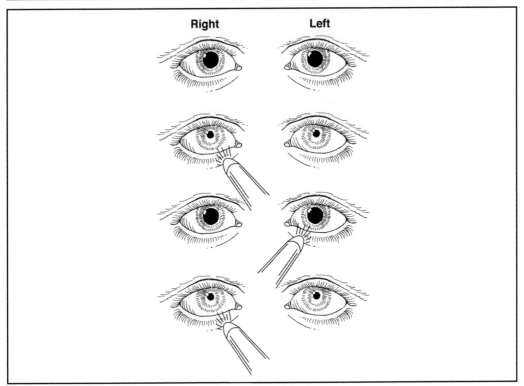

Right   **Left**

Figure 8-5. RAPD in the left eye using a swinging flashlight test. The pupils constrict when the light is shined in the right eye; however, when the flashlight is swung back to the left eye, both pupils dilate.

    b.   No change in pupil size initially, followed by dilation of the pupils (1+ to 2+ RAPD)

    c.   Initial constriction, but greater escape to a larger intermediate size than when the light is swung back to the normal eye (trace RAPD)

2.   When the light is swung back to the normal eye, the pupil demonstrates the normal pattern of brisk constriction (of short latency) with subsequent escape to an intermediate size

3.   Optic neuropathy (must be unilateral or markedly asymmetric) will usually present with a significant RAPD; if a bilateral optic neuropathy exists, there may not be an RAPD

4.   An RAPD can be quantified using neutral density filters (0.3, 0.6, 0.9, 1.2 log unit values). Appropriate amount of filter is placed before the normal eye to neutralize the afferent pupillary defect so that pupils constrict equally and reach the same final resting size

5.   Opacities of the ocular media (corneal scar, cataract, vitreous hemorrhage) are not expected to cause an RAPD if a strong enough flashlight is used

6.   Maculopathy, or amblyopic "lazy eye," will not cause an RAPD unless it is very extensive (< 20/200 acuity) and then it will only be a 1+ RAPD compared to a 3+ to 4+ if the 20/200 acuity was due to an optic neuropathy

7.   Extensive retinal damage will cause a significant RAPD

8.   Amaurotic pupil: the maximum RAPD imaginable; seen in patients with "blind eye"

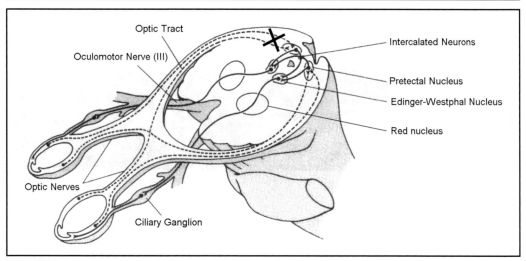

Figure 8-6. Location of lesion ("X") causing a RAPD without visual field loss.

9. There is no such thing as "bilateral" RAPD; there may be bilaterally reduced direct response of the pupils to light, resulting in "light-near" dissociation, but the RAPD requires asymmetry of the afferent light transmission, hence the "relative" in RAPD

10. Isolated, unilateral optic neuropathy does not cause the ipsilateral pupil to be larger; the pupils remain the same size because of the consensual reflex. Unilateral amaurotic mydriasis does not exist

11. Detection of the RAPD requires only one "working" pupil. If one pupil is mechanically or pharmacologically nonreactive, one can simply perform a swinging flashlight test observing the reactive pupil. If the abnormal eye is the eye with a fixed pupil, then the pupil of the normal eye will constrict briskly when the light is shined directly in it and will dilate when the light is shined in the opposite eye. If the abnormal eye is the eye with the reactive pupil, then the pupil will constrict when light is shined in the opposite eye and will dilate when light is shined directly in it. This is the so-called "reverse RAPD," but there is really nothing reverse about it and the term is not really an accurate description of this phenomena

12. Rarely, an RAPD occurs without visual acuity loss or a visual field defect. Due to lesion involving pupillomotor fibers traversing brachium of SC while sparing visual fibers in the optic tract (Figure 8-6)

13. Amblyopia: small proportion of amblyopes have a reduced pupillary contraction amplitude in the affected eye, as established by pupillographic recordings. Amblyopia should not cause a significant RAPD

B. Adie tonic pupil

1. Idiopathic, benign cause of internal ophthalmoplegia

2. Eighty percent unilateral initially; tends to become bilateral at a rate of 4% per year

3. Female predilection (70% female; 30% male)

4. Young adults: 20 to 40 years of age

5. Dilated pupil with poor to absent light reaction

6. Slow constriction to prolonged near-effort and slow redilation (tonic response) after near effort

7. Most patients initially have accommodative paresis, which usually resolves over several months

8. Primary finding of segmental palsy of iris sphincter muscle (if detected, look for iris atrophy and transillumination defects at slit lamp, which may indicate iris trauma or ischemia)

9. Adie pupil frequently (80% of cases) demonstrates cholinergic supersensitivity to weak pilocarpine solutions (0.125% or 0.10%)

10. Etiology in most cases is unknown. Lesion causing tonic pupil located in the ciliary ganglion or short posterior ciliary nerves; aberrant regeneration of more numerous fibers innervating the ciliary muscle (97%) into those subserving the iris sphincter muscle (3%)

11. Adie syndrome: pupillary abnormalities occurring in a patient with associated diminished deep tendon reflexes

12. As the patient ages, the pupil tends to get smaller (miotic) "little old Adie"

C. Argyll Robertson pupils

1. Miotic, irregular pupils

2. Absence of pupillary light response associated with normal anterior visual pathway function

3. Brisk pupillary constriction to near stimuli

4. Poor dilation in the dark and in response to mydriatic agents

5. Condition is usually bilateral, but is often asymmetric and may be unilateral

6. Etiology: major consideration is neurosyphilis. Other reported causes include diabetes mellitus, chronic alcoholism, multiple sclerosis, sarcoidosis

7. Site of lesion: most likely in the region of the Sylvian aqueduct in the rostral midbrain interfering with the light reflex fibers and supranuclear inhibitory fibers as they approach the EW nuclei. More ventrally located fibers for near response are spared (see Figure 8-2)

D. Light-near dissociation of the pupils

1. Better pupillary response to "near" than to "light"

2. Differential diagnosis

   a. Optic neuropathy or severe retinopathy (probably most common cause)

   b. Adie tonic pupil

   c. Argyll Robertson pupils

   d. Dorsal midbrain syndrome (Parinaud syndrome; see Chapter 2)

   e. Aberrant regeneration of III nerve; defective response to light with aberrant hook-up of medial rectus fibers to the pupillary fibers, resulting in pupillary constriction during adduction

   f. Miscellaneous causes: amyloidosis, diabetes mellitus, Dejerine-Sottas, Charcot-Marie-Tooth

E. The pupils of coma

1. Hutchinson pupil

   a. Comatose patient with unilaterally dilated, poorly reactive pupil

   b. Probably due to ipsilateral, expanding, intracranial, supratentorial mass (eg, tumor, subdural hematoma) that is causing downward displacement of hippocampal gyrus and uncal herniation across the tentorial edge with entrapment of the III nerve (see Figure 5-5)

   c. The pupillomotor fibers travel in the peripheral portion of the III nerve (near the perineurium) and are subject to early damage from compression

2. Miosis

   a. During the early stages of coma, the cortical inhibitory input to the EW nucleus is diminished and the pupils are small but reactive to light

      b.   Remember pharmacologic miosis
         i.   Morphine
        ii.   Pilocarpine: if the patient is being incidentally treated for glaucoma

F.   Pharmacologic blockade
   1.   Unilaterally dilated, fixed pupil
   2.   Due to inadvertent contact with mydriatic agent, most commonly atropine in hospital personnel or transdermal scopolamine patches used for nausea

G.   Traumatic pupil
   1.   Contusion injury of the eye may cause miosis or mydriasis
   2.   Miosis may be due to sphincter spasm seen with iritis
   3.   Mydriasis may be due to contusion injury (or actual rupture) of the iris sphincter muscle
      a.   Irregular pupil
      b.   Poorly responsive to 1% pilocarpine

H.   Pharmacologic differentiation of the causes of a fixed, dilated pupil
   1.   The patient is tested first with 0.1% pilocarpine, then, if necessary, 1% pilocarpine
   2.   If the pupil constricts to 0.1% pilocarpine, then this suggests a tonic pupil; if there is no response to 0.1% pilocarpine, then proceed to 1%
   3.   If 1% pilocarpine constricts the involved pupil, then the patient may have a III nerve paresis
   4.   If 1% pilocarpine fails to constrict the involved pupil, or does so poorly, the patient has either pharmacologic blockade or a traumatic pupil

I.   Horner syndrome (oculosympathetic paralysis)
   1.   Three neuron pathways (see Figure 8-3)
   2.   Clinical signs:
      a.   Miosis of the affected pupil, which is more marked in dim illumination (evoking dilation) than in bright illumination
      b.   Ptosis of the upper lid; usually 2 to 3 mm
      c.   Upside-down ptosis of the low lid (due to paresis of inferior tarsal muscle), causing the lower lid to rest 1 to 2 mm higher on the affected side
      d.   Apparent enophthalmos due to narrow palpebral fissure
      e.   Anhidrosis of the affected side of the face. This occurs only if the lesion involves the sympathetic pathway proximal to the bifurcation of the common carotid artery since the sudomotor fibers travel with the external carotid artery
      f.   Heterochromia of the affected iris. Characteristic of congenital Horner with the affected eye having a lighter color
      g.   Transient findings:
         i.   Dilated conjunctival and facial vessels
        ii.   Decreased intraocular pressure
       iii.   Increased accommodation
   3.   Diagnostic steps in suspected Horner syndrome
      a.   Amount of anisocoria should increase in dim versus bright illumination. If this step seems inconclusive, then proceed to pharmacologic testing
      b.   Cocaine test
         i.   Cocaine (4% to 10%) eye drops creating sympathomimetic effect by blocking the reuptake of norepinephrine at the myoneural junction, thereby prolonging the action of norepinephrine upon the dilator muscle
        ii.   Therefore, cocaine requires release of norepinephrine at the myoneural junction by a normal functioning oculosympathetic pathway

          iii.   Cocaine drops result in dilation of the normal pupil

          iv.   If there is a lesion involving any of the 3 neurons, pupillary inequality will increase, and the presence of Horner syndrome is confirmed

          v.   Anisocoria of 1 mm or more following instillation of cocaine drops suggests Horner syndrome

   c.   Paredrine test

          i.   Paredrine (1% hydroxyamphetamine) eye drops create a sympathomimetic effect by causing release of norepinephrine from the nerve endings at the myoneural junction, thereby stimulating the dilator muscle

          ii.   Paredrine requires that the third-order (postganglionic) neuron be intact and have normal axoplasmic activity, including formation and transfer of norepinephrine to the nerve ending at the myoneural junction

          iii.   Paredrine drops result in dilation of the normal pupil

          iv.   If there is a lesion of the third-order neuron, there will be subnormal dilation of the pupil by Paredrine

          v.   Pupillary dilation to Paredrine drops will be normal if the Horner syndrome is due to lesions of the first- or second-order neurons

   d.   Therefore, cocaine serves to confirm the presence of Horner syndrome and Paredrine serves to identify Horner syndrome due to lesions of the third-order neuron

   e.   Apraclonidine drops (1% or 0.5%) may also help in establishing diagnosis of Horner syndrome

          i.   Causes reversal of anisocoria with dilation of Horner pupil and no effect on size of normal pupil

          ii.   Likely due to denervation hypersensitivity of α-1 receptors of pupillary dilator muscle ipsilateral to the Horner syndrome

          iii.   False negative results have been reported

          iv.   More validation testing is needed

          v.   Use with caution in infants

   f.   Beware of pseudo-Horner syndrome: ipsilateral ptosis and miosis of unrelated cause

4.   Differentiation of causes of Horner syndrome

   a.   First-order neuron lesion (brainstem and spinal cord)

          i.   Cerebrovascular accident (Wallenberg syndrome)

          ii.   Neck trauma

          iii.   Neoplasm

          iv.   Demyelinating disease

          v.   Syringomyelia

   b.   Second-order neuron lesion (preganglionic)

          i.   Chest lesions: occult carcinoma of the lung apex (Pancoast tumor), mediastinal mass, cervical rib

          ii.   Neck lesions: trauma, abscess, thyroid neoplasm, lymphadenopathy

          iii.   Surgery: thyroidectomy, radical neck surgery, carotid angiography (direct carotid puncture)

   c.   Third-order neuron lesion (postganglionic)

          i.   Lesion may be extracranial (similar etiologies as listed for second-order neuron neck lesions) or cause may be intracranial

          ii.   Migraine variants: cluster headaches, Raeder paratrigeminal neuralgia

        iii. Complicated otitis media

        iv. Cavernous sinus/superior orbital fissure lesion

        v. Internal carotid artery dissection

        vi. Carotid-cavernous fistula

        vii. Nasopharyngeal carcinoma

    5. Horner syndrome in children

        a. Horner syndrome present at birth is usually benign and associated with heterochromia

        b. Usually idiopathic (30% to 70%); may be associated with birth trauma (brachial plexus injury); rarely due to intrauterine neuroblastoma

        c. Second-order neuron lesion (eg, chest tumor) often behaves pharmacologically like third-order neuron lesion (fails to dilate to hydroxyamphetamine). Probably due to transsynaptic degeneration of preganglionic neuron

        d. Acquired Horner syndrome in first 5 years of life is a more ominous occurrence; often due to neuroblastoma involving sympathetic chain in chest or neck

        e. Rarely, acquired pediatric Horner syndrome may manifest variable and fluctuating signs including ptosis and miosis

        f. In both congenital and acquired Horner syndrome, a pediatric evaluation is warranted

  J. Oculomotor palsy (see Chapter 5)

        a. Oculomotor cranial nerve palsy owing to an aneurysm at or near the junction of the internal carotid and posterior communicating arteries may initially demonstrate normal pupillary size and reactivity in up to 14% of patients (especially with partial somatic involvement), but pupillary involvement may develop in the ensuing 7 to 10 days

        b. To be judged "pupil-sparing" III cranial nerve palsy, the isocoric and reactive pupil must be seen in a setting of complete ptosis and complete involvement of the muscles innervated by the oculomotor nerve. If there is not complete ptosis and the correct pattern and severity of oculomotor nerve-related ophthalmoplegia, then "all bets are off"

        c. In addition, ischemic oculomotor cranial nerve palsies have been reported to be "pupillary involving" in up to 32% of cases, and the associated anisocoria may be as great as 2.5 mm

        d. Pain may be present with both compressive and ischemic causes and therefore not very helpful in distinguishing between these 2 entities

IV. Evaluation of a patient with anisocoria (Figure 8-7)

V. Rare pupillary disorders

  A. Benign episodic pupillary dilatation ("springing pupil")

    1. Young, healthy adults

    2. Variable history of migraine

    3. Characteristics:

        a. One pupil widely dilated for minutes to hours

        b. Mild blurring of vision

        c. May have associated periocular discomfort

        d. Headache occurring following episode

    4. Must exclude accidental pharmacologic blockade

    5. Uniformly benign condition

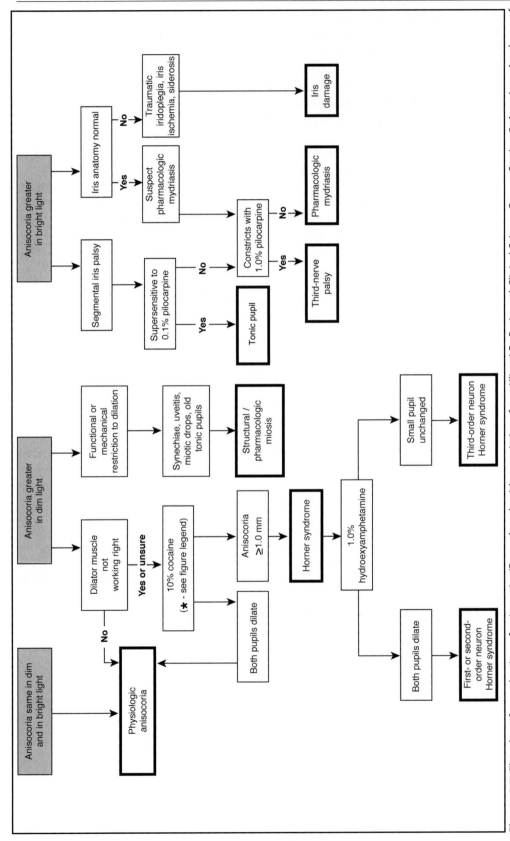

Figure 8-7. Flowchart for evaluation of anisocoria. (Reproduced, with permission, from Kline LB, *Basic and Clinical Science Course, Section 5,* American Academy of Ophthalmology, 2011-2012. © 2017 American Academy of Ophthalmology. Courtesy of Lanning B. Kline, MD.)[3] *Apraclonidine drops may be used. (See page 138, III, I, 3, e.)

    B.   Tadpole pupils
1. Sectoral pupillary dilation lasting for a few minutes, then returning to normal
2. Occurs multiple times per day for several days or 1 week and then disappears
3. Unusual periocular sensation draws attention to the pupil
4. Patient may have history of migraine
5. Possibly due to segmental spasm of iris dilator muscle
6. Benign condition

    C.   Midbrain corectopia
1. Eccentric or oval pupil seen in patients with rostral midbrain disease
2. Thought to be due to selective inhibition of iris sphincter tone
3. Oval pupils may also be seen with midbrain dysfunction due to extrinsic compression from shift of midline supratentorial structures

    D.   Paradoxical pupils
1. Pupillary constriction in darkness
2. Initially felt to be a sign of retinal disease (congenital stationary night blindness, congenital achromatopsia)
3. Also observed in anomalies of optic nerve development (optic nerve coloboma, optic nerve hypoplasia), congenital nystagmus, and a variety of retinal disorders (retinitis pigmentosa, Best disease, macular dystrophy, albinism)
4. Mechanism of phenomenon unknown

REFERENCES

1. Miller NR. *Walsh and Hoyt's Clinical Neuro-Ophthalmology.* 4th ed. Vol 2. Baltimore, MD: Williams & Wilkins; 1985:421.
2. Slamovits TL, Glaser JS. The pupils and accommodation. In: Tasman W, Jaeger E, eds. *Duane's Clinical Ophthalmology.* Vol 2. Lippincott Williams & Wilkins; 1994.
3. Kline LB. *2011-2012 Basic and Clinical Science Course, Section 5: Neuro-Ophthalmology.* San Francisco, CA: American Academy of Ophthalmology; 2011.

BIBLIOGRAPHY

Burde RM, Savino PJ, Trobe JD. Anisocoria. In: *Clinical Decisions in Neuro-Ophthalmology.* 3rd ed. St. Louis, MO: Mosby; 2002:246-271.

Cremer SA, Thompson HS, Digre KB, Kardon RH. Hydroxyamphetamine mydriasis in Horner's syndrome. *Am J Ophthalmol.* 1990;110:66-70.

Fang C, Leavitt JA, Hodge DO, Holmes JM, Mohney BG, Chen JJ. Incidence and etiologies of acquired third nerve palsy using a population based method. *JAMA Ophthalmol.* 2017;135:23-28.

Freedman KA, Brown SM. Topical apraclonidine in the diagnosis of suspected Horner syndrome. *J Neuroophthalmol.* 2005;25:83-85.

Girkin CA, Perry JO, Miller NR. A relative afferent pupillary defect without any visual sensory deficit. *Arch Ophthalmol.* 1998;116:1544-1545.

Jacobson DM. Benign episodic unilateral mydriasis: clinical characteristics. *Ophthalmology.* 1995;102:1623-1627.

Jeffery AR, Ellis FJ, Repka MX, Buncic JR. Pediatric Horner's syndrome. *J AAPOS.* 1998;2:159-167.

Kardon RH. Anatomy and physiology of the autonomic nervous system. In: Miller NR, Newman NJ, eds. *Walsh and Hoyt's Clinical Neuro-Ophthalmology.* 6th ed. Vol 1. Philadelphia, PA: Lippincott Williams & Wilkins; 2005:649-714.

Kardon RH, Denison CE, Brown C, Thompson HS. Critical evaluation of the cocaine test in the diagnosis of Horner's syndrome. *Arch Ophthalmol*. 1990;108:384-387.

Kawasaki A, Borruat FX. False negative aproclonidine test in two patients with Horner syndrome. *Klin Monbl Augenheilkd*. 2008;225:520-522.

Levitan P. Pupillary escape in disease of the retina or optic nerve. *Arch Ophthalmol*. 1959;62:768-779.

Liu GT, Volpe NJ, Galetta SL. Pupillary disorders. In: *Neuro-Ophthalmology: Diagnosis and Management*. 2nd ed. New York, NY: Saunders Elsevier; 2010:415-447.

Loewenfeld IE. "Simple, central" anisocoria: a common condition, seldom recognized. *Trans Sect Ophthalmol Am Acad Ophthalmol Otolaryngol*. 1977;83:832-839.

Loewenfeld IE. *The Pupil: Anatomy, Physiology and Clinical Applications*. Boston, MA: Butterworth-Heinemann; 1999.

Miki A, Iijima A, Takagi M, et al. Pupillography of automated swinging flashlight test in amblyopia. *Clin Ophthalmol*. 2008;2:781-786.

Pollard ZF, Greenberg MF, Bordenca M, Lange J. Atypical acquired pediatric Horner syndrome. *Arch Ophthalmol*. 2010;128:937-940.

Smith SJ, Diehl N, Leavitt JA, Mahoney BG. Incidence of pediatric Horner syndrome and the risk of neuroblastoma. *Arch Ophthalmol*. 2010;128:324-329.

Thompson BM, Corbett JJ, Kline LB, et al. Pseudo-Horner's syndrome. *Arch Neurol*. 1982;39:108-111.

Thompson HS. Adie's syndrome: some new observations. *Trans Am Ophthalmol Soc*. 1977;75:587-626.

Thompson HS, Newsome DA, Lowenfeld IE. The fixed dilated pupil: sudden iridoplegia or mydriatic drops? A simple diagnostic test. *Arch Ophthalmol*. 1971;86:21-27.

Thompson HS, Pilley SEJ. Unequal pupils. A flow chart for sorting out the anisocorias. *Surv Ophthalmol*. 1976;21:45-48.

Thompson HS, Zackon DH, Czarnecki JSC. Tadpole-shaped pupils caused by segmental spasm of the iris dilator muscle. *Am J Ophthalmol*. 1983;96:467-472.

Vaphiades MS, Roberson GH. Imaging of oculomotor (third) cranial nerve palsy. *Neurol Clin*. 2017;35:101-113.

CHAPTER 9

The Swollen Optic Disc

ROD FOROOZAN, MD

I. **DEFINITIONS**
   A. Optic disc edema, swollen disc, "choked" disc: general terms used to describe the optic nerve head affected by a variety of local and systemic causes (Table 9-1)
   B. Papilledema: edema of the optic discs due to increased intracranial pressure being transmitted to the optic nerves by the CSF in the subarachnoid space

II. **PATHOPHYSIOLOGY OF OPTIC DISC EDEMA**
   A. Axonal (axoplasmic) transport along ganglion cell axons that form the optic nerve occurs in anterograde (cell body to LGN) and retrograde (geniculate nucleus to cell body) direction
   B.

Axonal Transport Type	Motor Protein
Anterograde	Kinesin
Fast: 50 to 400 mm/day	
Slow:	
Type a: 0.3 to 3 mm/day	
Type b: 2 to 8 mm/day	
Retrograde	Dynein
Fast: 200 to 400 mm/day	

   C. Anterograde flow mainly involves transport of neurally synthesized proteins, while retrograde transport is concerned with movement of endosomes and lysosomes
   D. Accumulation of axoplasmic flow, especially slow anterograde component, at the lamina cribrosa produces optic disc swelling and NFL opacification
   E. In papilledema, increased perineural pressure results in damming of the axoplasmic transport. Other causes of interrupted axonal transport include inflammation (eg, papillitis) and ischemia (eg, ION)
   F. Secondary associated phenomena include dilated retinal veins, exudates, hemorrhages, cotton-wool spots (microinfarcts of the NFL)

III. **PAPILLEDEMA**
   A. Ophthalmoscopic features
      1. Bilateral disc edema (may be asymmetric; rarely unilateral)
      2. Opacification of peripapillary NFL

Foroozan R, Vaphiades MS. *Kline's Neuro-Ophthalmology Review Manual, Eighth Edition (pp 143-161)*.
© 2018 SLACK Incorporated.

Table 9-1
CAUSES OF OPTIC DISC EDEMA

Ocular Disease

Uveitis
Hypotony
Vein occlusion

Vascular

Ischemic neuropathy
Arteritis, giant cell arteritis, collagen
Radiation vasculopathy

Infiltrative

Lymphoma
Reticuloendothelial

Disc Tumors

Hemangioma
Glioma
Metastatic

Inflammatory

Papillitis
Neuroretinitis
Papillophlebitis

Elevated Intracranial Pressure

Mass lesion
Pseudotumor cerebri
Hypertension

Metabolic

Dysthyroidism
Juvenile diabetes mellitus
Proliferative retinopathies

Orbital Tumors

Perioptic meningioma
Glioma
Sheath "cysts"
Retrobulbar mass

Systemic Disease

Anemia
Hypoxemia
Hypertension
Hypotension
Uremia

Adapted from Glaser JS. *Neuro-Ophthalmology.* 3rd ed. Philadelphia, PA: Lippincott Williams & Wilkins; 1999:138.[1]

3. Hyperemia of disc (superficial capillary telangiectasias)
4. Absent venous pulsations (if venous pulsations are present, then the CSF pressure is probably < 200 mm of water, 20% of normal patients have absent venous pulsations; therefore, the phenomenon of venous pulsations is helpful only if present)
5. Splinter hemorrhages (ie, hemorrhages within the NFL)
6. Exudates (may form a macular star)
7. Chorioretinal folds
8. Cotton-wool spots
9. Haziness of the retinal vessels at the disc margins due to swelling of the NFL in which the retinal vessels course
10. Circumferential retinal folds (Paton lines) in peripapillary region
11. Obliterated central cup—usually a late finding in papilledema

B. Degree of optic disc edema may be graded based on funduscopic findings or measures with ancillary studies such as OCT

C. Diagnosis of papilledema typically constitutes a medical emergency (see also Chapter 20)
1. Cranial CT or MRI to exclude a mass lesion
2. Computed tomography venography (CTV) or MRV also performed to exclude cerebral venous sinus thrombosis (see page 147, IV, H)
3. If no mass is discovered, there is no significant Chiari malformation, and the ventricles are not dilated, LP with CSF analysis to measure opening pressure and look for infectious, inflammatory, or neoplastic cause

    D.   Visual loss in chronic papilledema
1. Typically in early papilledema, and in the absence of optic atrophy, the visual dysfunction parallels the degree of optic disc edema
2. Enlarged blind spots on visual field examination
3. Transient obscurations of vision, unilateral or bilateral "blacking out" or "graying out" of vision lasting 10 to 15 seconds and recurring many times per day; often precipitated by sudden changes in posture and likely related to transient ischemia of the optic nerve
4. Small, glistening hard exudates become apparent in the superficial disc substance ("pseudodrusen"); may represent chronic axoplasmic stasis
5. Gradually, progressive visual field loss, usually beginning nasally and leading to generalized constriction
6. Chronic atrophic papilledema with eventual loss of central visual function including acuity

IV. IDIOPATHIC INTRACRANIAL HYPERTENSION (ALSO KNOWN AS *PSEUDOTUMOR CEREBRI*)

    A.   Diagnostic criteria have been revised from symptom based to more quantifiable criteria
1. Awake and alert patient
2. Signs and symptoms of increased intracranial pressure (headache, nausea, vomiting, transient visual obstructions, papilledema, diplopia)
3. Absence of localizing findings (except those expected from elevated intracranial pressure) on neurologic examination
4. Neuroimaging studies demonstrate normal brain parenchyma, ventricular system, and cerebral venous sinuses
5. LP reveals increased CSF pressure (>25 cm water in adults and >28 cm water in children)
6. No other cause of increased intracranial pressure present

    B.   In addition to papilledema, ophthalmologic findings may include the following:
1. VI nerve palsy (see Chapter 4, III on page 96)
2. Visual field changes (large blind spots, generalized constriction)

    C.   It has been suggested that IIH has been overdiagnosed in the absence of papilledema

    D.   Patients are frequently young adult, obese women

    E.   In one study,[2] MRI showed the following subtle signs:
1. Flattening of the posterior sclera (80%)
2. Empty sella (70%)
3. Enhancement of the prelaminar optic nerve (50%)
4. Distention of the perioptic subarachnoid space (45%)
5. Vertical tortuosity of the orbital optic nerve (40%)
6. Intraocular protrusion of the prelaminar optic nerve (30%)

Each neuroimaging sign was detected in 5% of control subjects, except for enhancement of the prelaminar optic nerve, which was not detected in control subjects.

    F.   Other MRI signs:
1. Stenosis of the cerebral venous sinuses
2. Cerebellar tonsillar herniation
3. Meningocele

    G.   Management
1. Weight loss: as little as 6% reduction has beneficial effect, including on papilledema
2. Medication: acetazolamide, furosemide, corticosteroids, analgesics

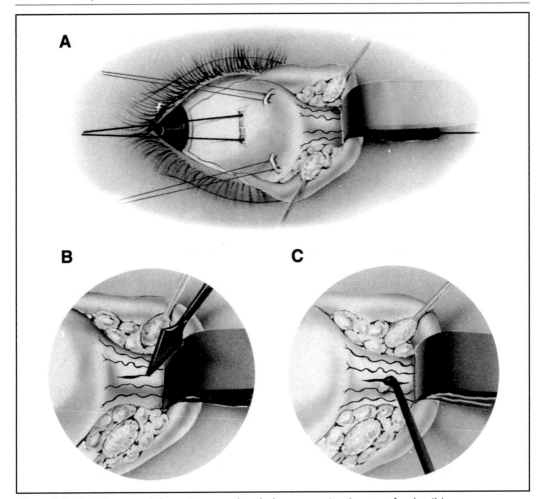

Figure 9-1. Medial approach for optic nerve sheath decompression (see text for details).

3. The Idiopathic Intracranial Hypertension Treatment Trial (IIHTT) was a multi-center, randomized, double-masked, placebo-controlled trial designed to determine the efficacy of acetazolamide compared with placebo in IIH patients with mild visual loss (mean deviation between -2 to -7 dB in the worse eye)

    a. At 6 months, the mean deviation in the acetazolamide group had improved slightly more than the placebo group. Significant difference in improvements between the acetazolamide and placebo group was also reported for the fellow eye mean deviation, papilledema grade, CSF opening pressure, and quality-of-life measures

    b. The IIHTT provides class 1 evidence that acetazolamide use provides a modest improvement in visual field function in patients with IIH with mild visual loss.

4. Optic nerve sheath decompression, neurosurgical shunting procedure (CSF diversion)

    a. Some patients who do not respond to one type of surgical procedure may require another depending on the clinical course

5. Performing an optic nerve sheath decompression (Figure 9-1)

    a. The orbital optic nerve can be approached surgically either medially or laterally

b. The medial approach is preferred, since it is technically easier, is typically faster, and avoids removal of the lateral bony orbital wall

c. A speculum is used to open the lids, and a lateral canthotomy is performed

d. A medial conjunctival peritomy is made, the medial rectus muscle is isolated on a muscle hook, a double-armed 6-0 coated Vicryl suture (Ethicon J-570) is passed through the muscle close to its insertion, and the muscle is disinserted from the globe

e. Another double-armed 6-0 Vicryl suture (J-556) is woven through the stump of the medial rectus insertion, and this suture is used to pull the eye into an abducted position (see Figure 9-1A)

f. Single-armed 5-0 Dacron sutures (Davis & Geck 2919-23) are passed through partial-thickness sclera in the superonasal and inferonasal quadrants (see Figure 9-1A)

g. The 2 Dacron sutures are pulled firmly to position the eye in full abduction (see Figure 9-1A)

h. A malleable orbital retractor is placed between the disinserted medial rectus muscle and the globe to expose the optic nerve immediately behind the globe

i. Cotton-tipped applicators and cottonoids are used to retract orbital fat

j. The intrascleral course of the long posterior ciliary artery leads directly to the optic nerve

k. Once exposed, an avascular segment of the nerve sheath is selected for fenestration

l. Incision of the sheath is made with a sharp blade (MVR Untitome 5560, Beaver Surgical) and extended approximately 5 mm (see Figure 9-1B)

m. A gush of CSF is often seen with the initial incision

n. Adhesions between the meninges and optic nerve are broken by passing a tenotomy or nerve hook into the fenestration (see Figure 9-1C)

o. Two to 4 fenestrations are made routinely, with lysis of the underlying adhesions

p. Meticulous attention to hemostasis is required

q. The traction sutures are removed and the medial rectus is reattached at its original insertion

r. The medial conjunctival incision is closed with an absorbable suture

6. Other procedures

a. Transverse sinus stenting

i. Largely experimental stenting procedure when a pressure gradient is noted along the transverse sinus

ii. Has been performed in patients failing other treatment methods

b. Repeated LP and lumbar drain

i. May be helpful to temporarily lower the intracranial pressure while awaiting more definitive treatment

H. Other settings associated with increased intracranial pressure in the absence of a CNS mass lesion are as follows:

1. Cerebral venous sinus thrombosis—detected with CTV or MRV and often treated with anticoagulation

2. Variety of other systemic disorders (Table 9-2)

3. These settings lead to "secondary" pseudotumor cerebri syndromes

I. Close follow-up with ophthalmology, neurology, or neuro-ophthalmology is important to monitor visual function and symptoms

Table 9-2

CONDITIONS ASSOCIATED WITH INCREASED INTRACRANIAL PRESSURE AND PAPILLEDEMA

1. Obstruction or impairment of intracranial venous drainage

Dural sinus thrombosis	Radical neck surgery	Obstruction of vena cava or large venous vessels
Chronic respiratory insufficiency	Mediastinal mass	

2. Endocrine and metabolic dysfunction

Eclampsia	Diabetic ketoacidosis	Hypoparathyroidism
Menarche	Addison disease	Hyperthyroidism
Scurvy	Obesity	Pregnancy
Oral progestational agents		

3. Exogenously administered agents

Heavy metals: lead, arsenic	Nalidixic acid	Vitamin A
Prolonged steroid therapy	Tetracycline	Steroid withdrawal
Amiodarone	Isotretinoin	

4. Systemic illness

    Chronic uremia

    Infectious disease

        Bacterial: subacute bacterial endocarditis (SBE), meningitis

        Viral: meningitis, Guillain-Barré syndrome

        Parasitic: trypanosomiasis, torulosis

        Contiguous infection (middle ear, mastoid)

    Neoplastic disease

        Carcinomatous meningitis

        Leukemia

        Spinal cord tumors

    Hematologic disease

        Hypercoagulable states

        Infectious mononucleosis

        Anemia

        Hemophilia

        Idiopathic thrombocytopenic purpura

    Miscellaneous

        Lupus erythematosus

        Sarcoidosis

        Syphilis

        Paget disease

        Whipple disease

        Obstructive sleep apnea

V. OPTIC NEURITIS

  A. Primary inflammation of the optic nerve

  B. Two clinical forms of optic neuritis:

    1. Papillitis: intraocular form in which disc swelling is present

    2. Retrobulbar optic neuritis: optic disc appears normal and inflammatory lesion along course of optic nerve is behind globe

  C. Acute impairment of vision

  D. Usually unilateral, although may be bilateral, especially in children

  E. Occurs in young adults (ages 14 to 45 years); females outnumber males (5:1)

  F. Pain occurs in over 90%: periocular, retrobulbar, tenderness of the globe, pain especially with eye movement

  G. An RAPD is present if optic neuritis is unilateral

  H. Visual field defects: usually central scotoma, but may be any type expected from optic neuropathy, including centrocecal or NFB defects (see Chapter 1)

  I. Cells in vitreous with papillitis, often suggestive of a cause other than demyelination

  J. Chronological pattern of visual loss: rapid decrease in vision during the first 2 or 3 days; stable level of decreased vision for 7 to 10 days, then gradual improvement of vision, frequently returning to near normal levels within 2 to 3 months

  K. Uhthoff symptom: dimming of vision in affected eye with elevation of body temperature (eg, exercise, hot shower, fever) in a patient with optic neuritis

  L. Etiologies of optic neuritis:

    1. Idiopathic

    2. Multiple sclerosis

    3. Neuromyelitis optica (NMO; Devic syndrome)

      a. Bilateral optic neuritis associated with transverse myelitis

      b. Propensity for children and young adults

      c. Diagnostic criteria for NMO have been revised multiple times based on clinical, laboratory, and neuroimaging criteria

      d. Broadened recognition of clinical manifestation of NMO: NMO spectrum disorders (NMOSD) which has included limited forms (single or recurrent attacks of myelitis or optic neuritis), optic neuritis or myelitis with systemic autoimmune disease (eg, lupus, Sjögren syndrome), and optic neuritis or myelitis with other brain lesions (eg, hypothalamus, corpus callosum, periventricular, brainstem)

      e. Often associated with NMO-IgG (antibodies to aquaporin-4 [AQP4])

      f. Diagnostic criteria for NMOSD with AQP4-IgG (modified from Wingerchuk et al[3]):

        i. At least 1 core clinical characteristic (optic neuritis, acute myelitis, area postrema syndrome [episode of otherwise unexplained hiccups, nausea and vomiting], acute brainstem syndrome, symptomatic narcolepsy, or acute diencephalic clinical syndrome with NMOSD–typical diencephalic MRI lesions or symptomatic cerebral syndrome with NMOSD–typical brain lesions)

        ii. Positive test for AQP4-IgG using best available detection method

        iii. Exclusion of alternative diagnoses

      g. Diagnostic criteria for NMOSD without AQP4-IgG or NMOSD with unknown AQP4-IgG status:

        i. At least 2 core clinical characteristics occurring as a result of one or more clinical attacks and meeting all of the following requirements:

at least 1 core clinical characteristic must be optic neuritis, acute myelitis with longitudinally extensive transverse myelitis (LETM), or area postrema syndrome; dissemination in space (2 or more different core clinical characteristics); fulfillment of additional MRI requirements, as applicable; negative tests for AQP4-IgG using best available detection method, or testing unavailable; exclusion of alternative diagnoses

    h. Additional MRI requirements for NMOSD without AQP4-IgG and NMOSD with unknown AQP4-IgG status:

        i. Acute optic neuritis: requires brain MRI showing (a) normal findings or only nonspecific white matter lesions, or (b) optic nerve MRI with T2-hyperintense lesion or T1-weighted gadolinium enhancing lesion extending over ≥ 0.5 optic nerve length or involving optic chiasm

        ii. Acute myelitis: requires associated intramedullary MRI lesion extending over ≥ 3 contiguous segments or ≥ 3 contiguous segments of focal spinal cord atrophy in patients with a history compatible with acute myelitis

        iii. Area postrema syndrome: requires associated dorsal medulla/area postrema lesions

        iv. Acute brainstem syndrome: requires associated periependymal brainstem lesions

    i. Typically worse clinical course for visual and neurologic recovery than multiple sclerosis and may relapse quickly after tapering corticosteroid therapy

    j. Treatment:

        i. Often more aggressively treated than multiple sclerosis

        ii. Corticosteroids, immunosuppressive agents (eg, azathioprine), plasmapheresis, intravenous immunoglobulin

        iii. Some evidence suggestive that typical treatments for multiple sclerosis, including interferon β, may worsen the course of NMOSD

4. Viral infections: childhood (eg, mumps, measles, chicken pox), adult (eg, zoster)

5. Postviral syndrome

6. Intraocular inflammation (eg, uveitis)

7. Contiguous inflammation (eg, meninges, orbit, sinuses)

8. Systemic illness including infectious causes (eg, sarcoid, syphilis, tuberculosis)

M. Optic Neuritis Treatment Trial (ONTT)

    1. Prospective, randomized study of 457 patients with optic neuritis

    2. Three treatment groups:

        a. Oral prednisone (1 mg/kg/day) for 14 days

        b. Intravenous methylprednisolone (1000 mg/day) for 3 days, followed by oral prednisone (1 mg/kg/day) for 11 days

        c. Oral placebo for 14 days

    3. Fastest recovery for intravenous group, but at 1-year follow-up and thereafter, no significant difference in visual recovery among 3 groups

    4. At 1-year follow-up, 91% to 95% of patients in 3 groups regained acuity of 20/40 or better

    5. Patients treated with oral prednisone had significantly higher rates of new attacks of optic neuritis

    6. Group receiving intravenous regimen and having 2 or more typical demyelinating white matter lesions on MRI had a significantly lower rate of developing multiple sclerosis within 2 years of follow-up than did the placebo or prednisone groups. However, this benefit was no longer measurable after 3 years of follow-up

7. Visual prognosis for optic neuritis generally good. ONTT at 15-year follow-up:
   a. 20/25 or better: 89%
   b. 20/30 to 20/40: 4%
   c. 20/50 to 20/200: 5%
   d. Worse than 20/200: 2%
8. Overall probability of developing clinically definite multiple sclerosis (CDMS) at 5 years = 30%, 10 years = 38%, 15 years = 50%
9. MRI findings are the strongest predictor of developing CDMS at 15-year follow-up:
   a. No MRI lesions: 25%
   b. One or more lesions: 72%
   c. Greater number of lesions on MRI increases the likelihood of developing multiple sclerosis
10. At 15-year follow-up: NFB defects (arcuate, paracentral) were the most common localized visual field abnormalities
11. Combination of the following substantially decreases the likelihood of developing multiple sclerosis (atypical for demyelinating optic neuritis):
    a. Lack of periocular pain
    b. Severe optic disc edema
    c. No light perception (NLP)

N. Multiple studies have shown benefit in treating patients with a first clinical event (including optic neuritis) suggestive of multiple sclerosis and in treating patients with multiple sclerosis with disease-modifying therapies

O. Controlled High-Risk Subjects Avonex Multiple Sclerosis Prevention Study (CHAMPS)
   1. Prospective, randomized study of 383 patients with first acute demyelinating event (optic neuritis, myelitis, brainstem, cerebellum) and at least 2 MRI white matter signal abnormalities
   2. Treatment groups:
      a. ONTT protocol IV/oral steroids (see page 150, V, M, 2, b) followed by weekly intramuscular injection of 30 micrograms of interferon ß-1a (Avonex)
      b. ONTT protocol IV/oral steroids followed by weekly intramuscular injection of placebo
   3. Results: 3-year follow-up
      a. Development of CDMS significantly lower in interferon ß-1a group
      b. Reduction in volume of brain lesions in interferon ß-1a group
      c. Fewer new or enlarging lesions and fewer gadolinium enhancing lesions in interferon ß-1a group
      d. Trial terminated because of clear benefit of therapy over placebo
   4. 5-year follow-up
      a. Controlled High-Risk Avonex Multiple Sclerosis Prevention Study in Ongoing Neurologic Surveillance (CHAMPIONS study)
      b. Continued beneficial effect of intramuscular interferon ß-1a after first demyelinating effect
      c. Immediate institution of treatment yields greatest benefits

P. Early Treatment of Multiple Sclerosis (ETOMS) Study Group
   1. Prospective, randomized, multicenter, double-masked study of 300 patients experiencing first episode of neurologic dysfunction suggesting multiple sclerosis within the previous 3 months and strongly suggestive brain MRI findings

    2. Treatment groups:
- a. Interferon ß-1a (Rebif) 22 micrograms subcutaneously once per week
- b. Placebo injected subcutaneously once per week

    3. Results: 2-year follow-up
- a. Fewer patients developed CDMS (34%) versus the placebo group (45%; $P = 0.047$)
- b. For 30% of each group to convert to CDMS required 569 days in treatment group versus 252 in placebo group ($P = 0.034$)
- c. Annual relapse rate in treatment group was 0.33 versus 0.43 with placebo ($P = 0.045$)
- d. Number and total volume of new T2-weighted MRI lesions lower in treatment group

Q. Betaseron in Newly Emerging Multiple Sclerosis for Initial Treatment (BENEFIT) trial

    1. Prospective, randomized, multicenter, double-masked study of 468 patients experiencing first clinical demyelinating event (monofocal or multifocal) and at least 2 brain MRI lesions

    2. Treatment group:
- a. Interferon ß-1b (Betaseron) 250 micrograms subcutaneously every other day
- b. Placebo injected subcutaneously every other day

    3. Results: diagnosis of CDMS established or follow-up of 2 years
- a. Reduction of development of CDMS over 2 years from 45% (placebo) to 28% (treatment)
- b. Similar significant reduction at 2 years if McDonald criteria (combines clinical and MRI findings) used: 51% (placebo) versus 28% (treatment)
- c. At the 25th percentile, time to develop CDMS was delayed from 255 (placebo) to 618 days (treatment)

R. PreCISe study (early glatiramer acetate treatment in delaying conversion to CDMS subjects presenting with a clinically isolated syndrome)

    1. Randomized double-masked trial involving 481 patients (80 sites in 16 countries) presenting with the following:
- a. Clinically isolated syndrome
- b. Two or more T2 brain lesions (≥ 6 mm)

    2. Treatment protocol:
- a. Glatiramer acetate (Copaxone): 20 mg subcutaneous injection/day
- b. Placebo-subcutaneous injection
- c. Endpoint: up to 36 months or conversion to CDMS

    3. Results:
- a. Glatiramer acetate reduced risk of developing CDMS by 45%
- b. Time for 25% of patients to convert to CDMS prolonged from 336 to 722 days, if treated with glatiramer acetate
- c. At 5-year follow-up, 41% reduced conversion rate to CDMS for treated patients. Also, reduction in number of T2 white matter lesions and T2 lesion volume

S. Other disease modifying treatments used in multiple sclerosis

    1. Natalizumab (Tysabri), a recombinant humanized monoclonal antibody given as a monthly intravenous infusion, and interferes with leukocyte migration across the blood-brain barrier
- a. Associated with progressive multifocal leukoencephalopathy (PML)

Table 9-3

AMERICAN COLLEGE OF RHEUMATOLOGY CRITERIA FOR CLASSIFICATION OF GIANT CELL ARTERITIS

1. Age at onset of 50 years or older
2. Onset of new headache
3. Temporal artery abnormality (tender or reduced pulsation)
4. Elevated erythrocyte sedimentation rate (ESR) defined as > 50 mm/hour using Westergren method
5. Abnormal artery biopsy showing necrotizing vasculitis with predominant mononuclear cell infiltration or granulomatous inflammation

Sensitivity 93.5%, specificity 91.2% for diagnosis with at least 3 of 5 criteria met.

2. Alemtuzumab (Lemtrada), a humanized monoclonal antibody targeting CD52, a cell-surface marker found on a variety of immune cells, including mature B and T lymphocytes, monocytes, and macrophages
   a. Has been associated with autoimmune conditions including thyroid disease
3. Fingolimod (Gilenya), an orally administered sphingosine-1-phosphate (S1P) receptor modulator that impairs lymphocyte egress from lymph nodes
   a. Associated with cystic maculopathy
4. Teriflunomide (Aubagio) effects lymphocyte proliferation through blockade of de novo pyrimidine synthesis
   a. Classified as category X in pregnancy
5. Dimethyl fumarate (Tecfidera), thought to effect factors that result in transcription of antioxidative genes, stimulating the natural anti-inflammatory response of immune cells
   a. Associated with lymphopenia and flushing
6. Ocrelizumab has been approved for the treatment of adult patients with relapsing or primary progressive forms of multiple sclerosis
   a. It is contraindicated in patients with active hepatitis B infection

VI. ISCHEMIC OPTIC NEUROPATHY
A. Ischemic infarction of the anterior portion (anterior ION [AION]) or posterior portion (posterior ION [PION]) of the optic nerve
B. Acute visual loss, typically in patients over the age of 60 years
C. Clinical settings in which ION is seen:
1. Arterial disease
   a. Arteritis
      i. Giant cell arteritis (Table 9-3)
      ii. Collagen vascular diseases
      iii. Herpes zoster
   b. Nonarteritic AION (NAION)—"unknown etiology"—by far the most common form of ION
   c. Diabetes mellitus
   d. Malignant hypertension
   e. Embolic disease
   f. Vasospastic (migraine)
   g. Post-irradiation

	Table 9-4	
	MAJOR CAUSES OF ISCHEMIC OPTIC NEUROPATHY	
	NAION	**Giant Cell Arteritis**
Age Peak	60 to 70 years	70 to 80 years
Visual Loss	Minimal to severe	Usually severe
Involvement of Second Eye	Approximately 40%	Approximately 75%
Acute Fundus	Swollen disc	Swollen disc, may be pallid
Other Ophthalmologic Presentations		Central retinal artery occlusion, choroidal infarction, anterior segment ischemia
Systemic	Hypertension (approximately 50%)	Headache, scalp tenderness, malaise, weakness, weight loss, fever, jaw claudication, polymyalgia
ESR (Westergren, mm/hour)	Up to 40	Typically high (50 to 120)
C-Reactive Protein (CRP, mg/L)*	Normal	Elevated
Temporal Artery Biopsy	May show arteriosclerotic change	Granulomatous inflammation, multinucleated giant cells, disruption of internal elastic lamina
Response to Steroids	None	Relief of systemic symptoms, infrequent return of vision, protect other eye

*Normal range established by individual laboratory.

Adapted from Glaser JS. *Neuro-Ophthalmology.* 3rd ed. Philadelphia, PA: Lippincott Williams & Wilkins; 1999:163.[1]

2. Hypotension/hypovolemia
    a. Massive blood loss
    b. Cardiac insufficiency
    c. Surgical hypotension, particularly spine and cardiac surgery
    d. Anemia
3. Other
    a. Post–cataract surgery
        i.   May occur in the immediate postoperative period where elevated intraocular pressure was thought to be a risk factor
        ii. Epidemiologic studies suggest an increased risk months to years after cataract surgery as well
    b. Amiodarone
        i.   Controversial
        ii. Often bilateral
    c. Phosphodiesterase type 5 inhibitors
        i.   Increased risk of NAION in a case-control study
    d. Sleep apnea
D. Differential diagnosis involves arteritic (giant cell arteritis) versus nonarteritic as major causes of ION (Table 9-4)
E. AION is always accompanied by disc swelling in the acute stage, while there is no optic disc edema in PION

F. Optic disc edema in AION, which may occur before the onset of visual symptoms, typically lasts weeks before resolving

G. Optic disc in the unaffected eye in NAION is commonly full and cupless ("disc at risk")

H. Visual defect is usually maximal in onset. On occasion, field abnormality may progress within the first month. Subsequent improvement may occur in up to 40% of patients with NAION

I. With arteritic ION, may see marked delay in choroidal perfusion with fluorescein angiography: signifies involvement of posterior ciliary arteries

J. Recognition of giant cell arteritis is essential; prompt steroid therapy may restore some degree of vision, avert visual loss in the fellow eye, and improve long-term systemic morbidity and mortality. Tocilizumab, an inhibitor of interleukin-6, has been approved for the treatment of giant cell arteritis

K. Performing a temporal artery biopsy

1. The temporal artery is a terminal branch of the external carotid artery. Because of its ready accessibility and high frequency of involvement in giant cell arteritis, it is most often biopsied to establish the diagnosis

2. The artery lies in front of the ear over the zygomatic process of the temporal bone. It divides into a posterior parietal branch and anterior frontal branch (Figure 9-2A). The frontal branch lies above the temporalis fascia and follows a tortuous course across the forehead to an anastomosis with the supraorbital and supratrochlear branches of the ophthalmic artery

3. The frontal branch is usually chosen for biopsy. The artery is classically described as being nodular and tender when involved. However, the vessel may feel and look normal, yet prove abnormal on histologic examination

4. After the frontal branch is identified, the area should be prepared by shaving the overlying skin

5. The shaved area is scrubbed with Betadine (povidone-iodine) solution for 5 minutes with 4×4s. The area is then dried and a sterile plastic eye drape is applied to the biopsy area

6. The vessel is carefully palpated and its course marked for 4 to 5 cm

7. Plain 2% xylocaine is used for local infiltration. Epinephrine should be avoided because of its vasospastic potential. Five to 10 cc should be injected 1 cm to either side of the artery and parallel to, but not directly over, the artery itself

8. The skin incision is made with a No. 15 Bard-Parker blade (Becton, Dickinson and Company) directly along the skin mark. Traction at each end of the incision site is used when making the full-thickness incision through the skin. 4×4s can then be used at the incision edges to control bleeding. Rarely is cautery or ligature needed

9. Subcutaneous blunt dissection is done using a hemostat or small blunt-nosed scissors. Dissection with sharp instruments is typically avoided. The frontal branch is identified above the temporalis fascia (Figure 9-2B)

10. If pulsations were obtained at the beginning of the procedure, the dissection bed is repeatedly palpated to identify the course of the artery

11. If the pulse disappears, several drops of proparacaine can be instilled on the wound, reducing vasospasm

12. Two 4-0 black silk sutures are passed below the artery, one proximally and one distally to permit manipulation without the use of instruments that could cause crush artifact. At least 3 cm of artery should be isolated and freed from surrounding tissue. Branches of the artery are ligated with 4-0 chromic sutures. The artery is ligated as far proximally and distally as possible. Three square knots should be placed with the silk sutures and the ends not cut too closely. Some prefer a double ligature proximally and distally (Figure 9-2C)

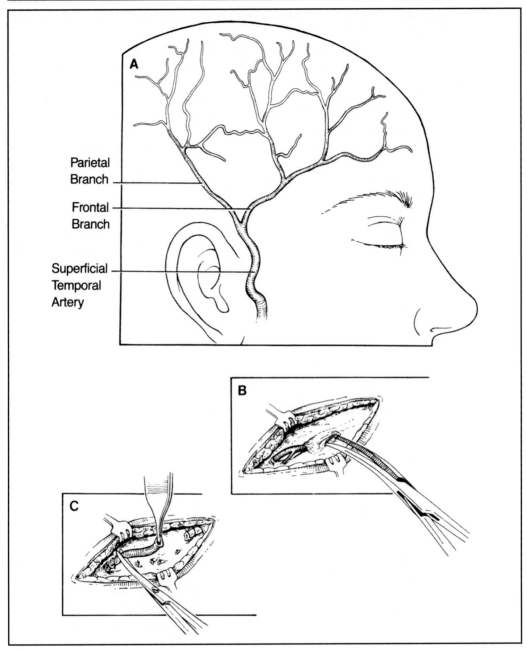

Figure 9-2. Steps in performing a superficial temporal artery biopsy. (A) Localization. (B) Blunt dissection. (C) Removal of biopsy specimen.

13. Once bleeding is controlled, the wound is closed with 6-0 nylon sutures. A pressure dressing is applied for 24 hours

14. The most common late complication is hemorrhage. There is one case report of a patient with asymptomatic internal carotid occlusion who suffered a stroke during biopsy of the ipsilateral temporal artery because of interruption of collateral flow. It may be prudent to compress the vessel for several minutes to ensure that critical collateral flow will not be compromised if it is removed

15. Skin sutures are removed in 5 days

VII.   MISCELLANEOUS CAUSES OF SWOLLEN OPTIC DISC

A.   Orbital disease

    1.   Optic nerve or arachnoid cyst

    2.   Orbital tumor

    3.   Dysthyroid optic neuropathy (see Chapter 11, V on page 179)

        a.   Unilateral or bilateral progressive visual loss

        b.   Patient may have only mild to moderate congestive, orbital signs with resistance to retropulsion of the globes

        c.   Visual field loss typically central scotoma, sometimes combined with inferior depression

        d.   Optic disc may appear swollen, normal, or pale

        e.   Optic neuropathy typically occurs due to compression of optic nerve by enlarged extraocular muscles at orbital apex and rarely from distension and stretching of the optic nerve

        f.   Treatment: systemic steroids and other immunosuppressives, radiotherapy, orbital decompression surgery

B.   Intraocular disease: uveitis, retinal vein occlusion, disc tumor, hypotony

C.   Diabetic papillopathy ("acute disc swelling in juvenile diabetes mellitus")

    1.   Onset: second to eighth decades (average: 50 years of age)

    2.   Type 1 or 2 diabetics of some chronicity (average: 10 to 12 years of age)

    3.   Commonly bilateral but may be unilateral

    4.   Disc edema with prominent telangiectatic change without neovascularization

    5.   May not correlate with degree of diabetic retinopathy

    6.   Frequently asymptomatic or modest acuity loss to 20/50; occasionally more profound loss

    7.   Visual field defects include enlarged blind spot and arcuate defects

    8.   Generally good visual prognosis with return of normal acuity in 3 months to 1 year

    9.   Visual improvement precedes disappearance of disc swelling

    10.   Disc usually regains normal appearance, although may also develop diffuse or segmental pallor

    11.   Some feel this is not distinguishable from NAION

D.   Papillophlebitis (retinal vasculitis, optic disc vasculitis, big blind spot syndrome)

    1.   Usually unilateral disc edema often with vitreous cells

    2.   Young, healthy adults

    3.   Vague visual complaints of blurred vision with minimal impairment of acuity (typically no worse than 20/30)

    4.   Typically no RAPD

    5.   Only visual field abnormality is enlargement of blind spot

    6.   Disc swelling with associated engorged retinal veins and occasional retinal hemorrhages

    7.   Spontaneous, usually complete recovery within several months to 1 year

    8.   Pathologic examination reveals inflammation of the retinal veins, although etiology of inflammation is unknown

E.   LHON (see Table 10-1)

    1.   Most often, but not exclusively, affects males in the second or third decade of life

    2.   Progressive monocular visual loss to a variable level (20/200 or worse)

    3.   Second eye usually affected within weeks

      4.   In acute phase, optic disc may appear normal or have typical triad of findings

         a.   Circumpapillary telangiectatic microangiopathy

         b.   Prominent NFL around disc

         c.   Absence of dye leakage on fluorescein angiography from the disc or peripapillary region (ie, not true disc edema)

      5.   Visual field abnormality is centrocecal scotoma

      6.   Ultimately, the patient develops either temporal or generalized disc pallor

      7.   Maternal inheritance pattern in LHON

         a.   Disorder of mitochondrial, not chromosomal, DNA

         b.   Chromosomal DNA follows Mendelian pattern of inheritance, but mitochondrial DNA is inherited exclusively from the mother

         c.   Leber optic neuropathy linked with several point mutations in mitochondrial DNA, most commonly 11778, but also 14484, 3460

         d.   Mitochondrial DNA is essential for oxidative phosphorylation, the energy-producing cycle in the cell

         e.   Heteroplasmy: intracellular mitochondrial DNA is a mixture of mutant and normal forms; provides basis for variable clinical expression of mutation

      8.   Electrocardiogram obtained to exclude potential cardiac conduction defect

      9.   Fat suppressed contrast-enhanced MRI may show optic nerve enhancement.

      10. No definitive treatment—eliminate use of tobacco, alcohol

      11. Rarely, spontaneous recovery of vision may occur (frequency based on genetic mutation: 14484 > 3460 > 11778)

      12. Trials with gene therapy have been encouraging

F.   Spheno-orbital meningioma

      1.   Chronic compression of the intraorbital or intracanalicular optic nerve (see Chapter 10, VII, B on page 170)

      2.   Clinical triad:

         a.   Visual loss

         b.   Optic disc swelling that resolves into optic atrophy

         c.   Appearance of optociliary shunt vessels

      3.   The clinical picture may also be seen with optic nerve glioma, chronic papilledema, craniopharyngioma

G.   Optic disc edema with macular star

      1.   Descriptive term that describes clinical findings and includes several different disease processes

      2.   Main clinical settings:

         a.   Inflammatory papillitis

         b.   Vascular disorders (hypertension, diabetes mellitus)

         c.   Papilledema

         d.   Infectious/immune mediated

      3.   Neuroretinitis is a general description often applied to infectious/immune-mediated cause

      4.   Leber idiopathic stellate neuroretinitis

         a.   Triad: visual loss, optic disc edema, macular star

         b.   Children and young adults

         c.   Antecedent viral illness in up to 50% of patients

         d.   Generally benign, self-limited condition

         e.   Resolution of disc edema in 3 months; up to 1 year for macular star to resolve

         f.   Visual prognosis usually good

5. Neuroretinitis may be due to organisms other than virus
    a. Cat scratch disease (*Bartonella henselae*)
    b. Toxoplasmosis
    c. Toxocariasis
    d. Histoplasmosis
    e. Spirochetoses (syphilis, Lyme disease)
    f. Rocky Mountain Spotted Fever (*Rickettsia rickettsii*)

H. Paraneoplastic optic neuropathy
1. Subacute, progressive, usually bilateral visual loss without pain
2. Optic disc usually edematous; may be normal
3. Usually part of paraneoplastic brainstem or cerebellar syndrome
4. Reported with variety of cancers, including the following:
    a. Small-cell lung carcinoma
    b. Hodgkin and non-Hodgkin lymphoma
    c. Neuroblastoma
    d. Nasopharyngeal cancer
    e. Thymoma
5. Must rule out direct compression or infiltration of the optic nerve
6. Check serum for collapsin response-mediated protein-5 (CRMP-5) antibodies: IgG antibodies directed against antigen expressed in neural tissues and associated neoplasms
7. Paraneoplastic antibodies may be detected in the blood or CSF
8. Pathology: perivascular inflammation, axonal loss, demyelination
9. Significant visual improvement may occur following chemotherapy and/or radiation therapy

I. Autoimmune optic neuropathy
1. Acute to subacute visual loss may be associated with pain
2. There may be predisposing autoimmune disease or propensity (positive ANAs)
3. Often responsive to corticosteroids and other immunosuppressives
4. May be associated with auto-antibodies to optic nerve and retina
5. May be chronic and relapsing (chronic relapsing idiopathic optic neuropathy [CRION])

VIII. **PSEUDOPAPILLEDEMA (ANOMALOUS ELEVATION OF THE DISC; CONGENITALLY FULL DISC)**
A. Ophthalmoscopic features
1. Disc is not hyperemic and there are no dilated capillaries on its surface
2. Despite disc elevation, surface arteries are not obscured (no peripapillary NFL opacification)
3. Physiologic cup usually absent
4. May see anomalous branching and tortuosity of retinal vessels (abnormally large number of branches at disc margin)
5. May see drusen (hyaline bodies) buried in disc of patient or relatives
6. No hemorrhages (rare exceptions)
7. No exudates or cotton-wool spots
8. Disc usually has irregular border with pigment epithelial defects in peripapillary retina
9. Visual field testing may show enlarged blind spots and NFB defects
B. If exam is suggestive of buried disc drusen, may use orbital ultrasonography, CT, fundus autofluorescence, and OCT to "visualize" them

References

1. Glaser JS. *Neuro-Ophthalmology.* 3rd ed. Philadelphia, PA: Lippincott Williams & Wilkins; 1999:138.
2. Brodsky MC, Vaphiades M. Magnetic resonance imaging in pseudotumor cerebri. *Ophthalmology.* 1998;105:1686-1693.
3. Wingerchuk DM, Banwell B, Bennett JL, et al. International consensus diagnostic criteria for neuro-myelitis optica spectrum disorders. *Neurology.* 2015;85:177-189.

Bibliography

Bennett JL. Finding NMO: the evolving diagnostic criteria of neuromyelitis optica. *J Neuroophthalmol.* 2016;36:238-245.

Bennett JL, Nickerson M, Costello F, et al. Re-evaluating the treatment of acute optic neuritis. *J Neurol Neurosurg Psychiatry.* 2015;86:799-808.

Bidot S, Saindane AM, Peragallo JH, Bruce BB, Newman NJ, Biousse V. Brain imaging in idiopathic intracranial hypertension. *J Neuroophthalmol.* 2015;35:400-411

Comi G, Fillipi M, Barkhof F, et al. Effect of early interferon treatment on conversion to definite multiple sclerosis: a randomized study. *Lancet.* 2001;357:1576-1582.

Comi G, Martinelli V, Rodegher M, et al. For the PreCISe study group. Effect of glatiramer acetate on conversion to clinically definite multiple sclerosis in patients with clinically isolated syndrome (PreCISe study): a randomized, double-blind, placebo-controlled trial. *Lancet.* 2009;374:1503-1511.

Eckstein C, Bhatti MT. Currently approved and emerging oral therapies in multiple sclerosis: an update for the ophthalmologist. *Surv Ophthalmol.* 2016;61:318-332.

Evans J, Steel L, Borg F, Dasgupta B. Long-term efficacy and safety of tocilizumab in giant cell arteritis and large vessel vasculitis. *RMD Open.* 2016;2:e000137.

Flippi M, Rovaris M, Ingles M, et al. Interferon beta-1a for brain tissue loss in patients at presentation with syndrome suggestive of multiple sclerosis: a randomized, double-blind, placebo-controlled trial. *Lancet.* 2004;364:1489-1496.

Friedman DI, Liu GT, Digre KB. Revised diagnostic criteria for the pseudotumor cerebri syndrome in adults and children. *Neurology.* 2013;81:1159-1165.

Hayreh SS, Zimmerman MB. Non-arteritic anterior ischemic optic neuropathy: role of systemic corticoste-roid therapy. *Graefes Arch Clin Exp Ophthalmol.* 2008;245:1029-1046.

Ischemic Optic Neuropathy Decompression Trial Research Group. Optic nerve decompression surgery for nonarteritic ischemic optic neuropathy is not effective and may be harmful. *JAMA.* 1995;273:625-632.

Jacobs LD, Beck RW, Simon JH, et al. Intramuscular interferon beta 1-a therapy initiated during a first demyelinating event in multiple sclerosis. CHAMPS study group. *N Engl J Med.* 2000;343:898-904.

Kappos L, Polman CH, Freedman MS. Treatment with interferon beta-1b delays conversion to clinically definite and McDonald MS in patient with clinically isolated syndromes. *Neurology.* 2006;67:1-8.

Keltner JL, Johnson CA, Cello KE, et al. Visual field profile of optic neuritis: a final follow-up report from the optic neuritis treatment trial from baseline through 15 years. *Arch Ophthalmol.* 2010;128:330-337.

Kline LB, Foroozan R, eds. *Optic Nerve Disorders. Ophthalmology Monographs Volume 10.* San Francisco, CA: American Academy of Ophthalmology; 2007.

Liu GT, Volpe NJ, Galetta SL. Visual loss: optic neuropathies. In: *Neuro-Ophthalmology: Diagnosis and Management.* 2nd ed. New York, NY: Saunders Elsevier; 2010:103-236.

Merle H, Olindo S, Bonnan M, et al. Natural history of the visual impairment of relapsing neuromyelitis optica. *Ophthalmology.* 2007;114:810-815.

Mollan SP, Ali F, Hassan-Smith G, Botfield H, Friedman DI, Sinclair AJ. Evolving evidence in adult idiopathic intracranial hypertension: pathophysiology and management. *J Neurol Neurosurg Psychiatry.* 2016;87:982-992.

Optic Neuritis Study Group. High- and low-risk profiles for the development of multiple sclerosis within 10 years after optic neuritis. *Arch Ophthalmol.* 2003;121:944-949.

Optic Neuritis Study Group. Multiple sclerosis risk after optic neuritis: final optic neuritis treatment trial follow-up. *Arch Neurol*. 2008;65:727-732.

Optic Neuritis Study Group. Visual function 15 years after optic neuritis. *Ophthalmology*. 2008;115:1079-1082.

Rahimy E, Sarraf D. Paraneoplastic and non-paraneoplastic retinopathy and optic neuropathy: evaluation and management. *Surv Ophthalmol*. 2013;58:430-458.

Vaphiades MS. Rocky Mountain Spotted Fever as a cause of macular star figure. *J Neuroophthalmol*. 2003;23:276-278.

Vaphiades MS, Newman NJ. Optic nerve enhancement on orbital magnetic resonance imaging in Leber's hereditary optic neuropathy. *J Neuroophthalmol*. 1999;19:238-239.

Wall M, McDermott MP, Kieburtz KD, et al. Effect of acetazolamide on visual function in patients with idiopathic intracranial hypertension and mild visual loss: the idiopathic intracranial hypertension treatment trial. *JAMA*. 2014;311:1641-1651.

Zhang J, Foroozan R. Optic disc edema from papilledema. *Int Ophthalmol Clin*. 2014;54:13-26.

CHAPTER 10

The Pale Optic Disc
Optic Atrophy

ROD FOROOZAN, MD AND MICHAEL S. VAPHIADES, DO

I. **OPTIC DISC PALLOR VERSUS OPTIC ATROPHY**

    A. Ophthalmoscopic appearance of disc pallor alone does not establish the presence of optic atrophy

    B. Frequently, the temporal side of the normal disc has less color than the nasal side

    C. Optic atrophy is a pathologic description of optic nerve shrinkage from any process that produces degeneration of axons in the anterior visual system (retinogeniculate) pathway

    D. The clinical diagnosis of optic atrophy is based on the following:

        1. Ophthalmoscopic abnormalities of color and structure of the disc with associated changes in retinal vessels and NFL

        2. Defective visual function (acuity, color vision, fields, visual evoked response), which can be localized to the optic nerve

    E. Axons with cell bodies in the retinal ganglion cell layer extend to the LGN before a synapse occurs

        1. Therefore, optic disc pallor may result from lesions involving the following:

            a. Retina

            b. Optic nerve

            c. Optic chiasm

            d. Optic tract

        2. Optic disc pallor may be seen from cortical lesions (periventricular leukomalacia) in utero or around the time of birth because of transsynaptic degeneration. Increasing evidence, particularly with retinal imaging, suggests that transsynaptic degeneration may also occur in adults, although rarely causing optic disc pallor

    F. Patients with optic atrophy may develop inner retinal changes suggestive of cysts with imaging such as OCT

II. **HISTOPATHOLOGIC CONSIDERATIONS**

    A. When a visual axon is severed, its ascending (to the brain) segment disintegrates and disappears in approximately 7 days. This is termed *Wallerian degeneration*

    B. The portion of the axon still connected to the ganglion cell body remains viable for 3 to 4 weeks but then rapidly degenerates by 6 to 8 weeks. This is called *descending (to the eye) degeneration*

Foroozan R, Vaphiades MS. *Kline's Neuro-Ophthalmology Review Manual, Eighth Edition (pp 163-174).* © 2018 SLACK Incorporated.

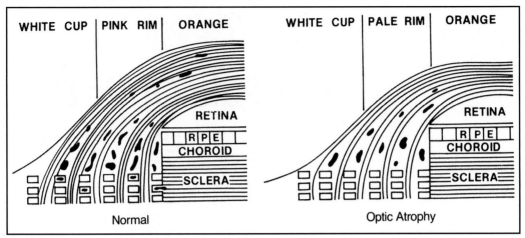

Figure 10-1. Schematic drawing of the longitudinal section of normal and atrophic optic discs. In optic atrophy, there is a decrease in the number of nerve fibers and capillaries, but the proportion of capillaries per unit volume is unchanged. (Adapted from Quigley HA, Anderson DR. The histologic basis of optic disc pallor in experimental optic atrophy. *Am J Ophthalmol.* 1977;83:709-717.)[1]

C. With the completion of descending degeneration of axons, optic disc pallor appears. Currently, there are 2 major theories to explain acquired disc pallor:

    1. Vascular-glial theory: when the optic nerve degenerates, its blood supply is reduced and smaller vessels, recognizable in the normal disc, disappear from view. In addition, formation of glial tissue at the nerve head is said to occur with optic atrophy

    2. NFL theory (Figure 10-1): with degeneration of visual axons, there is alteration in the thickness and cytoarchitecture of NFBs passing between glial columns containing capillaries. Alteration of light conducted along the NFBs leads to the appearance of pallor, and there is no reduction in blood supply to the optic disc

III. OPHTHALMOSCOPIC FEATURES OF OPTIC ATROPHY

A. As a general rule, fundus signs are not specific for any particular etiology of optic atrophy, and the diagnosis must be obtained from clinical, nonophthalmoscopic findings

B. In the early stages of atrophy, the optic disc loses its reddish hue, and the substance of the disc slowly melts away to leave a pale, shallow concave meniscus—the exposed lamina cribrosa

C. Ipsilateral attenuation of the retinal arterioles is frequently a sign of old retinal artery occlusion

D. Healed papillitis or ION may cause narrowing of retinal arterioles, but typically only in their peripapillary segment, after which they appear to enlarge slightly in caliber as they traverse the fundus ("reverse taper sign")

E. Pathologic disc cupping may develop, along with disc pallor, in patients without glaucoma. Etiologies include ischemic, compressive, inflammatory, hereditary, toxic, and traumatic optic neuropathies. Findings that suggest optic disc excavation is nonglaucomatous include the following:

    1. Decreased visual acuity out of proportion to amount of cupping or visual field loss

    2. Acquired dyschromatopsia

    3. Visual field defects out of proportion to degree of cupping

    4. Visual field defects not typical of glaucoma (central scotoma; defects align along vertical meridian)

    5. Optic disc pallor out of proportion to the degree of cupping

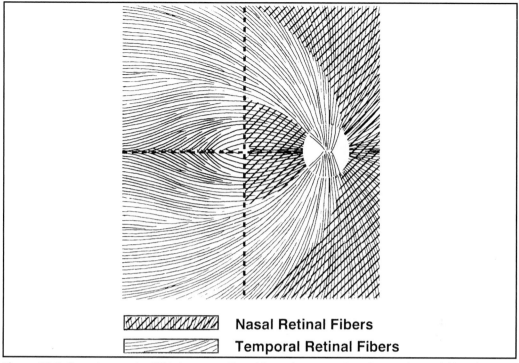

Nasal Retinal Fibers
Temporal Retinal Fibers

Figure 10-2. Bow-tie atrophy. With long-standing chiasmal compression, the nasal retinal fibers become atrophic, and pallor is seen in a pattern corresponding to the location of the fibers in the optic disc. (Adapted from Newman NJ. Chiasm, parachiasmal syndromes, retrochiasm and disorders of higher visual function. In: Slamovits TL, Burde RM, eds. *Neuro-Ophthalmology.* St Louis, MO: Mosby-Year Book; 1994:4-7.)[2]

F. During funduscopic examination, NFL defects should be carefully looked for when suspecting optic atrophy. They appear as dark slits or wedges and are most easily identified in the superior and inferior arcuate regions where the NFL is particularly thick. Also, vessels in this area, having lost their surrounding nerve fiber covering, appear darker than normal and stand out sharply

1. Red-free (green) light may be helpful in demonstrating defects of the NFL
2. Imaging modalities of the optic disc and retinal NFL including OCT, scanning laser polarimetry, and scanning laser ophthalmoscopy can help quantitate the degree of NFL and ganglion cell loss
3. In general, the degree of optic disc pallor and reduction of retinal NFL thickness correlate with level of visual dysfunction

G. "Bow-tie" or "band" optic atrophy (Figure 10-2)

1. Specific patterns of NFL and optic atrophy from optic chiasmal and retrochiasmal-pregeniculate lesions
2. With temporal field defects, loss of nerve fibers from ganglion cells nasal to the fovea results in atrophy of nasal and temporal portions of the disc, with relative sparing of superior and inferior arcuate bundles
3. Arcuate bundles are spared since they arise from ganglion cells both temporal and nasal to the fovea
4. OCT has shown diffuse NFL loss and a band pattern in patients with chiasmal syndromes
   a. Preserved NFL may be predictive of visual improvement in patients with compressive optic neuropathy and chiasmal syndromes

IV. **CONGENITAL OPTIC DISC ABNORMALITIES**

A. Optic nerve hypoplasia
  1. Incomplete development of the optic nerve
  2. Unilateral or bilateral
  3. Variable acuity depending on degree of development
  4. Double ring sign: hypoplastic disc surrounded by ring of sclera and ring of hyperpigmentation
  5. Clinical settings:
      a. Unilateral: isolated or accompanied by strabismus and/or nystagmus
      b. Bilateral: forebrain malformation and endocrinologic defects
          i. Septo-optic dysplasia
          ii. Short stature
          iii. Absence of septum pellucidum, corpus callosum
          iv. Endocrine deficits: growth hormone, hypothyroidism, sexual development, diabetes insipidus
          v. Association with cortical migration disorders: schizencephaly, pachygyria, cortical heterotopias
  6. Associated conditions:
      a. Maternal diabetes mellitus
      b. Fetal alcohol syndrome
      c. Use during pregnancy of LSD, quinine, anti-seizure drugs
  7. Patient evaluation (most commonly done for bilateral cases)
      a. Cranial MRI: with endocrine abnormalities, often find posterior pituitary ectopia or absence of posterior pituitary infundibulum
      b. Endocrinologic and neurologic evaluations

B. Homonymous hemioptic hypoplasia
  1. Optic disc findings in patients with congenital cerebral hemiatrophy, presumably due to fetal vascular insufficiency
  2. Fundus ipsilateral to hemispheric defect shows slightly small optic disc with temporal pallor and loss of NFL of ganglion cells temporal to the fovea
  3. Fundus contralateral to hemispheric defect shows small disc with "band" atrophy
  4. Associated findings include intellectual disabilities, seizures, congenital hemiplegia, and complete homonymous hemianopia

C. Superior segmental optic hypoplasia
  1. Ophthalmoscopic findings:
      a. Bilateral
      b. Superior entrance of central retinal artery into optic disc
      c. Pallor of superior disc
      d. Superior peripapillary halo
      e. Thinning of superior NFL
  2. Inferior visual field deficits of which patient may be unaware
  3. Often found in children of diabetic mothers

D. Morning Glory disc anomaly
  1. Ophthalmoscopic findings:
      a. Unilateral
      b. Enlarged, funnel-shaped, excavated optic disc with central glial tuft and radial array of the retinal vessels emanating from the disc
      c. Surrounded by annulus of chorioretinal pigmentary disturbance

2. Vision usually poor

3. May lead to retinal detachment

4. Occurrence:

    a. Isolated

    b. Basal encephalocele

    c. Pituitary dwarfism

    d. Moyamoya disease

    e. Neurofibromatosis—type 2

E. Papillorenal (renal-coloboma) syndrome

    1. Triad of the following:

        a. Optic disc "coloboma"—multiple cilioretinal vessels

        b. Renal hypoplasia/insufficiency

        c. PAX 2 genetic mutation

    2. Additional clinical features:

        a. May develop retinal detachment

        b. CNS abnormalities: microcephaly, intellectual disabilities

        c. Auditory: high-frequency hearing loss

F. Optic disc coloboma

    1. Excavation of the optic disc (typically inferiorly) due to failure or incomplete closure of the fetal (choroidal) fissure as the eye develops

        a. May occur sporadically or inherited (autosomal dominant)

        b. May be associated with CHARGE syndrome (coloboma, heart defects, atresia of the choanae, retardation of growth, genitourinary abnormalities, and ear abnormalities)

G. Optic disc pit

    1. Not true optic atrophy; they are small excavations of the optic disc, usually temporally or inferiorly, resulting from abnormal closure of the fetal (choroidal) fissure

        a. May lead to subretinal fluid extending into the macula

H. Perinatal infections, such as that from Zika virus, have been associated with optic atrophy, often with other associated funduscopic lesions

V. HEREDITARY OPTIC NEUROPATHIES

A. These forms of optic nerve disease often cause insidious, bilateral, symmetric loss of central visual function

B. Table 10-1 summarizes the major forms of hereditary optic nerve disease

C. LHON (see Table 10-1)

    1. Most often, but not exclusively, affects males in the second or third decade of life

    2. Rapid (within weeks) monocular visual loss to a variable level (20/200 or worse)

    3. Second eye usually affected within days or weeks

    4. In the acute phase, optic disc may appear normal or have typical triad of findings:

        a. Circumpapillary telangiectatic microangiopathy

        b. Prominent NFL around disc

        c. Absence of dye leakage from the disc or peripapillary region with fluorescein angiography

    5. Visual field abnormality is centrocecal scotoma

    6. Ultimately, the patient develops either temporal or generalized disc pallor

    7. Maternal inheritance pattern in LHON

        a. Disorder of mitochondrial, not chromosomal, DNA

Table 10-1				
HEREDITARY OPTIC NEUROPATHIES				
	Disorders of Chromosomal DNA			**Disorders of Mitochondrial DNA**
	Dominant	**Recessive**		**Maternal**
	Juvenile (infantile)	**Early infantile (congenital); simple**	**Behr type; complicated**	**DIDMOAD; Wolfram syndrome**	**LHON disease**
Age at Onset	Childhood (4 to 8 years)	Early childhood* (3 to 4 years)	Childhood (1 to 9 years)	Childhood (6 to 14 years)	Early adulthood (18 to 30 years, up to sixth decade)
Visual Impairment	Mild/moderate (20/40 to 20/200)	Severe (20/200 to HM)	Moderate (20/200)	Severe (20/400 to FC)	Moderate/severe (20/200 to FC)
Nystagmus	Rare**	Usual	In 50%	Absent	Absent
Optic Disc	Mild temporal pallor ± temporal excavation	Marked diffuse pallor ± arteriolar attenuation†	Mild temporal pallor	Marked diffuse pallor	Moderate diffuse pallor. Disc swelling in acute phase
Color Vision	Blue-yellow dyschromatopsia	Severe dyschromatopsia/achromatopsia	Moderate to severe dyschromatopsia	Severe dyschromatopsia	Dense central scotoma for colors
Course	Variable, slight progression	Stable	Stable	Progressive	Acute visual loss, then usually stable, may improve/worsen
Genetic Testing	OPA1 gene; most commonly Chromosome 3q		OPA1 gene for some	WFS1 gene Chromosome 4p	Mitochondrial mutations; most commonly 11778, 3460, 14484

DIDMOAD = diabetes insipidus, diabetes mellitus, optic atrophy, deafness; FC = finger counting; HM = hand motions.

*Difficult to assess in infancy, but visual impairment usually manifests by age 4 years.
**Presence of nystagmus with poor vision and earlier onset suggests separate congenital or infantile form.
†Distinguished from tapetoretinal degenerations by normal ERG.

Adapted from Glaser JS. *Neuro-Ophthalmology*. 3rd ed. Philadelphia, PA: Lippincott Williams & Wilkins; 1999:128.[3]

b. Chromosomal DNA follows Mendelian pattern of inheritance, but mitochondrial DNA is inherited exclusively from the mother
c. LHON linked with several point mutations in mitochondrial DNA, most commonly 11778, but also 14484, 3460
d. Mitochondrial DNA is essential for oxidative phosphorylation, the energy-producing cycle in the cell
e. Heteroplasmy: intracellular mitochondrial DNA is a mixture of mutant and normal forms; provides basis for variable clinical expression of mutation

8. Electrocardiogram obtained to exclude potential cardiac conduction defect

9. MRI with contrast may rarely show optic nerve or chiasmal enhancement

10. Eliminate use of tobacco, alcohol (potential toxins, which have included medications such as antiretroviral agents)

11. Spontaneous recovery of vision may occur (frequency based on genetic mutation: 14484 > 3460 > 11778)

12. Genetic reconstitution of defective mitochondrial transport proteins has shown potential. Idebenone 900 mg/day has shown benefit in both prevention of visual loss and recovery

D. Dominant optic atrophy

1. The most common hereditary optic neuropathy (1:50,000)

2. Inheritance pattern is autosomal dominant

3. Most common mutations involve *OPA1* gene on chromosome 3

4. Symptoms generally begin in the first decade of life with mild to moderate reduction of central vision

    a. Cecocentral scotomas are typical

    b. Dyschromatopsia often with tritanopia (blue-yellow)

    c. Temporal optic disc pallor with disc excavation in the area of pallor over time

5. Visual loss typically progresses slowly or stabilizes by the third to fourth decade

6. No effective treatment

VI. TOXIC AND DEFICIENCY OPTIC NEUROPATHIES

A. Particular forms of medical therapy or exposure to specific toxins may lead to bilateral retrobulbar optic neuropathy, characterized by visual loss, severe dyschromatopsia, central field defects with occasional peripheral field constriction, and initially normal-appearing optic discs that may gradually become pale

B. Medication-induced toxic optic neuropathies

1. Antibiotics

    a. Ethambutol

    b. Isoniazid

    c. Streptomycin

    d. Rifampin

    e. Halogenated hydroquinolones

    f. Linezolid

2. Immunosuppressants/immunomodulators

    a. Cyclosporine

    b. Tacrolimus

    c. Interferon-α

    d. Infliximab and other tumor necrosis factor antagonists

3. Chemotherapeutic agents

    a. Cisplatinum

    b. Carboplatinum

    c. Nitrosoureas: 1, 3-bis (2-chloroethyl)-1-nitrosourea (BCNU) and 1-(2-chloroethyl)-3-cyclohexyl-1-nitrosourea (CCNU)

    d. Vincristine

4. Cardiac medications

    a. Amiodarone

5. Miscellaneous

    a. Disulfiram

    b. Chlorpropamide

C. Many other potential toxins have been listed to cause an optic neuropathy, including the following:
    1. Arsenic
    2. Lead
    3. Hexachlorophene (Phisohex)
    4. Methanol
    5. Lysol (Reckitt Benckiser Inc)
    6. Quinine
    7. Ethylene glycol
    8. Toluene
    9. Cobalt
D. Deficiency optic neuropathies
    1. Clinical picture of progressive bilateral visual loss, with central or centrocecal scotomas and some degree of temporal disc pallor and atrophy of the papillomacular NFL
    2. Vitamin deficiencies that may be responsible for optic atrophy include the following:
        a. Vitamin B_{12} (cobalamin)
        b. Vitamin B_6 (pyridoxine)
        c. Vitamin B_1 (thiamine)
        d. Niacin
        e. Vitamin B_2 (riboflavin)
        f. Folic acid
        g. Copper
E. Tobacco-alcohol amblyopia
    1. Similar clinical picture to deficiency optic neuropathies listed previously
    2. Continuing controversy regarding whether this represents a form of toxic (cyanide) or deficiency (vitamin) optic nerve disease
    3. In general, prognosis for recovery of vision is good except in the most chronic cases

VII. Primary optic nerve neoplasms
A. Optic glioma
    1. Two major forms: childhood (benign) and adulthood (malignant; Table 10-2)
    2. Childhood form
        a. Patient presents with visual loss, proptosis, occasionally monocular nystagmus ("spasmus nutans"; see Chapter 3)
        b. One/both optic nerves and/or chiasm
        c. Up to 25% may have neurofibromatosis (see Chapter 19, II on page 261)
        d. Neuroimaging: double-intensity tubular thickening and kinking of orbital optic nerve(s), enlargement of chiasm, infiltration of hypothalamus
        e. Visual pathway gliomas may remain stable, enlarge, or regress (post-biopsy or spontaneously)
        f. Treatment controversial: observation, surgery, radiation therapy, chemotherapy
    3. Adult form
        a. Rapid onset of visual loss and relentless deterioration
        b. Usually begins in the optic chiasm
        c. Neuroimaging: suprasellar mass with edema
        d. Treatment: radiation only palliative
B. Optic nerve sheath meningioma
    1. Typically occurs in young to middle-aged women

	Table 10-2	

PRIMARY GLIOMAS OF THE OPTIC NERVE AND CHIASM

	Childhood	**Adulthood**
Age at Onset of Symptoms	4 to 8 years	Middle age
Presentation	Visual loss, proptosis	Rapid severe visual loss
Course	Relatively stable, nonprogressive	Rapid bilateral visual deterioration, other intracranial signs (eg, confusion, lethargy)
Prognosis	Compatible with long life	Death within months to 2 years
Neurofibromatosis	Associated in up to 25% of cases	No relationship
Histology	Pilocytic astrocytoma	Malignant astrocytoma (glioblastoma); may metastasize

Adapted from Glaser JS. *Neuro-Ophthalmology.* 3rd ed. Philadelphia, PA: Lippincott Williams & Wilkins; 1999:218.[3]

2. Insidious, progressive visual loss
3. Most commonly unilateral, but may be bilateral
4. May be associated with neurofibromatosis type 2
5. Optic disc may be chronically swollen, becomes pale, with appearance of optociliary shunt vessels
6. Neuroimaging
   a. CT: "tram-track" appearance due to calcification
   b. MRI: enhancement with intravenous gadolinium; able to detect intracranial spread through optic canal
7. Treatment: radiation therapy; surgery with evidence of intracranial progression

VIII. INFILTRATIVE OPTIC NEUROPATHY
  A. Optic disc initially swollen or normal; ultimately becomes pale
  B. Often acute visual loss
  C. Etiology may be benign (often inflammatory) or malignant
    1. Sarcoidosis
    2. Lymphoma
    3. Leukemia
    4. Plasmacytoma
    5. Malignant histiocytosis

IX. CARCINOMATOUS OPTIC NEUROPATHY
  A. Fundus typically normal at onset of visual loss, with disc gradually becoming pale
  B. Patient may or may not have history of known malignancy
  C. Optic neuropathy may be isolated or accompanied by other neurologic defects
  D. Visual loss typically acute, progressive, and devastating
  E. Unless large intraparenchymal CNS spread has occurred, radiologic studies (CT, MRI, angiography) are often normal
  F. May see meningeal enhancement with cranial MR scanning following IV contrast
  G. Careful CSF analysis with cytologic examination for malignant cells
  H. Due to microscopic infiltrates of the nerve and its sheaths

X.   RADIATION OPTIC NEUROPATHY

A.   Due to delayed radionecrosis of optic nerve and chiasm

B.   Follows radiation therapy (external beam, gamma knife) for perisellar tumor, such as pituitary adenoma, craniopharyngioma, invasive sinus carcinoma

C.   Diagnostic criteria:

1.   Acute to subacute (over days to weeks) visual loss (monocular or binocular)

2.   Visual field defects indicating optic nerve or chiasmal dysfunction

3.   Optic disc edema usually absent (see Chapter 9, VI on page 153)

4.   Onset typically delayed months after radiation therapy and within 3 years of therapy (peak: 1 to 1.5 years)

5.   Neuroimaging studies demonstrate no evidence of anterior visual pathway compression

6.   MR scanning most commonly demonstrates contrast-enhancement in optic nerves and/or chiasm

D.   Pathology: fibrinoid necrosis of blood vessels, demyelination, necrosis

E.   Treatment: none of proven efficacy

XI.   NEURODEGENERATIVE DISORDERS

A.   Many disorders may cause neurodegeneration and optic disc pallor. The more common causes of neurodegeneration such as Alzheimer disease and Parkinson disease have been associated with decreased retinal thickness without frank optic atrophy

1.   Adrenoleukodystrophy

2.   Spinocerebellar ataxia

XII. TRAUMATIC OPTIC NEUROPATHY

A.   Three categories:

1.   Evulsion

2.   Direct injury

3.   Indirect injury

B.   Optic nerve evulsion

1.   Dislocation of optic nerve from scleral canal

2.   Partial or complete

3.   As early vitreous hemorrhage clears optic disc partially or totally absent

4.   May be confirmed with imaging studies (ultrasound, CT, MRI)

5.   Treatment: none

C.   Direct injury

1.   Impact on optic nerve or its sheaths by a blunt or sharp object

2.   With anterior injury, may see fundus picture of central retinal artery occlusion (CRAO)

3.   More posterior involvement leads to normal fundus appearance followed by optic atrophy within 4 to 8 weeks

4.   Multiple pathophysiologic mechanisms

a.   Laceration

b.   Bone deformation/fracture

c.   Vascular insufficiency

d.   Hemorrhage

5.   Imaging studies: CT, MRI (contraindicated with ferromagnetic foreign body)

6.   Treatment individualized:

a.   Megadose corticosteroids—no proven benefit

i.   Corticosteroids toxic to optic nerve in some animal models

        ii. Increased mortality in patients with concomitant head trauma treated with corticosteroids in Corticosteroid Randomization for Acute Head Trauma (CRASH) trial

    b. Surgery

        i. May be helpful to relieve impingement from bony fragment with fracture

        ii. May be helpful to relieve compressive effects of intrasheath hemorrhage of the optic nerve

D. Indirect injury

    1. Blunt trauma to orbit or cranium with lines of force transmitted to orbital apex

    2. Most common form of traumatic optic neuropathy

    3. Canalicular optic nerve is site of injury

    4. Fundus initially typically normal with appearance of optic atrophy in 2 to 4 weeks

    5. Imaging studies may be normal or demonstrate optic canal fracture

    6. Pathophysiologic mechanisms, as with direct injury (see page 172, XII, C, 4)

    7. Treatment: none of proven efficacy (see page 172, XII, C, 6, a for concern using corticosteroids)

REFERENCES

1. Quigley HA, Anderson DR. The histologic basis of optic disc pallor in experimental optic atrophy. *Am J Ophthalmol*. 1977;83:709-717.
2. Newman NJ. Chiasm, parachiasmal syndromes, retrochiasm and disorders of higher visual function. In: Slamovits TL, Burde RM, eds. *Neuro-Ophthalmology*. St Louis, MO: Mosby-Year Book; 1994:4-7.
3. Glaser JS. *Neuro-Ophthalmology*. 3rd ed. Philadelphia, PA: Lippincott Williams & Wilkins; 1999:128.

BIBLIOGRAPHY

Al-Mohtaseb Z, Foroozan R. Congenital optic disc anomalies. *Int Ophthalmol Clin*. 2012;52:1-16.

Avery RA, Fisher MJ, Liu GT. Optic pathway gliomas. *J Neuroophthalmol*. 2011;31:269-278.

Borchert M. Reappraisal of the optic nerve hypoplasia syndrome. *J Neuroophthal*. 2012;32:58-67.

Chun BY, Rizzo JF, 3rd. Dominant optic atrophy: updates on the pathophysiology and clinical manifestations of the optic atrophy 1 mutation. *Curr Opin Ophthalmol*. 2016;27:475-480.

Feuer WJ, Schiffman JC, Davis JL, et al. Gene therapy for Leber hereditary optic neuropathy: initial results. *Ophthalmology*. 2016;123:558-570.

Fraser CL, White AJ, Plant GT, Martin KR. Optic nerve cupping and the neuro-ophthlamologist. *J Neuroophthalmol*. 2013;33:377-389.

Fraser JA, Biousse V, Newman NJ. The neuro-ophthalmology of mitochondrial disease. *Surv Ophthalmol*. 2010;55:299-334.

Grzybowski A, Zulsdorff M, Wilhelm H, Tonagel F. Toxic optic neuropathies: an updated review. *Acta Ophthalmol*. 2015;93:402-410.

Jonas JB, Budde WM, Panda-Jonas S. Ophthalmoscopic evaluation of the optic nerve head. *Surv Ophthalmol*. 1999;43:293-320.

Kersten HM, Roxburgh RH, Danesh-Meyer HV. Ophthalmic manifestations of inherited neurodegenerative disorders. *Nat Rev Neurol*. 2014;10:349-362.

Kline LB, Foroozan R. *Optic Nerve Disorders*. 2nd ed. Oxford University Press New York, New York, 2007

Lyseng-Williamson KA. Idebenone: a review in Leber's hereditary optic neuropathy. *Drugs*. 2016;76:805-813.

Meier PG, Maeder P, Kardon RH, Borruat FX. Homonymous ganglion cell layer thinning after isolated occipital lesion: macular OCT demonstrates transsynaptic retrograde retinal degeneration. *J Neuroophthalmol*. 2015;35:112-116.

Miller NR. Primary tumours of the optic nerve and its sheath. *Eye*. 2004;18:1026-1037.

O'Neill EC, Danesh-Meyer HV, Kong GX, et al. Optic disc evaluation in optic neuropathies: the optic disc assessment project. *Ophthalmology*. 2011;118:964-970.

Pollock BE, Link MJ, Leavitt JA, Stafford SL. Dose-volume analysis of radiation-induced optic neuropathy after single-fraction stereotactic radiosurgery. *Neurosurgery*. 2014;75:456-460.

Shapey J, Sabin HI, Danesh-Meyer HV, Kaye AH. Diagnosis and management of optic nerve sheath meningiomas. *J Clin Neurosci*. 2013;20:1045-1056.

Steinsapir KD, Goldberg RA. Traumatic optic neuropathy: an evolving understanding. *Am J Ophthalmol*. 2011;151:928-933.

Vaphiades MS. Magnetic resonance findings in the pregeniculate visual pathways in Leber hereditary optic neuropathy. *J Neuroophthalmol*. 2011;31:194.

Myasthenia and Ocular Myopathies

ROD FOROOZAN, MD

I. MYASTHENIA AND OCULAR MYOPATHIES

A. These disorders produce ocular motor dysfunction due to involvement of the extraocular muscles and the neuromuscular junction

B. Some of these entities may simulate isolated or combined ocular motor cranial nerve palsies

II. MYASTHENIA GRAVIS

A. Disease characterized clinically by muscle weakness and fatigue

B. It is the most common disorder affecting the neuromuscular junction

C. Myasthenia involves skeletal and not visceral musculature; therefore, the pupil and ciliary muscle are clinically unaffected. Major ophthalmologic complaints are ptosis and diplopia

D. Ocular involvement eventually occurs in 90% of myasthenics and accounts for the initial complaint in 75%. Approximately 80% of patients with ocular onset progress to involvement of other muscle groups (usually within 2 years), while 20% have only ocular complaints

E. Impaired neuromuscular transmission of myasthenia is due to the presence of antibodies, including to acetylcholine receptors in the motor endplate of striated muscles. This leads to a reduction in the number of acetylcholine receptors

F. Clinical characteristics of ocular myasthenia:

1. Variability of muscle function within minutes, hours, days, or weeks

2. Remissions and exacerbations (often triggered by infection, increased body temperature, and trauma)

3. Onset at any age

4. Ptosis (unilateral or bilateral) worse at end of day, may "shift" from eye to eye

5. Extraocular muscle involvement follows no set pattern; any ocular movement pattern may develop and thus mimic any ocular motor cranial nerve palsy or central gaze disturbance (eg, gaze palsy, INO, gaze-evoked nystagmus)

6. Dysthyroidism is found in approximately 5% of myasthenics, also an increased incidence of thymoma and autoimmune disorders

Foroozan R, Vaphiades MS. *Kline's Neuro-Ophthalmology Review Manual, Eighth Edition (pp 175-183).*
© 2018 SLACK Incorporated.

G. Diagnosis of ocular myasthenia

1. Lid fatigue: with sustained upward gaze, ptosis becomes more marked

2. Lid-twitch sign (Cogan): the patient looks down for 10 to 15 seconds and is then asked to rapidly refixate in the primary position. A positive lid-twitch sign consists of an upward overshoot of the lid, which then falls to its previously ptotic position

3. Enhanced ptosis: if ptosis is asymmetric, the patient may use the frontalis muscle to elevate both lids, producing what appears to be lid retraction on one side. If the more ptotic lid is elevated, the previously retracted one will fall

4. Variability in measuring phorias or tropias during the same examination or at different times is very suggestive of myasthenia

5. Myasthenic ptosis is frequently associated with orbicularis oculi weakness

6. Tensilon (edrophonium chloride) test: one positive test establishes the diagnosis of myasthenia, yet myasthenia may exist even in the face of a negative Tensilon test

   a. Tensilon is supplied in a single dose, 10 mg/1 mL breakneck vial

   b. A definite endpoint must be selected. If the patient has no findings at the time of examination, testing should be postponed. If ptosis is present, it should be documented (typically photographically) before and after injection

   c. If diplopia is present, careful measurement of the deviation should be carried out before, immediately after, and 3 to 4 minutes following injection. Three types of responses may occur in myasthenic patients. Type 1 responses occur only in myasthenics, while type 2 and 3 responses may be seen in nonmyasthenic ophthalmoplegia

      i. Type 1: an improvement in alignment (large tropia becomes smaller)

      ii. Type 2: a worsening of alignment (a small tropia becomes a large tropia)

      iii. Type 3: a reversal of alignment (a left HT becomes a right HT)

   d. Procedure in adults:

      i. Tensilon should be drawn up in a 1-cc tuberculin syringe

      ii. 0.4 mg of injectable atropine should also be drawn up in another 1-cc tuberculin syringe

      iii. A 10-cc syringe is filled with injectable saline

      iv. A small gauge needle is placed in a dorsal arm or hand vein

      v. 1 mL of saline solution is injected and the patient observed for 1 minute

      vi. 0.2 mL of Tensilon is injected and the tubing flushed with 1 mL of saline, then observed for 1 minute

      vii. If no response, a bolus of 0.8 mL of Tensilon is injected and the tubing flushed with another 1 mL of saline; atropine is then connected to the tubing

      viii. Atropine (0.4 mg intramuscularly) may be used to pretreat all patients 15 minutes before Tensilon testing, or used intravenously only to avoid undesirable cholinergic side effects (eg, bradycardia, angina, bronchospasm)

   e. In children and uncooperative adults, 0.4 mg of atropine is given intramuscularly 15 minutes prior to the injection of neostigmine (Prostigmin) and the dose calculated as follows: weight (kg) ÷ 70 (kg) × 1.5 mg = dose. Patient is re-examined 30 to 45 minutes after injection

7. **Alert!** Rarely:

   a. Patient may have false-positive Tensilon test, or

   b. Positive Tensilon test and coexistent intracranial mass (patient has 2 diseases)

8. Sleep test
   a. Safe alternative to Tensilon test
   b. Resolution of ptosis or ophthalmoparesis after 30-minute period of sleep, with reappearance of sign 30 seconds to 5 minutes after awakening
9. Ice test
   a. Also safe alternative to Tensilon test
   b. Resolution of ptosis after 2-minute application of ice pack to involved eyelid
   c. High degree of sensitivity and specificity for myasthenic ptosis
   d. Eye movement disorder may improve after 5-minute application of ice packs
10. Patients with myasthenia gravis have an increased frequency of autoantibodies
    a. Acetylcholine receptor antibodies, if present, are diagnostic of myasthenia. However, only about 60% of patients with ocular myasthenia have detectable antibody levels
    b. Anti–muscle-specific kinase (MuSK), a tyrosine kinase receptor
    c. Antistriational antibody (present in almost all patients with thymoma) and anti-lipoprotein–related protein 4 (LRP4) antibody (found in approximately 10% of MG patients who are negative for both anti-AChR and anti-MuSK)
11. Electromyography (EMG): with repetitive supramaximal motor nerve stimulation, there is a decremental muscular response in myasthenia. Helpful if present, but may be a normal response in clinically uninvolved extremity musculature in patients with ocular myasthenia. Should be performed on orbicularis oculi as well. Single fiber EMG of the orbicularis oculi muscle is thought to be the most sensitive type of neuromuscular test for myasthenia

H. Certain drugs may cause the following:
   1. Unmasking or aggravation of myasthenia (eg, quinidine, propranolol, lithium)
   2. Further impairment of neuromuscular conduction—aminoglycosides
   3. Drug-induced myasthenia syndrome (eg, penicillamine, statins)

I. Treatment of ocular myasthenia
   1. Occlusion of one eye
   2. Prism spectacles
   3. Eyelid crutches
   4. Pyridostigmine (Mestinon)
   5. Systemic steroids
      a. Controversy: early treatment of ocular myasthenia gravis with corticosteroids and/or immunosuppression may delay or prevent the subsequent development of generalized disease
   6. Other immunosuppressive agents (cyclosporine, mycophenolate, azathioprine)

J. Treatment of systemic myasthenia
   1. Pyridostigmine (Mestinon)
   2. Immunosuppressants (steroids, cyclosporine, azathioprine)
   3. Plasmapheresis
   4. Intravenous immunoglobulin
   5. Thymectomy

III. **CHRONIC PROGRESSIVE EXTERNAL OPHTHALMOPLEGIA (CPEO)**
   A. Comprises a group of disorders characterized by insidiously progressive, symmetric immobility of the eyes, with lids typically ptotic, the orbicularis oculi weak, and the pupils spared
   B. The eye movements remain limited with doll's head and caloric stimulation

    C.   CPEO may occur in an isolated ocular form, may have a hereditary pattern, or may be part of a recognizable clinical entity

        1.   Oculopharyngeal muscular dystrophy (OPMD): dysphagia, family history of ophthalmoplegia, often of French-Canadian or Hispanic ancestry

            a.   OPMD is caused by expansions in a 6-guanine-cytosine-guanine trinucleotide repeat tract located in the first exon of the polyadenylate binding protein nuclear 1 gene (PABPN1)

        2.   Kearns-Sayre syndrome: triad of CPEO, cardiac conduction defect, pigmentary retinopathy

        3.   Ophthalmoplegia plus: term applied to instances in which CPEO is associated with the previously mentioned abnormalities plus a variety of others, including elevated CSF protein, spongiform degeneration of the cerebrum and brainstem, slow electroencephalogram (EEG), subnormal intelligence, hearing loss

    D.   Muscle biopsy (ocular or limb) will demonstrate mitochondrial accumulations beneath the plasma membrane and between myofibrils. Using a modified trichrome stain, these abnormal muscle fibers have been called "ragged red" fibers

    E.   CPEO in itself or as part of a multisystem disease may be associated with deletions in the mitochondrial DNA of skeletal muscle ("mitochondrial myopathy")

    F.   PSP, or *Steele-Richardson-Olszewski syndrome*, a neurodegenerative syndrome, which can simulate CPEO (Chapter 2, G, on page 78)

        1.   Vertical gaze is affected first, often with slowing of vertical saccades and paresis of downward gaze

        2.   Eventually, horizontal gaze is involved

        3.   Doll's head and caloric testing demonstrate full excursions until later in the course of disease

        4.   Additional clinical findings can overlap with Parkinson disease: dystonic rigidity of neck and trunk, masked face, dysarthria, dysesthesia, hyperreflexia, dementia, square-wave jerks, diplopia typically exotropia (convergence insufficiency), and apraxia of eyelid opening

        5.   Hummingbird sign, also known as the *penguin silhouette sign*, refers to the mid-sagittal MRI appearance of the brainstem

        6.   Pathologically there is neuronal loss, gliosis, neurofibrillary tangles, and demyelination centered in the brainstem reticular formation and ocular motor nuclei

        7.   Characterized by abnormal accumulation of microtubule-association protein, tau

        8.   Therapy: none of proven efficacy for underlying condition, patients often treated initially for Parkinson disease with limited response

            a.   Single-vision reading glasses and elevate reading material to obviate the need to look down

            b.   Prism spectacles and eye muscle surgery for ocular misalignment

IV. MYOTONIC DYSTROPHY

    A.   Autosomal dominant muscular dystrophy in which myotonia is accompanied by dystrophic changes in other tissues and organs

    B.   A trinucleotide repeat disorder, 2 genetic loci have been associated with the clinical phenotype: chromosome 19 (DM1) and chromosome 3 (DM2)

    C.   Myotonia is a phenomenon in which muscle fibers have a pathologically persistent activity after a strong contraction or are continuously active when they should be relaxed

    D.   Ophthalmologic signs:

        1.   Bilateral ptosis

        2.   Progressive external ophthalmoplegia

        3.   Myotonia of lid closure and gaze holding

Table 11-1
GRAVES' DISEASE SIGNS (MNEMONIC)

No signs or symptoms
Only signs of lid retraction, lid lag, stare
Soft tissue signs and symptoms:

> **R**esistance to retropulsion
> **E**dema of conjunctiva and caruncle
> **L**acrimal gland enlargement
> **I**njection over rectus muscle insertion
> **E**dema of eyelids
> **F**ullness of eyelids

Proptosis
Extraocular muscle enlargement
Corneal involvement secondary to exposure
Sight loss secondary to optic nerve compression

Adapted from Van Dyk HJ. Orbital Graves' disease. A modification of the NO SPECS classification. *Ophthalmology.* 1981;88:479-483.[1]

4. Orbicularis weaknesses
5. Polychromatophilic cataracts
6. Miotic pupils, sluggish to light and near
7. Retinal pigmentary degeneration

E. Multiple systemic findings include face, neck, and limb myopathy with atrophy, testicular atrophy, baldness, cardiac conduction defects

V. **THYROID EYE DISEASE (DYSTHYROID MYOPATHY OR GRAVES' DISEASE)**

A. A restrictive myopathy occurring commonly in middle-aged and elderly individuals, leading to ophthalmoparesis and diplopia

B. Lymphocytic and plasmacytic infiltration of extraocular muscles; leads to edema, activation of fibroblasts with production of acid mucopolysaccharide and fibrosis

C. Variety of ocular motility patterns produced

1. "Elevator palsy," a supraduction deficit due to fibrotic shortening of the inferior rectus
2. "Abduction weaknesses" due to involvement of the medial rectus, mimicking a VI nerve palsy
3. Superior and lateral rectus muscles less frequently involved
4. Frequency of clinical involvement of rectus muscles: mnemonic "**I'm slow**"— **i**nferior rectus > **m**edial rectus > **s**uperior rectus > **l**ateral rectus

D. Additional findings include the following:

1. Proptosis
2. Lids: retraction, lid lag on downward gaze (von Graefe sign), edema
3. Conjunctiva: injection over horizontal rectus muscles, chemosis
4. Cornea: keratopathy, erosions, ulceration
5. Five percent of patients with thyroid eye disease develop optic neuropathy, typically due to compression at orbital apex by enlarged extraocular muscles (see Chapter 9, VII, A, 3 on page 157)

E. Table 11-1 summarizes clinical findings with "NO SPECS" mnemonic classification and soft-tissue involvement with "RELIEF" mnemonic

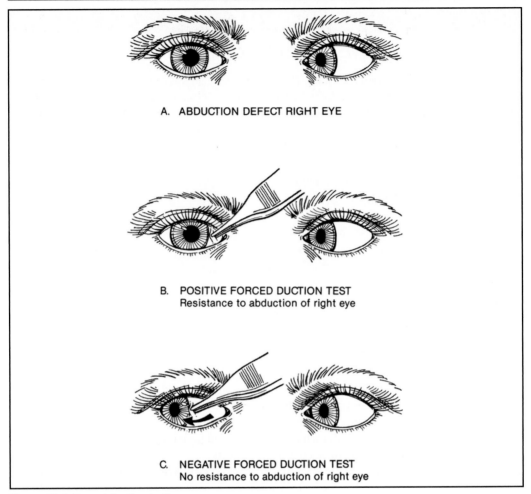

Figure 11-1. Forced duction testing.

F.   Diagnostic studies
1.   Forced duction testing (Figure 11-1)
a.   In patients with acquired diplopia and an incomitant deviation, forced duction testing can eliminate the need for extensive neurologic investigation if restriction is found. Remember, many patients with thyroid myopathy have only subtle or no other signs of classic thyroid eye disease
b.   Three drops of topical proparacaine solution are instilled in the inferior cul-de-sac of each eye. During this time, a cotton-tipped applicator is soaked with similar solution
c.   The patient is asked to look in the direction of gaze limitation. The cotton-tipped applicator is placed on the conjunctiva anterior to the presumed restricted muscle
d.   The conjunctiva is grasped with toothed forceps and the globe passively rotated in the direction of the limited duction
e.   The same procedure is carried out in the fellow eye and the relative limitation compared. In subtle cases, repeated comparisons between the 2 eyes may be necessary

      f. At times, with attempted forced ductions, the globe is displaced backward into the orbit. This phenomenon must be observed, or the examiner may believe the eye moves more easily than it actually does

      g. Occasionally, patients are not able to cooperate for forced duction testing. In these cases, measurement of the intraocular pressure in the primary position and again with the eyes moved into the direction of limited gaze is compared. A pressure rise of greater than 4 mm Hg in moving from one gaze position to another is felt to be suggestive of a restrictive process

  2. Ultrasonography to measure size of extraocular muscles

  3. Orbital CT or MRI

      a. Typically, enlargement of all extraocular muscles in both orbits

      b. Muscle tendon spared

  4. Thyroid function tests and thyroid antibodies

G. Association of dysthyroidism with myasthenia; 2 diseases may coexist and give a variety of ocular findings

H. Treatment

  1. Corticosteroids (in patients with active and severe disease, once weekly IV glucocorticoids appear to be more effective and better tolerated with less side effects than oral steroids)

      a. More effective when there is active orbital inflammation

  2. Orbital radiation

      a. Controversial as some feel it is not effective in thyroid eye disease

  3. Orbital decompression

      a. Typically performed for compressive optic neuropathy or severe proptosis

  4. Other immunosuppressives

      a. Rituximab

      b. Infliximab

  5. In patients with active ophthalmopathy, teprotumumab, an inhibitor of insulin-like growth factor 1 receptor, was more effective than placebo in reducing proptosis and the Clinical Activity Score

  6. Eye muscle surgery for ocular misalignment

      a. Typically rectus muscle recessions performed

      b. Eye muscle surgery should be performed after orbital decompression and before eyelid surgery

  7. Eyelid surgery

      a. Should be performed after eye muscle surgery as a shift in position of extraocular muscles may change the position of the eyelid

VI. Idiopathic orbital inflammation (orbital pseudotumor)

A. A syndrome occurring in any age group consisting of acute onset of orbital pain, chemosis, conjunctival injection, and frequently proptosis

B. If the inflammatory process affects one or more of the extraocular muscles, the term *orbital myositis* is employed. These patients typically complain of diplopia

C. Pathologic studies in such cases demonstrate orbital structures (blood vessels, muscles, lacrimal glands, etc) infiltrated with chronic inflammatory cells

D. In the vast majority of cases, the etiology of the inflammatory response is unknown, although it may occur with systemic disorders, including lupus erythematosus, rheumatoid arthritis, sarcoidosis, polyangiitis with granulomatosis (Wegener), dermatomyositis, amyloidosis

E. The sclerosing orbital variant can be less responsive to corticosteroids (see section VI, I, 1 next) and difficult to treat

F. Variant may be associated with elevated IgG4 immunoglobulin staining of involved tissue
1. Often more relentless course requiring more marked systemic immunosuppression

G. Diagnostic studies
1. Orbital ultrasonography
2. Orbital CT scanning
   a. Usually only 1 or 2 extraocular muscles enlarged in a single orbit (myositis)
   b. Muscle tendon enlarged as well
3. Orbital biopsy may be helpful to exclude other inflammatory and infiltrative conditions other than idiopathic orbital inflammation. For example:
   a. Immunostaining for IgG4
   b. Congo red stain for amyloidosis

H. Intracranial spread (may be similar pathology to idiopathic hypertrophic pachymeningitis) occurs in 5% to 10% of cases; patient may or may not have symptoms of CNS involvement

I. Treatment modalities
1. Systemic steroids usually produce dramatic improvement of symptoms in 24 to 48 hours with clearing of signs over 1 to 4 weeks
2. Orbital radiation therapy: 1000 to 2000 cGy
3. Chlorambucil, cyclophosphamide, cyclosporine, and other immunosuppressives have been used for chronic, recurrent orbital pseudotumor

J. It may be difficult to distinguish between idiopathic orbital inflammation and orbital lymphoma, both clinically and pathologically. All patients with idiopathic orbital inflammation must be followed carefully. An initial salutary response to steroid therapy by no means excludes a malignant process

Reference

1. Van Dyk HJ. Orbital Graves' disease. A modification of the NO SPECS classification. *Ophthalmology*. 1981;88:479-483.

Bibliography

Bahn RS. Graves' ophthalmopathy. *N Engl J Med*. 2010;362:726-738.

Bhatti MT, Dutton JJ. Thyroid eye disease: therapy in the active phase. *J Neuroophthalmol*. 2014;34:186-197.

Fraser JA, Biousse V, Newman NJ. The neuro-ophthalmology of mitochondrial disease. *Surv Ophthalmol*. 2010;55:299-334.

Gilbert ME, Savino PJ. Ocular myasthenia gravis. *Int Ophthalmol Clin*. 2007;47:93-103.

Gorman CA, Garrity JA, Fatourechi V, et al. A prospective, randomized, double-blind, placebo-controlled study of orbital radiotherapy for Graves' ophthalmopathy. *Ophthalmology*. 2001;108:1523-1534.

Harrad R. Management of strabismus in thyroid eye disease. *Eye (Lond)*. 2015;29:234-237.

Kahaly GJ, Pitz S, Hommel G, Dittmar M. Randomized, single blind trial of intravenous versus oral steroid monotherapy in Graves' orbitopathy. *J Clin Endocrinol Metab*. 2005;90:5234-5240.

Kazim M, Goldberg RA, Smith TJ. Insights into the pathogenesis of thyroid-associated orbitopathy. *Arch Ophthalmol*. 2002;120:380-388.

Kubis KC, Danesh-Meyer HV, Savino PJ, Sergott RC. The ice test versus the rest test in myasthenia gravis. *Ophthalmology*. 2000;107:1995-1998.

Lopez G, Bayulkem K, Hallett M. Progressive supranuclear palsy (PSP): Richardson syndrome and other PSP variants. *Acta Neurol Scand*. 2016;134:242-249.

Rootman J. *Diseases of the Orbit*. 3rd ed. Philadelphia, PA: Lippincott Williams & Wilkins; 2003.

Sanders DB, Wolfe GI, Benatar M, et al. International consensus guidance for management of myasthenia gravis: Executive summary. *Neurology*. 2016;87:419-425.

Shan SJ, Douglas RS. The pathophysiology of thyroid eye disease. *J Neuroophthalmol*. 2014;34:177-185.

Smith TJ, Kahaly GJ, Ezra DG, et al. Teprotumumab for thyroid-associated ophthalmopathy. *N Engl J Med*. 2017;376:1748-1761.

Verschuuren JJ, Huijbers MG, Plomp JJ, et al. Pathophysiology of myasthenia gravis with antibodies to the acetylcholine receptor, muscle-specific kinase and low-density lipoprotein receptor-related protein 4. *Autoimmun Rev*. 2013;12:918-923.

Wallace ZS, Khosroshahi A, Jakobiec FA, et al. IgG4-related systemic disease as a cause of "idiopathic" orbital inflammation, including orbital myositis, and trigeminal nerve involvement. *Surv Ophthalmol*. 2012;57:26-33.

CHAPTER 12

V Nerve (Trigeminal) Syndromes

ROD FOROOZAN, MD AND MICHAEL S. VAPHIADES, DO

I.   **ANATOMICAL CONSIDERATIONS (FIGURE 12-1)**
  A.   The trigeminal nerve is a mixed nerve
    1.   Sensory: ipsilateral side of face
    2.   Motor: ipsilateral muscles of mastication (masseter, temporalis, pterygoids)
  B.   Nuclear complex
    1.   Sensory portion of trigeminal nerve extends from the midbrain to the upper cervical cord
    2.   Mesencephalic (rostral) nucleus: proprioception and deep sensation from tendons and muscles of mastication
    3.   Main sensory nucleus
      a.   Located in pons
      b.   Subserves light touch
    4.   Spinal nucleus
      a.   Extends from pons to upper cervical cord
      b.   Subserves pain and temperature
      c.   Divided into segments that correspond to dermatomes that are concentric around the mouth
  C.   Peripheral nerve
    1.   The trigeminal nerve supplies sensation to the ipsilateral side of the face via 3 branches:
      a. V^1—Ophthalmic division: frontal, lacrimal, and nasociliary
      b. V^2—Maxillary division: cheek and lower eyelid
      c. V^3—Mandibular division: area of mandible (but not angle of mandible), lower lip, tongue
    2.   Motor nucleus lies in pons medially to main sensory nucleus and axons travel with mandibular (V^3) division
    3.   Three divisions of trigeminal nerve converge at trigeminal (gasserian) ganglion, which lies in the Meckel cave of temporal bone
    4.   Fibers then travel through main sensory root to brainstem

Foroozan R, Vaphiades MS. *Kline's Neuro-Ophthalmology Review Manual, Eighth Edition* (pp 185-190).
© 2018 SLACK Incorporated.

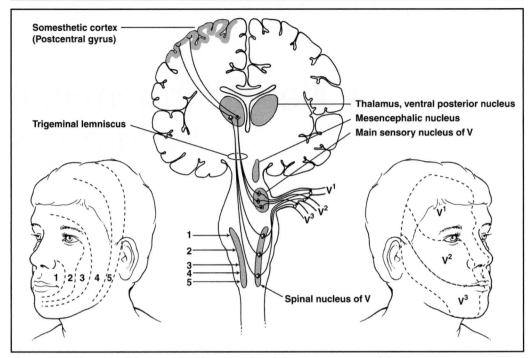

Figure 12-1. Diagram of the central pathways and peripheral innervation of the V nerve.

II. OCULOFACIAL HYPESTHESIA (SEE FIGURE 12-1)

A. Distribution of facial numbness or paresthesias helps determine central or peripheral origin

1. Concentric perioral numbness/paresthesia: central (nuclear) origin (eg, ischemia, demyelination)

2. Band of numbness/paresthesia: peripheral origin (ie, V^1, V^2, V^3)

3. Such somatotopic hypesthesia (eg, V^1 only, or V^2 and V^3 with sparing of V^1) suggests that the lesion is more likely to be in the middle cranial fossa (cavernous sinus) or orbit

B. Differential diagnosis of diminished sensation in the trigeminal distribution[1]

1. Corneal

   a. Herpes simplex

   b. Herpes zoster

   c. Ocular surgery

   d. Cerebellopontine angle tumors

   e. Dysautonomia

   f. Congenital

2. Ophthalmic division

   a. Neoplasm, orbital apex

   b. Neoplasm, superior orbital fissure

   c. Neoplasm, cavernous sinus

   d. Neoplasm, middle fossa

   e. Aneurysm, cavernous sinus

   3. Maxillary division

      a. Orbital floor fracture

      b. Maxillary antrum carcinoma

      c. Perineural spread of skin carcinoma (see page 190, III, B, 5)

      d. Neoplasm, foramen rotundum, sphenopterygoid fossa

   4. Mandibular division (inferior alveolar nerve, lingual nerve, and mental nerve)

      a. Nasopharyngeal tumor

      b. Middle fossa tumor

      c. Numb chin syndrome

         i. Involvement of mental nerve (terminal branch of inferior alveolar nerve)

        ii. Frequently due to systemic cancer: breast, lymphoproliferative disorders. It may also occur as a complication from chin implantation surgery or mucocele resection (mental nerve) or third molar (wisdom tooth) removal (inferior alveolar nerve). These nerves are very resilient but take a very long time to recover. Initially, numbness and tightness occurs, then an itching and burning sensation follows. Paresthesia and dysesthesia finally predominate as the numbness resolves. This entire process takes months to years to fully recover

       iii. Contrast: enhanced imaging (CT or MRI) of head including skull base and mandible

   5. All divisions

      a. Nasopharyngeal carcinoma

      b. Cerebellopontine angle tumors

      c. Brainstem lesions (dissociated sensory loss)

      d. Intracavernous aneurysm

      e. Demyelination

      f. Middle fossa or Meckel cave tumor

      g. Benign sensory neuropathy

      h. Tentorial meningioma

      i. Toxins (eg, trichloroethylene)

      j. Trigeminal neurofibroma

III. OCULOFACIAL PAIN

  A. Differential diagnosis of relatively common entities associated with ocular and facial pain on the basis of clinical findings

    1. Typically with ophthalmic findings

      a. Most commonly with an abnormal anterior segment examination

         i. Corneal and conjunctival abnormalities

        ii. Uveitis and ocular inflammation

       iii. Dry eye syndrome

       iv. Chronic ocular hypoxia, carotid occlusive disease

       v. Angle-closure glaucoma

      b. Often with a normal anterior segment examination

         i. Glaucoma, including intermittent angle-closure glaucoma

        ii. Posterior scleritis

       iii. Uveitis

       iv. Intraocular tumor

       v. Optic neuropathy

       vi. Ocular motor palsy

      c. Ocular pain with orbitopathy
- i. Orbital fracture
- ii. Orbital hemorrhage
- iii. Subperiosteal hemorrhage
- iv. Subperiosteal abscess
- v. Orbital cellulitis
- vi. Thyroid eye disease
- vii. Idiopathic orbital inflammation (orbital pseudotumor)

2. Can occur with or without ophthalmic findings
   a. Primary headache syndromes including migraine and cluster headaches
   b. Raeder paratrigeminal neuralgia (see page 189, III, B, 4)
   c. Herpes zoster—nasociliary nerve involvement indicated by vesicular eruption on side or tip of nose (Hutchinson sign)
      i. May be followed by postherpetic neuralgia
   d. Referred (dural) pain, including occipital infarction
   e. Tic douloureux (infrequent in V^1)
   f. Paranasal sinus disease
   g. Dental disease
   h. Temporomandibular syndrome
   i. Nasopharyngeal carcinoma
   j. Cavernous sinus syndromes (see Chapter 7)
      i. Tumors
      ii. Tolosa-Hunt syndrome
   k. Arteriovenous fistula
   l. Arteriovenous malformation (AVM)
   m. Elevated intracranial pressure and IIH
   n. Intracranial hypotension

3. Miscellaneous
   a. Atypical facial neuralgias
   b. Pain with medullary lesions (eg, Wallenberg syndrome)
   c. Giant cell arteritis (see Chapter 9)
   d. Occipital neuralgia can sometimes be confused with other causes of head and facial pain
   e. Trochleitis and trochlear migraine
   f. Nonorganic pain

B. Specific trigeminal syndromes
1. Referred pain
   a. Any intracranial process irritating the dural sensory fibers, which may be supplied by recurrent branches of V nerve
   b. Neck pain (eg, from osteoarthritis in the cervical spine) may be referred to the eye because of the cervical sensory fibers traveling with the trigeminal fibers of the spinal tract of V, which extends to C-2 level
2. Trigeminal neuralgia (tic douloureux)
   a. Paroxysmal pain in the distribution of one or more of the divisions of V ($V^3 > V^2 > V^1$)
   b. Recurring, lancinating, "lightning" hemifacial pain lasting 20 to 30 seconds
   c. Pain may be so intense that the facial muscles contract and distort the face during an attack. Frequently "triggered" by touching certain areas of the face or scalp; asymptomatic or mild headache between episodes

    d. No neurologic deficits (including normal corneal reflex)

    e. Neuralgia of more persistent nature and associated with neurologic deficits may resolve from compressive, demyelinative, or inflammatory lesion of the V nerve

    f. Medical treatment

       i. Anticonvulsants carbamazepine and gabapentin

       ii. Lioresal (baclofen)

       iii. Tricyclic antidepressants

       iv. There has been some success with the injection of onabotulinumtoxinA in the treatment of refractory trigeminal neuralgia

    g. Surgical treatment

       i. Microvascular decompression of aberrant vessel at V nerve root entry zone

       ii. A rhizotomy of the gasserian ganglion may be performed for trigeminal pain using percutaneous radiofrequency, percutaneous glycerol injection, gamma knife radiosurgery, balloon compression, or combined treatment modalities. The patient is usually left with numbness or dysesthesia involving the cheeks, gums, teeth, or tongue. The loss of corneal reflex must be addressed

3. Herpetic neuralgia

    a. Pain of herpes zoster is described as severe, burning, aching in quality

    b. Pain occurs over distribution of a dermatome of cranial nerve, usually V^1, although it may involve the facial nerve (external ear) with ipsilateral facial palsy (Ramsay Hunt syndrome)

    c. Pain often precedes onset of typical rash by 4 to 7 days

    d. Pain usually regresses within 1 to 2 weeks, but may persist for months or years: postherpetic neuralgia

    e. Patients typically describe dysesthesias as "crawling" and "prickly" sensations

    f. Treatment frequently is difficult but may include the following:

       i. Gabapentin

       ii. Pregabalin

       iii. Tricyclic antidepressants

       iv. Topical lidocaine patch

       v. OnabotulinumtoxinA injection

    g. Treatment of herpes zoster with antiviral therapy may decrease the risk of postherpetic neuralgia

    h. A vaccine for herpes zoster has been helpful in limiting the morbidity of postherpetic neuralgia

4. Raeder paratrigeminal neuralgia

    a. V nerve distribution pain with ipsilateral Horner syndrome

    b. Almost exclusively in middle-aged or elderly male patients

    c. May be caused by migrainous dilation of the internal carotid artery with compression of the V nerve and sympathetic plexus in the middle cranial fossa

    d. If the pain is persistent (not of migrainous episodic nature) or if associated with cranial nerve palsy, then suspect a middle fossa tumor, aneurysm, or internal carotid artery dissection

    5.   Perineural spread of cancer

        a.   Initial involvement often limited to single nerve branch (especially infraorbital), but proximal spread leads to cavernous sinus involvement

        b.   Often signals recurrence of previously treated tumor, the treatment of which may be forgotten by the patient

        c.   Frequently due to squamous cell carcinoma of the face or oropharyngeal mucosa

        d.   Diagnosis established with contrast-enhanced MRI and tissue biopsy

Reference

1.   Glaser JS. Neuro-ophthalmologic examination: general considerations and special techniques. In: Glaser JS. *Neuro-Ophthalmology*. 3rd ed. Philadelphia, PA: Lippincott Williams & Wilkins; 1999:51-74.

Bibliography

Bartling R, Freeman K, Kraut RA. The incidence of altered sensation of the mental nerve after mandibular implant placement. *J Oral Maxillofac Surg*. 1999;57:1408-1412.

Biousse V, Toubol PJ, D'Anglejan–Chatillon J, et al. Ophthalmologic manifestation of internal carotid artery dissection. *Am J Ophthalmol*. 1998;126:565-577.

Brisman R. Surgical treatment of trigeminal neuralgia. *Semin Neurol*. 1997;17:367-372.

Clouston PD, Sharpe DM, Corbett AJ, et al. Perineural spread of cutaneous head and neck cancer: its orbital and central neurologic complications. *Arch Neurol*. 1990;47:73-77.

Eide PK, Stubhaug A. Relief of trigeminal neuralgia after percutaneous retrogasserian glycerol rhizolysis is dependent on normalization of abnormal temporal summation of pain, without general impairment of sensory perception. *Neurosurg*. 1998;43:462-472.

Fazzone HE, Lefton DR, Kupersmith MJ. Optic neuritis, correlation of pain and magnetic resoance imaging. *Ophthalmology*. 2003;110:1646-1649.

Harooni H, Golnik KC, Geddie B, et al. Diagnostic yield for neuroimaging in patients with unilateral eye or facial pain. *Can J Ophthalmol*. 2005;40:759-763.

Lee AG, Beaver HA, Brazis PW. Painful ophthalmologic disorders and eye pain for the neurologist. *Neurol Clin*. 2004;22:75-97.

Levin LA, Lessell S. Pain: a neuro-ophthalmic perspective. *Arch Ophthalmol*. 2003;121:1633.

Liu GT. The trigeminal nerve and its central connections. In: Miller NR, Newman NJ, eds. *Walsh and Hoyt's Clinical Neuro-Ophthalmology*. 6th ed. Vol 1. Philadelphia, PA: Lippincott Williams & Wilkins; 2005:1233-1274.

Martin TJ, Corbett JJ. Pain and sensation. In: *Neuro-Ophthalmology—The Requisites*. St Louis, MO: Mosby; 2000:223-232.

Mittal SO, Safarpour D, Jabbari B. Botulinum toxin treatment of neuropathic pain. *Semin Neurol*. 2016;36:73-83.

Pavan-Langston D. Herpes zoster: antivirals and pain management. *Ophthalmology*. 2008;115 2 Suppl:S13-S20.

Prasad S, Galetta S. Trigeminal neuralgia; historical notes and current concepts. *Neurologist*. 2009;15:87-94.

Rand RW. Leksell gamma knife treatment of tic douloureux. *Neurosurg Clin North Am*. 1997;8:75-78.

Ringeisen AL, Harrison AR, Lee MS. Ocular and orbital pain for the headache specialist. *Curr Neurol Neurosci Rep*. 2011;11:156-163.

Van Stavern GP. Headache and facial pain. In: Miller NR, Newman NJ, eds. *Walsh and Hoyt's Clinical Neuro-Ophthalmology*. 6th ed. Vol 1. Philadelphia, PA: Lippincott Williams & Wilkins; 2005:1275-1311.

Verma G. Role of botulinum toxin type-A (BTX-A) in the management of trigeminal neuralgia. *Pain Res Treat*. 2013:831094.

CHAPTER 13

The Seven Syndromes of the VII Nerve (Facial)

ROD FOROOZAN, MD AND MICHAEL S. VAPHIADES, DO

I. **ANATOMICAL CONSIDERATIONS**

  A. Figure 13-1 is a schematic representation of the course of the supranuclear and infra-nuclear fibers controlling the facial musculature. The fibers are accompanied by the nervus intermedius (tearing, salivation, taste), as well as sensory fibers from the external ear and the nerve to the stapedius muscle. The nerve leaves the pons and travels with the VIII cranial nerve through the internal auditory canal, leaving the canal through the fallopian canal, which courses inferiorly through the petrous bone, exiting through the stylomastoid foramen

II. **THE 7 SYNDROMES OF THE VII NERVE**

  A. Supranuclear facial palsy (see Figure 13-1, site 1) results in contralateral weakness of the lower two-thirds of the face, with some weakness of the orbicularis oculi, but not as severe as with peripheral VII nerve palsy (Figure 13-2); does not usually require tarsorrhaphy

  B. Anatomic studies in the primate suggest an alternate explanation for sparing of the upper one-third of the face with an upper motor neuron lesion; one subsector of the facial nucleus (M3 or rostral cingulate motor region) provides bilateral innervation to the upper facial region

  C. Cerebellopontine angle tumor (see Figure 13-1, site 2)

   1. Total ipsilateral facial weakness

   2. Decreased tearing (nervus intermedius)

   3. Hyperacusis (nerve to stapedius muscle)

   4. Decreased taste of anterior two-thirds of tongue (nervus intermedius and chorda tympani)

   5. Associated neurologic deficits: V, VI, VIII, Horner syndrome, gaze palsy, nystagmus, papilledema, cerebellar dysfunction

  D. Geniculate ganglionitis (Ramsay Hunt syndrome, zoster oticus [see Figure 13-1, site 3])

   1. Same findings as Figure 13-1, site 2; no associated neurologic deficits except for possibly a VIII nerve involvement (hearing loss, vestibular dysfunction)

   2. May see zoster vesicles in areas supplied by sensory portion of VII nerve: tympanic membrane, external auditory canal, pinna, buccal mucosa, neck

   3. Recovery is poorer than with Bell palsy (see page 192, II, F)

Foroozan R, Vaphiades MS. *Kline's Neuro-Ophthalmology Review Manual, Eighth Edition (pp 191-196)*. © 2018 SLACK Incorporated.

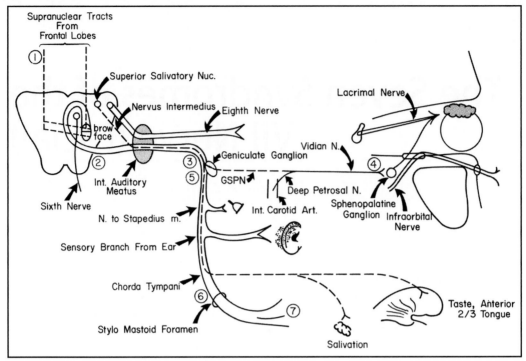

Figure 13-1. The seven syndromes of the VII nerve.

E. Isolated ipsilateral tear deficiency (see Figure 13-1, site 4)
    1. Nasopharyngeal carcinoma may affect the vidian nerve or sphenopalatine ganglion; often accompanying VI nerve palsy due to cavernous sinus involvement
F. Idiopathic (Bell) palsy (see Figure 13-1, site 5)
    1. Common idiopathic facial palsy, possibly due to viral infection and edema of VII nerve within fallopian canal
    2. Same findings as Figure 13-1, site 2 except for no associated neurologic deficits; tearing may be normal
    3. Complete recovery, within 60 days in 75% of patients; with steroid therapy, recovery over 90%
        a. May be subtle signs of aberrant regeneration, even with near complete recovery
    4. Treatment options:
        a. Medical
            i.   Antiviral agents often used: acyclovir, famciclovir
            ii. Corticosteroids: a large randomized trial found corticosteroids improved chances of recovery at 3 and 9 months. Antiviral therapy alone or in combination with corticosteroids did not add to the benefit
        b. Surgical decompression of facial nerve
G. Isolated total ipsilateral facial palsy (see Figure 13-1, site 6)
    1. Mastoidopathy, facial trauma, parotid gland surgery
H. Isolated partial ipsilateral facial palsy (see Figure 13-1, site 7)
    1. Only certain branches of VII nerve are affected
I. Cornea and ocular surface should be protected
    1. Topical lubricants
    2. Surgery: gold weight implantation, tarsorrhaphy

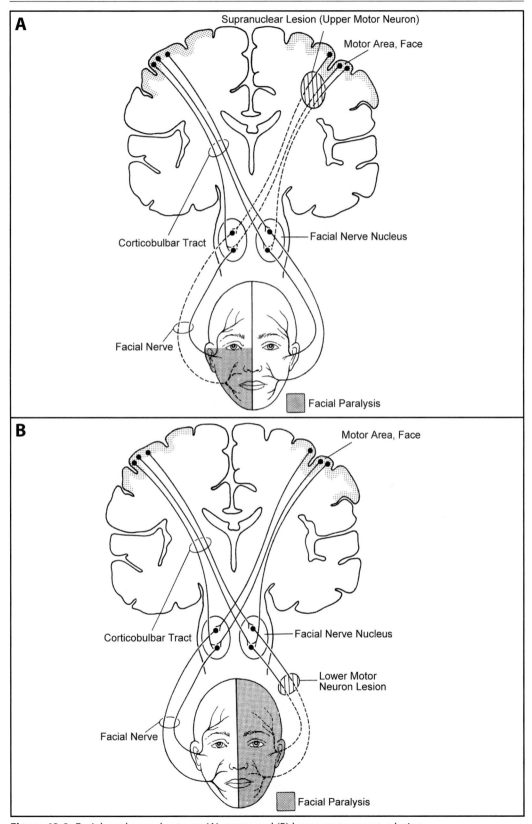

Figure 13-2. Facial weakness due to an (A) upper and (B) lower motor neuron lesion.

III. FACIAL DIPLEGIA
    A. Brainstem contusion
    B. Brainstem stroke (basilar artery)
    C. Brainstem glioma
    D. Möbius syndrome: aplasia of VII nerve nuclei in brainstem; often accompanied by the following:
        1. Bilateral VI nerve palsies
        2. Palatal and lingual palsy
        3. Deafness
        4. Deficiencies of pectoral and lingual muscles
        5. Extremity defects: syndactyly, supernumerary digits, absent fingers and toes
        6. Rarely inherited; defect on chromosome 3q
    E. Myasthenia gravis (see Chapter 11)
    F. Guillain-Barré syndrome
        1. Autoimmune acute peripheral neuropathy
        2. Subtypes:
            a. Acute inflammatory demyelinating polyneuropathy
                i. Motor weakness, often ascending, which progresses up to 4 weeks
                ii. Frequently preceded by flu-like episode or gastroenteritis
                iii. One-half of patients develop unilateral or bilateral facial weakness
                iv. Ophthalmoplegia
                v. Ptosis
                vi. Optic nerve involvement: papilledema (with very high CSF protein); optic neuritis
                vii. CSF: albuminocytologic dissociation (elevated protein without pleocytosis)
                viii. Treatment: plasma exchange; intravenous immunoglobulin
            b. Miller Fisher syndrome (see Chapter 7, V, G on page 127)
    G. Myotonic dystrophy (see Chapter 11, IV on page 178)
    H. Melkersson-Rosenthal syndrome
        1. Rare, idiopathic disorder
        2. Facial swelling
        3. Transversely fissured tongue
        4. Recurrent, alternating facial palsy
    I. Neoplastic: leukemia, meningeal carcinomatosis
    J. Inflammatory: sarcoidosis, porphyria
    K. Infectious: polio, AIDS, Lyme disease, botulism

IV. CROCODILE TEARS (GUSTO-LACRIMAL REFLEX)
    A. Any patient with VII nerve palsy that has affected the parasympathetic fibers stimulating tearing and salivation may experience tearing at mealtime due to aberrant regeneration or misdirection of fibers so that when neural stimulus for salivation is transmitted, it results in stimulation of tearing
    B. Treatment options:
        1. Anticholinergic gastrointestinal medication (eg, belladonna alkaloids)
        2. Botulinum toxin injection into lacrimal gland

V. SPASTIC PARETIC FACIAL CONTRACTURE (SEE CHAPTER 14, V, C, 6 ON PAGE 204)
    A. Unilateral spastic facial contracture with associated facial weakness
    B. May be indicative of intrinsic pontine disease (neoplasm, stroke, multiple sclerosis)

    C. Due to damage of VII nerve nucleus (facial paresis) and its supranuclear connections (facial spasticity)

    D. Other causes include extra-axial compression (cerebellopontine angle mass), Bell palsy, Guillain-Barré syndrome

VI. BLEPHAROSPASM

    A. Onset usually in adult life (sixth and seventh decade); 3:1 female predominance

    B. Bilateral, episodic, involuntary contractions of the orbicularis oculi

    C. At times, associated with involuntary spasm of the lower facial musculature: orofacial dyskinesia or Meige syndrome

    D. Etiology

        1. Adults

            a. Usually unknown ("essential" blepharospasm); possibly related to dysfunction of the basal ganglia and limbic system

            b. May occur in patients with Parkinson disease, PSP, Huntington disease, multiple sclerosis, and brainstem stroke

        2. Children

            a. Usually benign, self-limited habit

            b. Tourette syndrome

    E. Treatment

        1. Chemodenervation: botulinum toxin; treatment of choice (typically repeated every 3 to 6 months)

        2. Surgery: selective VII nerve sectioning; orbicularis myectomies

        3. Pharmacologic: clonazepam, lioresal

        4. Alleviating maneuvers such as facial touching to limit symptoms. The most commonly used maneuver was the touching of facial areas, other maneuvers included covering the eyes, singing, and yawning

    F. Apraxia of eyelid opening (see also Chapter 14, IV, C on page 203) is often confused with blepharospasm

        1. A nonparalytic movement disorder characterized by transient difficulty in initiating voluntary eyelid opening

        2. It is frequently observed in idiopathic Parkinson disease and other extrapyramidal diseases

        3. Treatment consists of botulinum toxin injection into the orbicularis oculi muscles

        4. Potential treatment aripiprazole, a drug that acts as a partial agonist on dopamine D2 receptors, D3 receptors, and serotonin 5-HT1A receptors, and as an antagonist on serotonin 5-HT2A receptors

VII. HEMIFACIAL SPASM

    A. Unilateral (rarely bilateral and asynchronous) spasm involving half of facial muscles, typically lasting several minutes at a time; persists during sleep

    B. Painless, no sensory loss

    C. Etiology

        1. Aberrant vascular loop (dolichoectasia) compressing VII nerve in subarachnoid space where it exits the pons

        2. Following Bell palsy (postparalytic hemifacial spasm)

    D. Treatment

        1. Chemodenervation: botulinum toxin; treatment of choice (typically repeated every 3 to 6 months)

        2. Pharmacologic: carbamazepine, lioresal, clonazepam, gabapentin

3. Surgery: posterior fossa craniotomy with insertion of inert material between vascular loop and VII nerve (neurovascular decompression)

4. Alleviating maneuvers (see page 195, VI).

VIII. FACIAL MYOKYMIA

A. Usually benign

1. Self-limited, particularly when confined to an isolated area such as one eyelid

B. If persistent and progressive, often involving multiple facial muscles, over weeks or months, then consider the following:

1. Multiple sclerosis

2. Brainstem glioma

3. Brainstem stroke

BIBLIOGRAPHY

Dutton JJ, Fowler AM. Botulinum toxin in ophthalmology. *Surv Ophthalmol*. 2007;52:13-31.

Foroozan R, Moster ML. Facial nerve disorders. In: Levin LA, Arnold AC, eds. *Neuro-Ophthalmology: The Practical Guide*. New York, NY: Thieme Medical Publishers Inc; 2005:392-399.

Hughes RA, Cornblath DR. Guillain-Barré syndrome. *Lancet*. 2005;366:1653-1666.

Kilduff CL, Casswell EJ, Salam T, Hersh D, Ortiz-Perez S, Ezra D. Use of alleviating maneuvers for periocular facial dystonias. *JAMA Ophthalmol*. 2016;134:1247-1252.

Liu GT, Volpe NJ, Galetta SL. Eyelid and facial nerve disorders. In: *Neuro-Ophthalmology: Diagnosis and Management*. St Louis, MO: WB Saunders; 2001:449-489.

Magaldi JA. Bell's palsy. *N Engl J Med*. 2005;352:416-418.

Morecraft RJ, Lovie JL, Herrick JL, et al. Cortical innervation of the facial nucleus in the non-human primate. *Brain*. 2001;124:176-208.

Rahman I, Sadiq SA. Ophthalmic management of facial nerve palsy: a review. *Surv Ophthalmol*. 2007;52:121-144.

Ross AH, Elston JS, Marion MH, Malhotra R. Review and update of involuntary facial movement disorders presenting in the ophthalmological setting. *Surv Ophthalmol*. 2011;56:54-67.

Sullivan FM, Swan IR, Donnan PT, et al. Early treatment with prednisolone or acyclovir in Bell's palsy. *N Engl J Med*. 2007;357:1598-1607.

Tokisato K, Fukunaga K, Tokunaga M, Watanabe S, Nakanishi R, Yamanaga H. Aripiprazole can improve apraxia of eyelid opening in Parkinson's disease. *Intern Med*. 2015;54:3061-3064.

CHAPTER 14

Eyelid Disorders

JENNIFER T. SCRUGGS, MD AND SAUNDERS L. HUPP, MD

I. **ANATOMICAL CONSIDERATIONS (FIGURE 14-1)**
   A. Eyelid opening (retraction) is mediated through the following:
      1. Levator muscle: primary elevator of upper eyelid
      2. Müller muscle: secondary elevator of upper eyelid
         a. Corresponding muscle in lower eyelid is known as *inferior tarsal muscle*
      3. Frontalis muscle: secondary elevator of upper eyelid
   B. Eyelid closing (protraction) is mediated through the following:
      1. Orbicularis oculi: primary closure of upper and lower eyelids
         a. Palpebral portion is active during spontaneous and reflexive blinking
         b. Orbital portion is active during voluntary blinking and forced or sustained lid closure
      2. Procerus muscle: secondary closure of upper eyelid
      3. Corrugator muscle: secondary closure of upper eyelid
   C. Innervation of eyelid opening
      1. Levator muscle: superior division of III nerve (see Figure 5-1)
      2. Müller muscle (and inferior tarsal muscle): oculosympathetic pathway, third order neuron (see Figure 8-3)
      3. Frontalis muscle: VII nerve
   D. Innervation of eyelid closing
      1. Orbicularis oculi: VII nerve (see Figure 13-2)
      2. Procerus muscle: VII nerve
      3. Corrugator muscle: VII nerve

II. **PHYSIOLOGY OF EYELID OPENING**
   A. Supranuclear control of eyelid opening
      1. Through both corticobulbar and extrapyramidal pathways
      2. Areas of the frontal, occipital, and temporal cortex have been associated with eyelid opening
      3. Arousal state of the brain influences palpebral fissure width through control of levator tone
         a. During sleep, levator function ceases

Foroozan R, Vaphiades MS. *Kline's Neuro-Ophthalmology Review Manual, Eighth Edition (pp 197-205).* © 2018 SLACK Incorporated.

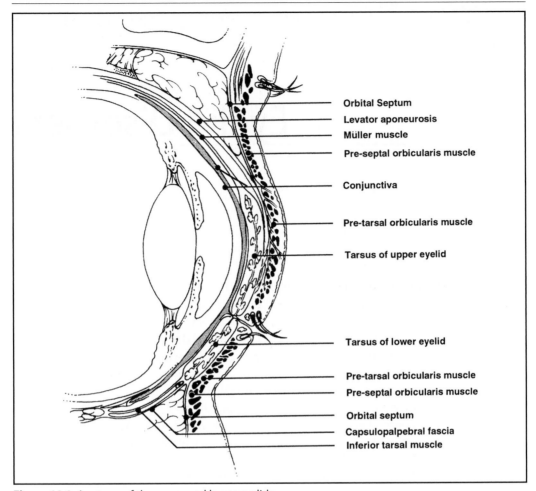

Figure 14-1. Anatomy of the upper and lower eyelids

    B.   Final common pathway for eyelid opening

        1.   Single midline central caudal subnucleus of III nerve nuclear complex provides innervation to both levator muscles

            a.   Conjugacy of lid opening likely arises at or near motoneuron level

        2.   Nerve fibers to the levator muscle travel with the superior division of III nerve

    C.   Physiologic synkineses link the activity of the levator muscles to related extraocular and facial muscles

        1.   Movements of the upper eyelids are identically coordinated, obeying the Hering law of equal innervation

        2.   Movements of the eyes, especially vertical gaze, are accompanied by lid movements: the lids lift with upgaze and lower with downgaze

III. PHYSIOLOGY OF EYELID CLOSURE

    A.   Normal blinking may be spontaneous, voluntary, or reflexive

        1.   With each blink, there is complete inhibition of levator tone just prior to the onset of orbicularis oculi contraction, causing lid closure

            a.   Indicates interconnections between the central caudal nucleus of III nerve and nucleus of VII nerve

Table 14-1

PHYSIOLOGIC SYNKINESES AND REFLEX BLINKING

Reflex	Clinical Examination
Orbicularis stress	Tap lateral orbicularis oculi
Corneal blink	Corneal touch (V^1 nerve)
Cochleopalpebral	Sudden noise
Auropalpebral	Stimulate EAC
Palatal palpebral	Touch palate
Bright flash	Rapid exposure to bright light

2. Spontaneous blinking
   a. Twelve to 16 blinks per minute in relaxed state
   b. Decreased with reading or concentration
   c. Increased with emotion (anxiety or arousal)
   d. Protects and nourishes avascular cornea
   e. Facilitates eye movement (saccade) to change the direction of gaze
3. Reflex blinking
   a. Mediated through a variety of physiologic synkineses with different afferent inputs into the VII nerve nuclei (Table 14-1)
   b. Elicited by various stimuli, including direct corneal or eyelid touch or air puff, light, sudden acoustic stimuli, and advancement of noxious stimuli toward the eye

B. Supranuclear control of eyelid closure
   1. Through both corticobulbar and extrapyramidal pathways
      a. Extrapyramidal pathways may be affected by emotional states and tension
      b. Extrapyramidal control may be absent in infants or synchronized with mouth movements, such as sucking

C. Final common pathway for eyelid closure
   1. Primarily ipsilateral motoneuron innervation from VII nerve nucleus to orbicularis (see Figure 13-1)
      a. Conjugacy of blinking likely mediated at supranuclear level

D. Physiologic synkineses link eyelid closure with eye movements
   1. Inverse relationship between superior rectus and eyelid movement during sleep and with forced eyelid closure
      a. Bell phenomenon: globe movement up and out as lids close

IV. **ABNORMALITIES OF EYELID OPENING**

A. Ptosis (blepharoptosis): insufficient eyelid opening from drooping of the upper eyelid. Ptosis may be congenital or acquired. Classification is based on etiology
   1. Myogenic ptosis—results from an abnormal levator muscle; may be congenital or acquired
      a. Typical features:
         i. Poor levator function (< 5 mm)
         ii. Poorly defined or absent upper lid crease

          iii. Poorly defined upper lid superior sulcus

          iv. Lid lag on downgaze

    b. Congenital myogenic ptosis—results from a poorly developed levator muscle with replacement of muscle fibers by fibrous and adipose tissue

          i. Most common cause of congenital ptosis

          ii. May be unilateral or bilateral

          iii. Most commonly is an isolated finding

          iv. Patients may have ocular or systemic associations

             1. Blepharophimosis syndrome: bilateral ptosis, horizontal phimosis of lid fissures, telecanthus, epicanthus inversus

             2. Congenital fibrosis of the extraocular muscles

             3. Double elevator palsy: myogenic ptosis and superior rectus weakness

             4. Coexistent strabismus or amblyopia

    c. Acquired myogenic ptosis—results from localized or diffuse muscular disease

          i. Rare cause of acquired ptosis

          ii. Patients commonly have ocular or systemic associations

             1. CPEO (see Chapter 11, III on page 177)

             2. Muscular dystrophy

             3. Myotonic dystrophy (see Chapter 11, IV on page 178)

             4. OPMD (see Chapter 11, III, C, 1 on page 178)

             5. Corticosteriod-induced ptosis—may be a localized form of steroid myopathy from long-term corticosteroid (including topical) therapy (uveitis)

2. Aponeurotic ptosis—results from attenuation, dehiscence, or disinsertion of the levator aponeurosis from its normal insertion on the anterior tarsus. Levator muscle function is normal

    a. Most common type of ptosis; also known as *involutional ptosis*

    b. Typical features:

          i. Good levator function (> 10 mm)

          ii. High upper lid crease

          iii. Deep upper lid superior sulcus

          iv. Lid position is lower in downgaze

    c. Contributing factors:

          i. Aging

          ii. Chronic inflammation

          iii. Blunt trauma

          iv. Repetitive traction on the lid (eye rubbing, contact lens use)

          v. Prior ophthalmic surgery

3. Neurogenic ptosis—results from innervational defects to the eyelid retractors; may be congenital or acquired

    a. Horner syndrome (see Chapter 8, III, I on page 137)—results from lesions of oculosympathetic pathway with paralysis of Müller muscle

          i. Ptosis is mild, usually < 3 mm

          ii. "Upside-down" ptosis of the lower lid: mild elevation of the lower lid with relaxation of the inferior tarsal muscle

    b. III nerve palsy (see Chapter 5)—results from lesions of III nerve with paralysis of the levator muscle

          i. Ptosis may be partial or complete

     c. Marcus Gunn jaw-winking phenomenon—a congenital synkinetic ptosis resulting from aberrant connections between the motor division of V nerve and III nerve

        i. Most common synkinetic movement associated with congenital ptosis

        ii. External pterygoid—levator synkinesis: elevation of lid with movement of mandible to opposite side, protruded forward, or wide opening of the mouth

        iii. Internal pterygoid—levator synkinesis: elevation of the lid with clenching of the teeth

     d. "Cortical ptosis"—results from interruption of supranuclear pathways from unilateral temporal, occipital, or bilateral frontal cortical lesions

        i. Unilateral or bilateral ptosis

        ii. Supranuclear ptosis may appear in patients with nonorganic disease (see Chapter 17)

     e. Paradoxic supranuclear inhibition of levator tone

        i. Ptosis may be isolated or associated with congenital horizontal or vertical eye movement abnormalities

        ii. Inverse Marcus Gunn phenomenon

            1. Eyelid closure during mouth opening

            2. With downward movement of the lower jaw, there is total inhibition of the levator with subsequent ptosis

     f. Ophthalmoplegic migraine (see Chapter 15, VII, I on page 217)

4. Neuromuscular ptosis—results from abnormalities of the neuromuscular junction

     a. Myasthenia gravis (see Chapter 11, II on page 175)—results from deficiency of acetylcholine receptors at the neuromuscular junction

        i. Ptosis is the most common presenting sign

            1. May be partial or complete, unilateral or bilateral

            2. Myasthenia involves skeletal and not visceral musculature; therefore, the pupil and ciliary muscle are clinically unaffected

        ii. Variable, typically worsens with fatigue

        iii. May be produced by having the patient sustain upgaze

        iv. Look for Cogan lid twitch sign

            1. Upper lid elevates excessively with an upward saccade from downgaze to primary gaze, then returns to its ptotic position

        v. Frequently associated with orbicularis weakness

        vi. May be accompanied by ocular motility disturbances

        vii. **Remember:** consider myasthenia gravis in all patients with onset of acquired isolated ptosis

     b. Botulism (see Chapter 7, V, F on page 126)

     c. Iatrogenic periocular botulinum toxin injections

        i. Transient ptosis from infiltration of toxin into levator muscle

5. Mechanical ptosis—results from excess weight of the lid that interferes with eyelid movement

     a. Dermatochalasis

     b. Brow ptosis

     c. Edema from blunt trauma or inflammation

     d. Eyelid tumors: large chalazion, basal cell carcinoma, squamous cell carcinoma, hemangioma, neurofibroma

     e. Eyelid infiltration: lymphoma, amyloidosis

      f.   Anterior orbital tumors

      g.   Cicatricial: damage following surgery, chemical or thermal injury, or inflammation (trachoma, ocular pemphigoid)

6.   Traumatic ptosis—results from blunt or sharp trauma to levator muscle or aponeurosis

      a.   Blunt trauma with levator dehiscence

      b.   Lid laceration

      c.   Occult lid or orbital foreign body

      d.   Orbital roof fracture

      e.   May rarely occur with blunt injury to the eyelid (presumably to the nerve to the levator) with spontaneous recovery

7.   Pseudoptosis—results from abnormalities of ocular, orbital, or facial anatomy with insufficient posterior support of the eyelid

      a.   Enophthalmos

      b.   Phthisis bulbi

      c.   Microphthalmos or anophthalmos

      d.   Hypotropia

      e.   Contralateral lid retraction

8.   Remember the Hering law of equal innervation (to both levator muscles):

      a.   With asymmetric ptosis, patient uses frontalis to elevate both lids—produces lid retraction on one side. With manual elevation (or use of phenylephrine drops to stimulate Müller muscle) of the more ptotic lid, the previously retracted lid falls—the phenomenon is termed *enhanced ptosis*

9.   Miller Fisher syndrome (see Chapter 7, V, G on page 127)

B.   Lid retraction: excessive eyelid opening characterized by sclera visible above superior corneal limbus when the eyes are directed straight ahead (superior scleral show)

    1.   Myopathic lid retraction

        a.   Most common form of lid retraction due to thyroid eye disease

           i.   Lid retraction is the most common presenting sign of thyroid eye disease

           ii.   Congenital transient lid retraction may be associated with maternal hyperthyroidism

        b.   Sympathomimetic drops (phenylephrine) stimulate Müller muscle

        c.   Hepatic cirrhosis

        d.   Maldevelopment of levator muscle

    2.   Neuropathic lid retraction

        a.   Supranuclear lid retraction

           i.   Often associated with lesions of the rostral dorsal midbrain in the region of the nucleus of the posterior commissure (Collier sign)

           ii.   Combination of lid retraction with downward displacement of eyes in infants produces the "setting sun" sign

           iii.   Periodic lid retraction may occur as an isolated myoclonic movement or as part of vertical nystagmus seen with ocular myoclonus (see Chapter 3)

           iv.   Comatose patient may demonstrate periodic lid retraction synchronous with breathing or head movements

        b.   Paradoxic levator excitation with lid retraction

           i.   Congenital lid retraction may be seen with abnormalities of horizontal gaze (Duane syndrome), jaw movements (Marcus Gunn phenomenon), or swallowing

ii.   Acquired lid retraction may be seen with aberrant regeneration following III nerve palsy (pseudo von Graefe sign)

iii. Pourfour du Petit syndrome is characterized by the unilateral appearance of mydriasis, lid retraction, and exophthalmos from oculosympathetic hyperactivity. It may be caused by trauma at the level of the proximal portion of the first dorsal root or in the cervical sympathetic chain

3. Physiologic lid retraction—results from physiologic response (Hering law) to ptosis of the contralateral eye

4. Eyelid lag—results from lack of inhibition of upper eyelids on downgaze

    a.   Most commonly associated with lid retraction due to thyroid eye disease

    b.   May occur without lid retraction in extrapyramidal syndromes with lesions of the midbrain involving the nucleus of the posterior commissure

       i.   Parkinson disease

       ii.   PSP

       iii. Thalamic-midbrain infarction

C. Apraxia of lid opening: nonparalytic inability to open eyes following voluntary or involuntary lid closure; no visible orbicularis oculi contraction

1. May occur in isolation

2. Majority of cases associated with benign essential blepharospasm

3. Other associations: basal ganglia disease, Huntington disease, Parkinson disease, PSP

4. Neuroanatomic basis and central pathophysiology unknown

5. Thought to be due to involuntary levator muscle inhibition and/or pretarsal orbicularis oculi contraction

6. Manual elevation of the lids may facilitate lid opening

V.   ABNORMALITIES OF EYELID CLOSURE

A. Insufficient eyelid closure

1. Neurogenic—results from innervational defects to eyelid protractors

    a.   Supranuclear facial palsy (see Chapter 13)

    b.   Peripheral VII nerve palsy (see Chapter 13)

       i.   Idiopathic (Bell palsy)

       ii.   Cerebellopontine angle tumor

       iii. Parotid tumors

2. Myogenic—results from decreased orbicularis oculi function

    a.   Myasthenia gravis—"peek" phenomenon: after sustained lid closure, lid opening occurs due to orbicularis fatigue

    b.   Muscular dystrophy

    c.   Myotonic dystrophy (see Chapter 11, IV on page 178)

    d.   CPEO (see Chapter 11, III on page 177)

3. Iatrogenic

    a.   After blepharoplasty with excessive skin or orbicularis excision

    b.   After surgery involving recession of the inferior rectus muscle with secondary lower lid retraction

B. Decreased blink rate

1. Parkinson disease

2. PSP

3. Thyroid eye disease

4. Infants in first few months of life

C. Excessive eyelid closure: pathologic blinking or blepharospasm
  1. Supranuclear blepharospasm
    a. Benign essential blepharospasm (see Chapter 13, VI on page 195)
      i. Bilateral, episodic, involuntary contractions of the orbicularis oculi, procerus, and corrugator muscles
      ii. Idiopathic
    b. Orofacial dyskinesia (Meige syndrome)
    c. Focal seizure
    d. Reflex blepharospasm (post-stroke)
    e. Response to ocular irritation and photophobia
    f. Associated with tardive dyskinesia
    g. Postencephalitis
    h. Habit spasms and tics (eg, Tourette syndrome)
    i. Nonorganic
  2. Peripheral VII disease
    a. Hemifacial spasm (see Chapter 13, VII on page 195)
      i. Unilateral, episodic contraction of muscles innervated by VII nerve including orbicularis oculi
      ii. "Idiopathic": high percentage of cases due to aberrant vascular loop of vertebral and/or basilar arteries with compression of VII motor nerve root at its brainstem exit
      iii. Infrequently results from neoplastic compression or inflammation of the nerve root
      iv. Postparalytic: aberrant regeneration following VII nerve palsy
  3. Pathologic blinking may occur in brainstem disease associated with decreased eye movements
    a. Blink facilitates saccade through a blink-saccade synkinesis
    b. May occur in Huntington disease, Gaucher disease, Parkinson disease, congenital ocular motor apraxia
  4. Primary brainstem disease
    a. Stroke
    b. Demyelinating disease
    c. Trauma
  5. Benign facial or eyelid myokymia
  6. Spastic paretic facial contracture (see Chapter 13, V on page 194)
    a. Facial myokymia with contracture plus weakness of facial muscles
    b. Etiologies:
      i. Intra-axial (pons): tumor, stroke, multiple sclerosis
      ii. Extra-axial: cerebellopontine angle mass, Bell palsy, Guillain-Barré syndrome
  7. Neuromuscular disease
    a. Tetany
    b. Strychnine poisoning
    c. Tetanus (risus sardonicus)
  8. Systemic disease
    a. Hypothyroidism
    b. Myotonic dystrophy (see Chapter 11, IV on page 178)
    c. Hyperkalemic familial paralysis
    d. Chondrodystrophic dystonia (Schwartz-Jampel syndrome)

D. Eyelid nystagmus
   1. Rhythmic oscillation of eyelids with a slow downward drift and a rapid upward phase
   2. Usually associated with the following:
      a. Convergence: seen in multiple sclerosis, Miller Fisher syndrome, brainstem lesion
      b. Gaze shifts: damage to brainstem or cerebellum
      c. Vertical nystagmus (eg, convergence-retraction nystagmus of dorsal midbrain syndrome; see Chapter 3, III, F on page 86)
      d. Oculopalatal tremor syndrome (see Chapter 3, III, J on page 87)

BIBLIOGRAPHY

Burde RM, Savino PJ, Trobe JD. Eyelid disturbances. In: Burde RM, Savino PJ, Trobe JD, eds. *Clinical Decisions in Neuro-Ophthalmology.* 3rd ed. St Louis, MO: CV Mosby; 2002:272-296.

de Figueiredo AR. Blepharoptosis. *Semin Ophthalmol.* 2010;25:39-51.

Kerty E, Eidal K. Apraxia of eyelid opening: clinical features and therapy. *Eur J Ophthalmol.* 2006;16: 204-208.

Kilduff CL, Casswell EJ, Salam T, Hersh D, Ortiz-Perez S, Ezra D. Use of alleviating maneuvers for periocular facial dystonias. *JAMA Ophthalmol.* 2016;134:1247-1252.

Landa M, Bedrossian EH. Blepharoptosis. In: Della Rocca RC, Bedrossian EH, Arthurs BP. *Ophthalmic Plastic Surgery: Decision Making and Techniques.* New York, NY: McGraw-Hill; 2002:77-89.

Liu GT, Volpe NJ, Galetta SL. Eyelid and facial nerve disorders. In: *Neuro-Ophthalmology: Diagnosis and Management.* 2nd ed. New York, NY: Saunders Elsevier; 2010:449-489.

Nerad JA. *Techniques in Ophthalmic Plastic Surgery.* New York, NY: Saunders Elsevier; 2010.

Ross AH, Elston JS, Marion MH, Malhotra R. Review and update of involuntary facial movement disorders presenting in the ophthalmological setting. *Surv Ophthalmol.* 2011;56:54-67.

Rucker JC. Normal and abnormal lid function. In: Kennard C, Leigh RJ, eds. *Neuro-Ophthalmology. Handbook of Clinical Neurology.* 3rd series. Vol 102. New York, NY: Elsevier; 2011:403-424.

Skarf B. Normal and abnormal eyelid function. In: Miller NR, Newman NJ, eds. *Walsh and Hoyt's Clinical Neuro-Ophthalmology.* 6th ed. Vol 1. Philadelphia, PA: Lippincott Williams & Wilkins; 2005:1177-1229.

SooHoo JR, Davies BW, Allard FD, Durairaj VD. Congenital ptosis. *Surv Ophthalmol.* 2014;59:483-492.

CHAPTER 15

Headache

John E. Carter, MD; Rod Foroozan, MD; and
Michael S. Vaphiades, DO

I. **CLASSIFICATION OF HEADACHE: THE INTERNATIONAL HEADACHE SOCIETY (IHS)**
   A. The IHS divides headache into 13 classifications (Table 15-1)
   B. Headache may be broadly divided into the primary headache syndromes such as migraine and the secondary headaches due to an underlying disorder such as giant cell arteritis, IIH, or brain tumor
   C. Primary headache disorders account for 90% of patients presenting with headache
   D. This chapter will concentrate on the primary and secondary headache syndromes with important neuro-ophthalmologic manifestations or implications

II. **ANATOMIC CONSIDERATIONS**
   A. Intracranial pain sensitive structures
      1. Large venous sinuses
      2. Dural and cerebral arteries at the base of the skull
      3. Pial arteries of the brain
   B. Extracranial sources of head pain
      1. Muscles, fascia, and galea
      2. Extracranial arteries and veins
      3. Mucous membranes, tympanic membrane
   C. Innervation of pain structures
      1. Ophthalmic division of the trigeminal nerve
      2. Posterior fossa by upper cervical nerve roots
      3. Pain may be referred to the eye or the suboccipital region
   D. Basic sources of intracranial headache and head pain
      1. Traction or displacement of tributary veins or venous sinuses
      2. Traction or dilation of major cerebral arteries
      3. Traction or dilation of dural arteries such as the middle meningeal artery
      4. Inflammation of pain sensitive structures
      5. Direct pressure on cranial or upper cervical nerves (V nerve above the tentorium; IX, X, XI, and XII nerves below the tentorium)

Foroozan R, Vaphiades MS. *Kline's Neuro-Ophthalmology Review Manual, Eighth Edition (pp 207-220).* © 2018 SLACK Incorporated.

Table 15-1

ABBREVIATED CLASSIFICATION OF HEADACHE

1. Migraine
   - 1.1 Migraine without aura
   - 1.2 Migraine with aura including typical aura without headache, familial hemiplegic migraine, and basilar-type migraine
   - 1.3 Childhood periodic syndromes that may be precursors to or associated with migraine
   - 1.4 Retinal migraine
   - 1.5 Complications of migraine
     - 1.5.1 Chronic migraine
     - 1.5.2 Status migrainosus
     - 1.5.3 Persistent aura without infarction
     - 1.5.4 Migrainous stroke
2. Tension-type headache
3. Cluster headache and other trigeminal autonomic cephalgias
   - 3.1 Cluster headache
   - 3.2 Paroxysmal hemicrania
   - 3.3 SUNCT—short-lasting unilateral neuralgiform headache attacks with conjunctival injection and tearing
4. Other primary headaches including cough headache, exertional headache, headache associated with sexual activity
5. Headache associated with head and/or neck trauma
6. Headache associated with vascular disorders
   - 6.1 Headache associated with stroke
   - 6.2 Unruptured vascular malformation including aneurysm, AVM, dural arteriovenous fistula
   - 6.3 Arteritis including giant cell arteritis
   - 6.4 Arterial dissection
   - 6.5 Cerebral venous thrombosis
   - 6.6 CADASIL—cerebral autosomal dominant arteriopathy with subcortical infarcts and leukoencephalopathy
   - 6.7 MELAS—mitochondrial encephalopathy, lactic acidosis, and stroke-like episodes
   - 6.8 Pituitary apoplexy
7. Headache associated with nonvascular intracranial disorders
   - 7.1 High CSF pressure
   - 7.2 Low CSF pressure
   - 7.3 Noninfectious inflammatory disease
   - 7.4 Intracranial neoplasm
8. Headache associated with drugs or their withdrawal
9. Headache attributed to infection
10. Headache attributed to disorder of homeostasis hypoxia/hypercapnia including high-altitude headache, diving headache, and sleep apnea headache; hypertension
11. Headache or facial pain associated with disorder of cranium, neck, eyes, ears, nose, sinuses, teeth, mouth, or other facial or cranial structure
12. Headache attributed to psychiatric disorder

(continued)

Table 15-1 (continued)

ABBREVIATED CLASSIFICATION OF HEADACHE

13.   Cranial neuralgias, nerve trunk pain, and deafferentation pain
    13.1   Trigeminal neuralgia
    13.2   Glossopharyngeal neuralgia
    13.3   Nervus intermedius neuralgia
    13.4   Occipital neuralgia
    13.5   Cold-stimulus headache
    13.6   Head or face pain due to Herpes zoster
    13.7   Tolosa-Hunt syndrome
    13.8   Ophthalmoplegic "migraine"

Adapted from the International Headache Society Classification of Headache.

III.   HISTORY IS THE KEY TO DIAGNOSIS; 95% OF HEADACHE PATIENTS HAVE A NORMAL EXAMINATION

  A.   Where is the pain?
  B.   How long does it last?
  C.   How often does it occur?
  D.   What kind of pain is it?
  E.   Does anything make it better or worse?
  F.   Are there any other symptoms that accompany the pain?

IV.   MIGRAINE

  A.   Paroxysmal disorder affecting approximately 15% of women and 5% of men in the United States
  B.   This compares to tension-type headache (muscle contraction headache), which affects about 80% of the population
  C.   Phases of migraine: migraine attacks have several phases and most patients experience more than one phase
    1.   Prodrome: premonitory symptoms occur hours to days before the onset of headache in 60% of patients
      a.   Psychological: depression, euphoria, irritability, restlessness and hyperactivity, drowsiness, mental fatigue, mental slowness
      b.   Neurologic: photophobia, phonophobia, hyperosmia
      c.   Constitutional: sluggishness, increased thirst and urination, fluid retention, food cravings, anorexia, diarrhea, constipation
    2.   Aura
      a.   Focal neurologic symptoms preceding or accompanying or rarely occurring after an attack of migraine
      b.   Experienced by 20% of migraineurs
      c.   Most develop in a progressive fashion over 5 to 20 minutes and last less than 60 minutes
      d.   Most frequently, aura consists of visual symptoms but sensory, motor, language, and brainstem symptoms may occur

       e.   Visual aura: bright, positive visual sensations often described as sparkles, zigzag fortification, flashes of color, or heat waves (Figure 15-1). Usually of a hemianopic in nature, lasts less than 1 hour, with typical "buildup" and "march." It obscures the visual field, there is movement, is present OU with the patient's eyes closed and is often ascribed to the eye with the larger hemifield despite its homonymous nature

       f.   Frequently, patients may experience aura without headache (acephalgic migraine)

   3. Headache phase

       a.   Headache is usually unilateral at onset and is characterized as throbbing

       b.   Headache often becomes pancephalic and the throbbing changes to a steady, aching pain

       c.   Nausea typically accompanies migraine without aura

       d.   Vomiting may occur at the height of the attack and signal the end of the headache phase or may begin an intensifying phase of the headache

       e.   Photophobia and phonophobia accompany the headache in most patients

       f.   Ocular symptoms and signs include conjunctival injection, periorbital swelling, and excessive tearing

       g.   Headache usually lasts from 4 to 24 hours. Headache lasting longer than 72 hours is called *status migrainosus*

   4. Postdrome phase

       a.   In some patients, especially migraine with aura, the headache resolves with a period of sleep

       b.   After the headache, the patient is often left with malaise for 24 to 48 hours

D. Pathophysiology of migraine: the trigeminovascular system and the neural hypothesis of migraine (Figure 15-2)

   1. The possible mechanisms of pain in migraine involve the cranial blood vessels, changes in the dura mater, and changes in the modulation of nociceptive input to the CNS

   2. Stimulation of cranial vascular afferents activates neurons of the brainstem and spinal cord (trigeminocervical complex), which project to the thalamus and out through the parasympathetic ganglia (trigemino-autonomic reflex)

   3. An axon reflex then reaches the cranial arteries, meningeal tissues, and dural arteries and sinuses, releasing neuropeptides that promote local vasodilatation and plasma extravasation, referred to as *neurogenic inflammation*. Throbbing pain may be the result of normal pulsations of cranial blood vessels or normal pulsations of CSF

   4. Serotonin (5-hydroxytryptamine or 5HT) is a key neurotransmitter in migraine

       a.   5HT receptors on cranial vessels have a vasoconstrictive action

       b.   5HT receptors on the terminals of trigeminal nerve axons have an inhibitory action

       c.   Drugs specifically effective in aborting migraine attacks, both ergots and triptans, are 5HT receptor agonists. Some prophylactic drugs useful in migraine are serotonergic

   5. Although controversial, there is increasing evidence for an increased state of excitability in the brains of migraineurs, not just during attacks, but also between attacks. This may be related to dysfunction in the serotonergic dorsal raphe nuclei of the brainstem

E. Migraine without aura (common migraine)

   1. Diagnostic criteria are shown in Table 15-2

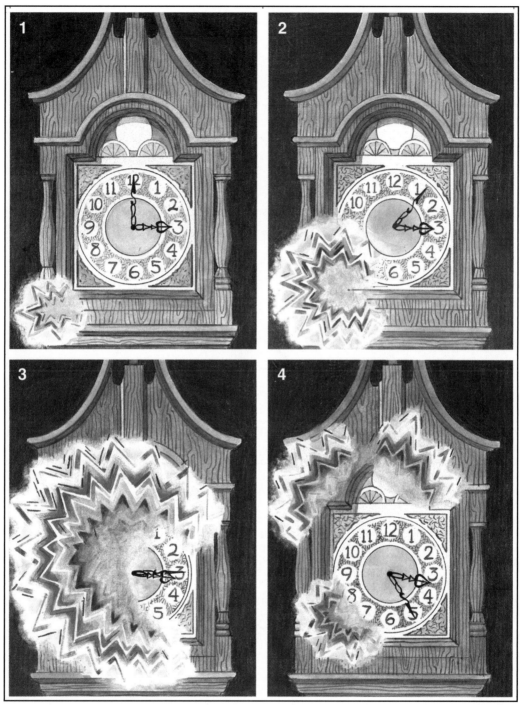

Figure 15-1. Scintillating fortification scotoma of migraine appears in one portion of the visual field, typically enlarges to cover central fixation, then "marches" toward the periphery and breaks apart. The entire phenomenon lasts 15 to 30 minutes. (Reprinted with permission from Hupp SL, Kline LB, Corbett JJ. Visual disturbances of migraine. *Surv Ophthalmol.* 1989;33:221-236.)[1] **Please see the 4-color tearout page at the back of the book.**

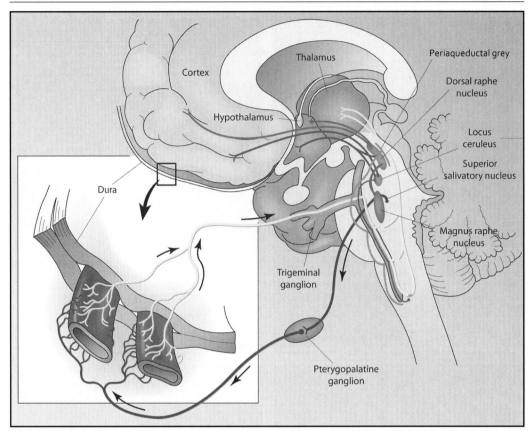

Figure 15-2. Pathophysiology of migraine. Migraine involves dysfunction of the brainstem pathways that normally modulate sensory input. Trigeminovascular input from the meningeal vessels passes through the trigeminal ganglion and synapses on second-order neurons in the trigeminocervical complex. These second-order neurons project to the thalamus. This trigeminal-autonomic reflex is present in normal persons and is expressed most strongly in patients with trigeminal-autonomic cephalgias, such as cluster headache and paroxysmal hemicrania; it may be active in migraine. Brain imaging studies suggest that important modulation of the trigeminovascular nociceptive input comes from the dorsal raphe nucleus, locus ceruleus, and nucleus raphe magnus in the brainstem. (From *Headache in Clinical Practice*. 2nd ed. Silberstein SD, Lipton RB, Goadsby PJ, © 2002 Martin Dunitz. Reproduced by permission of Taylor & Francis Books UK.)[2]

Table 15-2

DIAGNOSTIC CRITERIA FOR MIGRAINE WITHOUT AURA

A. Headache lasts 4 to 72 hours
B. Headache has at least 2 of the following characteristics:
    1. Unilateral location
    2. Pulsating quality
    3. Moderate or severe intensity inhibiting daily activities
    4. Aggravation by routine physical activity
C. At least one of the following occurs during headache:
    1. Nausea and/or vomiting
    2. Photophobia and phonophobia

Table 15-3

DIAGNOSTIC CRITERIA FOR MIGRAINE WITH AURA

A.   At least 3 of the following 4 characteristics are present:
1.   One or more fully reversible aura symptoms indicate focal cerebral cortical or brainstem dysfunction
2.   At least one aura symptom develops gradually over more than 4 minutes or 2 or more symptoms occur in succession
3.   No single aura symptom lasts more than 60 minutes
4.   Headache follows aura within 60 minutes or begins before or simultaneously with the aura
B.   Headache has at least 2 of the following characteristics:
1.   Unilateral location
2.   Pulsating quality
3.   Moderate or severe intensity inhibiting daily activities
4.   Aggravation by routine physical activity
C.   At least one of the following occurs during headache:
1.   Nausea and/or vomiting
2.   Photophobia and phonophobia

F.   Migraine with aura (classic migraine)
1.   Diagnostic criteria are shown in Table 15-3
2.   The features of migrainous visual aura are so characteristic as to be diagnostic
3.   Note that a diagnosis of migraine with aura can be made without the presence of headache even though that is uncommon
4.   Over a lifetime, a given patient may start with migraine with aura and later evolve to a migraine without aura pattern or vice versa
G.   Retinal (ocular) migraine is an uncommon form of migraine consisting of repeated attacks of monocular visual loss lasting < 1 hour and associated with headache
1.   Many patients experiencing homonymous visual field defects attribute the defect to the eye on the involved side. Confirmation of the monocular nature requires an observant patient testing each eye individually to confirm that the visual loss is limited to a single eye
2.   IHS criteria are at least 2 attacks of fully reversible monocular visual loss lasting < 60 minutes followed by a headache within 60 minutes but sometimes preceding the visual loss
3.   Typically patients are young (< 50 years) and already have a history of migraine with or without aura
4.   Patients with migraine and monocular visual loss have been described with arterial and venous retinal vascular occlusion, central serous retinopathy, vitreous hemorrhage, retinal hemorrhage, and anterior and posterior ION
5.   It has been suggested the term *retinal migraine* be replaced with more general designation of *retinal vasospasm*
6.   Because it is uncommon and because other conditions may mimic it, retinal migraine is a diagnosis of exclusion
7.   Treatment:
a.   Calcium channel blockers
b.   Beta-blockers

H. "Basilar-type" migraine
  1. Initially proposed by Bickerstaff and formerly referred to as *basilar artery migraine*, the IHS classification considers migraine patients with aura symptoms attributable to brainstem or cerebellar dysfunction as being another variant of migraine with aura
  2. Neurologic symptoms include ataxia, diplopia, dysarthria, vertigo, tinnitus, facial or limb paresthesias, and disturbance of vision
  3. Visual symptoms are bilateral and may include the following:
     a. Dimming or total loss of sight
     b. Visual hallucinations or unformed images
     c. Photopsias
I. Complications of migraine
  1. Migrainous stroke
     a. Patients may have migraine and stroke coincidentally
     b. Occasionally, patients with stroke experience migrainous symptoms such as positive neurologic symptoms or a buildup of the neurologic deficits, a migraine mimic. When occurring in an older patient who has continued to suffer from migraine, it may be difficult to distinguish from other forms of stroke and it requires a workup directed at causes of stroke
     c. When a migraineur has a typical aura during the course of a typical migraine but the neurologic deficit persists, then the stroke may be attributed to the migraine, but other causes of stroke still must be excluded by diagnostic studies
     d. It has been hypothesized that migraine-induced neurologic deficits are not the result of ischemia but of excitotoxicity caused by dysfunction of serotonergic pathways and fatal "neuronal overdrive," resulting in cell death with free radical formation and nitric oxide effects
     e. In young cohorts (<50 years) with stroke, 10% to 15% of patients have migraine; a majority of these are women who are also on oral contraceptives. Young women with migraine have a stroke risk several times their peers, and this risk is magnified by use of tobacco and oral contraceptives
  2. Persistent aura in migraine
     a. Rarely, patients with migraine experience positive visual symptoms during periods between migraine attacks. Besides supporting the concept of neuronal hyperexcitability in migraine, it is important to recognize these as related to migraine and to reassure the patients of their benign nature
J. Treatment of migraine
  1. Nonpharmacologic therapy
     a. Lifestyle changes: regular sleep, regular meals, exercise
     b. Dietary triggers may include alcohol, red wine, certain cheeses, and other foodstuffs
  2. Abortive therapies to treat the individual headaches are of 2 types:
     a. Nonspecific treatments such as aspirin, acetaminophen, nonsteroidal anti-inflammatory drugs, opiates, and combination analgesics
        i. May cause a rebound increase in headaches if used excessively
     b. Migraine-specific treatments
        i. Ergot derivatives (ergotamine, cafergot, dihydroergotamine [DHE])
        ii. Triptans

Table 15-4
DIAGNOSTIC CRITERIA FOR CLUSTER HEADACHE

A. Severe unilateral orbital, supraorbital, and/or temporal pain lasts 15 to 180 minutes untreated
B. Headache is associated with at least one of the following on the side of the pain:
   1. Conjunctival injection
   2. Lacrimation
   3. Nasal congestion
   4. Rhinorrhea
   5. Forehead and facial sweating
   6. Miosis
   7. Ptosis
   8. Eyelid edema
C. Frequency of attacks ranges from 1 every other day to 8 per day

3. Preventive therapy is indicated in patients experiencing more frequent attacks and should be considered in patients experiencing headache 1 or more days per week. A wide variety of drugs are used as prophylactic therapy, only some of which have been demonstrated effective in controlled clinical trials
   a. Beta-blockers (propranolol, metoprolol)
   b. Calcium-channel blockers (verapamil)
   c. Tricyclic antidepressants (amitriptyline, nortriptyline)
   d. Serotonin reuptake inhibitors (fluoxetine, paroxetine, sertraline)
   e. Trazodone
   f. Anticonvulsants: valproic acid, topiramate, gabapentin
   g. Botulinum toxin injections
   h. Acetaminophen, ibuprofen, and nasal-spray sumatriptan are all effective symptomatic pharmacologic treatments for episodes of migraine in children

V. **TENSION-TYPE HEADACHE (MUSCLE CONTRACTION HEADACHE)**
   A. Typical symptoms include bilateral headache, often with posterior neck tightness. The headache is dull and may be likened to pressure or a band-like or vise-like sensation
   B. Exercise does not worsen the pain and may relieve it
   C. Nausea and vomiting, photophobia, and phonophobia are not features of tension-type headache
   D. As migraine may be associated with psychological stress, occurring during or sometimes after relief of the stressful situation, so tension-type headache may occur during identifiable psychological stress
   E. There is substantial overlap in the pain experience of patients with migraine and tension-type headache:
      1. Tension-type headache may start or be worse on one side
      2. One-third of patients with migraine without aura have bilateral headache from the outset and many more have unilateral headache initially that subsequently generalizes
      3. The occiput and posterior neck is a common site of pain in both groups

VI. **CLUSTER AND OTHER TRIGEMINAL AUTONOMIC CEPHALGIAS**
   A. Diagnostic criteria for cluster headache are listed in Table 15-4
   B. Cluster (also known as *Horton headache*) is the most common trigeminal autonomic cephalgia

C. Five-to-one male sex predilection

D. Typically characterized by unilateral attacks of short-lived (< 60 minutes) but very severe pain associated with rhinorrhea, lacrimation, and Horner syndrome

E. Attacks may occur one or more times daily, often in the early morning and repeating the same pattern each day

F. In distinction to migraine, most patients with cluster become restless and move around during the attack

G. Clusters may last from weeks to months and may be seasonal

H. Individual headaches may be treated with oxygen, parenteral triptans, or DHE

I. Cluster periods are managed with corticosteroids and daily triptan administration, and methysergide, verapamil, and lithium have been used successfully as well

J. SUNCT—short-lasting unilateral neuralgiform headache attacks with conjunctival injection and tearing—is categorized as a trigeminal autonomic cephalgia

　　1. Projectile lacrimation may occur

　　2. Episodes usually last 5 seconds to 5 minutes but usually occur 25 times per day

　　3. Cranial MRI is necessary to exclude a secondary cause including pituitary adenoma and posterior fossa tumors, demyelinating disease, and vascular compression of the trigeminal nerve

　　4. Best treatment: anticonvulsants (topiramate, lamotrigine) and carbamazepine; SUNCT often worsens with corticosteroids and calcium channel blockers

VII. **Secondary headache syndromes**

A. Some secondary headaches have important neuro-ophthalmologic implications. Systemic symptoms and signs and past medical history are critical in directing laboratory evaluations in these patients

B. Giant cell arteritis

　　1. New onset of headache in a patient over age 50 years

　　2. Bitemporal

　　3. Scalp tenderness

　　4. Jaw claudication

　　5. Polymyalgia

　　6. Visual symptoms (see Chapter 9)

C. Carotid or vertebral arterial dissection

　　1. Ophthalmic manifestations: carotid dissection may cause an ipsilateral Horner syndrome and may be associated with retinal or optic nerve ischemia and occasionally ocular motor cranial nerve palsies and hemispheric stroke. Vertebral artery dissection may cause brainstem stroke

　　2. Associated symptoms and signs: ipsilateral neck or head pain with or without contralateral hemiparesis; dysgeusia

　　3. Diagnostic evaluation should include MRI, MRA, CTA, and possibly catheter angiography

　　4. Treatment: antiplatelet therapy; anticoagulation; carotid stenting

D. Cerebral venous sinus thrombosis

　　1. Ophthalmic manifestations: papilledema, diplopia including from VI nerve palsy

　　2. Associated symptoms and signs: seizures, contralateral hemiparesis from venous stroke, obtundation

　　3. Diagnostic evaluation should include MRI, MRV (see also Chapter 20)

E. Pituitary apoplexy

　　1. Pituitary adenoma may outgrow its blood supply and experience spontaneous hemorrhagic necrosis. Sudden increase in size of the mass compresses the optic

chiasm and extension into the cavernous sinuses damages the ocular motor cranial nerves

    2.   Ophthalmic manifestations: acute ophthalmoparesis, acute visual loss

    3.   Associated symptoms and signs include severe headache, photophobia, meningismus

    4.   Cranial MRI is important in establishing the correct diagnosis. Multiple different signals may be present from ischemia (often hypointensity) and hemorrhage (often hyperintensity). There is also typically sphenoid sinus mucosal thickening on enhanced T1-weighted MRI in both ischemic and hemorrhagic types of apoplexy

    5.   Treatment includes corticosteroids, endocrinologic support, and surgery

F.   Intracranial hypertension, papilledema, and IIH

    1.   Increased intracranial pressure may be due to obstructive hydrocephalus, a space-occupying lesion, AVM, dural arteriovenous fistula, or meningeal processes including infection and noninfectious inflammation. In the absence of one of these processes, the correct diagnosis is often IIH or pseudotumor cerebri (see Chapter 9, IV on page 145)

    2.   Headache of increased intracranial pressure

        a.   Usually appears quite suddenly

        b.   May be mild or intermittent initially, but progressively worsens

        c.   May be worse in head-down position and with coughing or straining

G.   Intracranial hypotension

    1.   Commonly seen after LP; patients experience headache present when upright and resolves when lying down

    2.   Syndrome of spontaneous intracranial hypotension is recognized by this same posture-dependent headache

    3.   MRI findings include the following:

        a.   Diffuse enhancement of the dura

        b.   Sagging of the brain with descent of the cerebellar tonsils into the foramen magnum

        c.   Decreased size of the CSF cisterns

        d.   Pituitary gland may be enlarged and the chiasm draped over it

        e.   Subdural fluid collections may develop

    4.   On LP, opening pressure may be normal but is usually low or unmeasurable

H.   Microvascular ocular motor cranial nerve infarcts

    1.   Ophthalmic manifestations: III (pupil-sparing), IV, or VI nerve palsy usually in setting of diabetes mellitus or hypertension (see Chapters 4 through 6)

    2.   Associated symptoms and signs include pain around the eye, possibly due to meningeal ischemia, which may precede the diplopia by up to 1 week

    3.   Pain resolves within 1 to 2 weeks

    4.   Severity of the pain is not a distinctive feature when comparing microvascular and aneurysmal III nerve palsy

I.   Ophthalmoplegic migraine (see Chapter 5)

    1.   Diagnostic criteria: at least 2 attacks of a migraine-like headache accompanied or followed within 4 days of onset by paresis of one or more of III, IV, or VI cranial nerves and not attributable to parasellar, superior orbital fissure, or posterior fossa lesions

    2.   Onset usually before age 10 years

    3.   III nerve affected 10 to 1 over VI nerve

    4.   Pupil and accommodation frequently involved

     5. Ophthalmoplegia occurs at height of headache, persisting when headache clears (may last days to weeks)

     6. Strict criteria for diagnosis

       a. Onset in first decade of life

       b. History of typical migraine

       c. Ophthalmoplegia ipsilateral to headache

       d. MRI: normal or enhancement of involved ocular motor cranial nerve

     7. MRI findings suggest condition may be due to structural lesion (schwannoma, angioma), ischemia, or demyelination of the involved cranial nerve rather than being a primary headache (ie, is not really migraine)

J. Herpes zoster ophthalmicus

     1. Ophthalmic manifestations:

       a. Keratitis

       b. Uveitis

       c. Ophthalmoplegia due to vasculitis of vasa nervorum of ocular motor cranial nerves or orbital myositis

       d. Optic neuritis—papillitis or retrobulbar

       e. Vasculitis involving cranial arteries may produce homonymous hemianopia due to stroke

     2. Associated symptoms and signs: pain followed within days by vesicular eruption in the distribution of the ophthalmic division of the trigeminal nerve

     3. Acute treatment:

       a. Corticosteroid

       b. Antiviral—acyclovir, famvir

     4. Postherpetic neuralgia

       a. Carbamazepine

       b. Gabapentin

       c. Pregabalin

       d. Lidocaine patch

K. Raeder paratrigeminal neuralgia

     1. In 1924, Raeder described 5 patients with facial pain, attributed to structural lesion in the trigeminal ganglion region, and a Horner syndrome sparing sweating

     2. Later authors used the term *Raeder paratrigeminal neuralgia Type 2* in describing patients who had cluster headache

     3. A Horner syndrome with any other cranial nerve deficit, including V1 sensory loss, may have a structural lesion underlying the condition and merits a neuroimaging evaluation

     4. A Horner syndrome with facial pain merits a neuroimaging evaluation

L. Other secondary headache syndromes

     1. Paranasal sinus disease

     2. Temporomandibular joint disorder

     3. Eyestrain

     4. Nonorganic pain

VIII. **TABLE 15-5 EMPHASIZES FINDINGS ACCOMPANYING HEADACHE THAT MAY SUGGEST THE NEED FOR ADDITIONAL EVALUATION AND IMPORTANT CONSIDERATIONS IN DIFFERENTIAL DIAGNOSIS. THESE CLINICAL FINDINGS ASSOCIATED WITH HEADACHE OFTEN PROMPT FURTHER PATIENT EVALUATION INCLUDING NEUROIMAGING**

Table 15-5	
RED FLAGS IN PATIENTS WITH HEADACHE	
Sudden onset headache	Subarachnoid hemorrhage, bleeding into AVM or neoplasm, posterior fossa mass with developing hydrocephalus
Progressive headache	Mass lesion, subdural hematoma, medication overuse
Systemic symptoms accompanying headache (fever, rash, neck stiffness, jaw or tongue pain)	Giant cell or other arteritis, meningitis, encephalitis, Lyme disease, systemic infection, collagen vascular disease
Focal neurologic symptoms other than typical visual or sensory aura of migraine or persistent focal neurologic symptoms or signs	AVM, mass lesion, collagen vascular disease, stroke
Papilledema	Intracranial mass or hemorrhage, encephalitis or meningitis, IIH
Triggered by cough, exertion, Valsalva maneuver, or head or neck movements	Carotid or vertebral dissection, subarachnoid hemorrhage, mass lesion
Headache during pregnancy or peripartum period	IIH, cortical vein or cerebral venous sinus thrombosis, carotid dissection, pituitary apoplexy
New headache in patients with the following:	
Cancer	Metastases
HIV	Opportunistic infection, lymphoma
Lyme disease	Meningoencephalitis

REFERENCES

1. Hupp SL, Kline LB, Corbett JJ. Visual disturbances of migraine. *Surv Ophthalmol*. 1989;33:221-236.
2. Silberstein SD, Lipton RB, Goadsby PJ. *Headache in Clinical Practice*. 2nd ed. Boca Raton, FL: CRC Press; 2002.

BIBLIOGRAPHY

Bousser MG. Estrogens, migraine, tobacco, and stroke. *Stroke*. 2004;35 Suppl 1:2652-2656.

Carlow TJ. Oculomotor ophthalmoplegic migraine: is it really migraine? *J Neuroophthalmol*. 2002;22:215-221.

Eggers AE. New neural theory of migraine. *Medical Hypotheses*. 2001;56:360-363.

Goadsby PJ. Recent advances in the diagnosis and management of migraine. *BMJ*. 2006;332:25-29.

Goadsby PJ, Lipton RB, Ferrari MD. Drug therapy: migraine—current understanding and treatment. *N Engl J Med*. 2002;346:257-270.

Headache Classification Subcommittee of the International Headache Society. *Cephalalgia: The International Classification of Headache Disorders*. 2nd ed. 2004;24 1 Suppl.

Lipton RB, Silberstein SD, Saper JR, Bigal ME, Goadsby PJ. Why headache treatment fails. *Neurology*. 2003;70:1064-1070.

Liu GT, Schatz NJ, Galetta SL, Volpe NJ, Skobieranda F, Kosmorsky GS. Persistent positive visual phenomena in migraine. *Neurology*. 1995;45:664-668.

Loder E. Triptan therapy in migraine. *N Engl J Med*. 2010;363:63-70.

May A, Goadsby PJ. Pharmacological opportunities and pitfalls in the therapy of migraine. *Curr Opin Neurol.* 2001;14:341-345.

Oleson J, Tfelt-Hanson P, Welch MA, et al. *The Headaches.* 3rd ed. Philadelphia, PA: Lippincott Williams & Wilkins; 2006.

Richer L, Billinghurst L, Linsdell MA, et al. Drugs for the acute treatment of migraine in children and adolescents. *Cochrane Database Syst Rev.* 2016;4:CD005220. doi: 10.1002/14651858.CD005220.pub2.

Silberstein SD, Lipton RB, Dodick DW, eds. *Wolff's Headache and Other Head Pain.* 8th ed. New York, NY: Oxford University Press; 2007.

Troost BT. Migraine and other headaches. In: Glaser JS, ed. *Neuro-Ophthalmology.* 3rd ed. Philadelphia, PA: Lippincott-Williams & Wilkins; 1999:553-587.

Van Stavern GP. Headache and facial pain. In: Miller NR, Newman NJ, eds. *Walsh and Hoyt's Clinical Neuro-Ophthalmology.* Vol 1. 6th ed. Philadelphia, PA: Lippincott Williams & Wilkins; 2005:1275-1311.

Vaphiades MS. The "pituitary ring sign": an MRI sign of pituitary apoplexy. *Neuro-ophthalmology.* 2007;31:111-116.

Vaphiades MS. Pituitary apoplexy. *Medscape.* http://emedicine.medscape.com/article/1198279-overview. Published March 23, 2015.

Winterkorn JM, Kupersmith MJ, Wirtschafter JD, Forman S. Treatment of vasospastic amaurosis fugax with calcium-channel blockers. *N Engl J Med.* 1993;329:396-398.

CHAPTER 16

Carotid Artery Disease and the Eye

ROD FOROOZAN, MD AND MILTON F. WHITE JR, MD

I. **GENERAL CONSIDERATIONS**
   A. Carotid artery arteriosclerosis accounts for around 20% of all strokes
   B. Cerebrovascular insufficiency is often accompanied by ocular signs and symptoms
   C. Depending on the clinical setting, there is a spectrum of stroke risk (Table 16-1)
   D. Patients with stroke are at high risk for subsequent vascular events, including recurrent stroke (highest risk), myocardial infarction, and death from vascular causes

II. **ANATOMY OF THE CAROTID SYSTEM**
   A. The first major branch of the aortic arch is the innominate artery, which gives rise to the right common carotid artery
   B. The left common carotid is the second major branch of the aortic arch
   C. Each common carotid artery divides into internal and external branches at the C4 level, about 3 cm below the angle of the mandible
   D. The internal carotid artery enters the skull through the carotid canal of the temporal bone, ascends along the side of the sella turcica, forms the carotid siphon as it passes through the cavernous sinus, then emerges intracranially
   E. The ophthalmic artery is its first major branch, and the internal carotid ultimately divides into the anterior and middle cerebral arteries
   F. Numerous connections between the external and internal carotid systems involve the ophthalmic artery (Figure 16-1)
   G. Third-order neuron (postganglionic) sympathetic fibers to the eye, orbit, and face travel in the posterior carotid sheath
   H. Cervical portion of carotid artery is surgically accessible

III. **OCULAR MANIFESTATIONS OF CAROTID DISEASE**
   A. Transient monocular visual loss (TMVL)
      1. Alternate terms: amaurosis fugax ("fleeting blindness"), transient monocular blindness
      2. Duration: 2 to 30 minutes
      3. Typically, a "shade" temporarily covers part or all of the visual field. Other descriptions include a "dark cloud," "a film," or generalized darkening
      4. Visual loss may include the entire visual field or only one-half or a quadrant of the field
      5. Positive visual phenomena may be described by one-third of patients

Foroozan R, Vaphiades MS. *Kline's Neuro-Ophthalmology Review Manual, Eighth Edition (pp 221-232)*. © 2018 SLACK Incorporated.

Table 16-1	
SPECTRUM OF STROKE RISK	
Patient Group	**Risk of Stroke Per Year (%)**
No carotid disease	0.1
Asymptomatic carotid bruit	0.1 to 0.4
TMVL	2.0
Asymptomatic carotid stenosis	2.5
Retinal infarcts, emboli	3.0
Transient cerebral ischemic attack	8.0
Adapted from Trobe JD. Carotid endarterectomy: who needs it? *Ophthalmology.* 1987;94:725-730.[1]	

6. TMVL associated with carotid stenosis is most commonly due to embolic disease (see section B next)

7. Less common pathophysiologic mechanisms include diminished blood flow (hypoperfusion) and vasospasm of the ophthalmic and/or central retinal artery. Vasospastic amaurosis is evaluated like typical TMVL, but the work-up is negative and calcium channel blockers are often an effective treatment.

8. Occasionally, TMVL can be precipitated by exposure to bright light (photostress: retinal vascular insufficiency to photoreceptors). Transient smartphone "blindness" is an entity that falls into this category. It is felt to be from differential bleaching of photopigment, with the viewing eye becoming light-adapted, while the eye blocked by the pillow was becoming dark-adapted

9. Natural history of TMVL when related to carotid disease:
   a. Risk of permanent visual loss: 1% per year
   b. Risk of stroke: 2% per year (20 times higher than a patient without carotid disease; see Table 16-1)
   c. Mortality rate: 2% to 4% per year
   d. Main causes of death: cardiac and cerebrovascular disease
   e. TMVL with associated visible retinal emboli: mortality rate increases to 4% to 6% per year
   f. No relationship between frequency or duration of visual symptoms and risk of stroke

10. A variety of other conditions, including vasculitis (giant cell arteritis), cause TMVL (Table 16-2). History often is important as many times patients will have no evidence of pathology on the eye examination

B. Retinal circulatory emboli (Table 16-3)
   1. Cholesterol
      a. Hollenhorst plaques
      b. Bright, orange-yellow, refractile
      c. Source: carotid and aortic atheroma
   2. Platelet-fibrin
      a. Fisher plugs
      b. White intra-arterial plugs lodge at bifurcations
      c. Source: internal carotid artery atheroma and ulceration

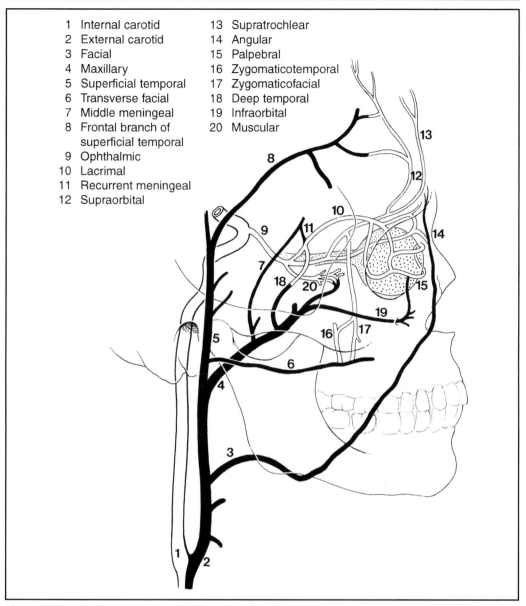

1	Internal carotid	13	Supratrochlear
2	External carotid	14	Angular
3	Facial	15	Palpebral
4	Maxillary	16	Zygomaticotemporal
5	Superficial temporal	17	Zygomaticofacial
6	Transverse facial	18	Deep temporal
7	Middle meningeal	19	Infraorbital
8	Frontal branch of	20	Muscular
	superficial temporal		
9	Ophthalmic		
10	Lacrimal		
11	Recurrent meningeal		
12	Supraorbital		

Figure 16-1. Anastomotic connections between the internal and external carotid arteries. Note the key position of the ophthalmic artery (9).

3. Calcium
    a. Gray-white, nonrefractile
    b. Usually lodge in retinal arterioles near or on the optic disc
    c. Source: cardiac valves or aortic wall
4. Septic vegetation—bacterial endocarditis
5. Fat—due to long bone fracture
6. Myxoma—heart
7. Amniotic fluid—uterus
8. Talc—intravenous drug use
9. Rare—mercury, air, paraffin

Table 16-2

CAUSES OF TRANSIENT MONOCULAR VISUAL LOSS

Typically Associated With Abnormal Eye Examination

Ocular Pathology (Nonvascular)

        Blepharospasm

        Tear film abnormalities

        Keratoconus

        Hyphema

        Uveitis-glaucoma-hyphema (UGH) syndrome

        Intermittent angle-closure glaucoma

        Vitreous debris

Orbitopathy

        Orbital masses and foreign bodies

        Gaze-evoked (typically intraconal mass)

Optic Nerve

        Papilledema

        Optic nerve drusen/Congenital optic disc anomalies

        Compressive lesions of the intraorbital optic nerve

        ION (particularly from vasculitis)

        Demyelinating disease

Retina

        Age-related macular degeneration

        Macular disease and photostress

        Impending CRAO

        Retinal detachment

Vascular Disease

        Ocular hypoperfusion (ocular ischemic syndrome)

        Internal/common carotid artery stenosis

        Embolic phenomenon

            Carotid

                Arterial dissection

            Cardiac

                Arrhythmia

                Valvular disease

            Great vessels

        Carotid artery dissection

        Vasculitis

        Anemia

            Sickle cell disease

        AVM

        Arterial vasospasm (during acute episode)

(continued)

Table 16-2 (continued)

CAUSES OF TRANSIENT MONOCULAR VISUAL LOSS

Hyperglycemia
Hypercoagulable state
    Thrombocytosis
    Polycythemia
    Antiphospholipid syndrome

Typically Associated With Normal Eye Examination

Vascular Disease

    Internal/common carotid artery stenosis
    Hypotension
    Hypertension

Neurologic

    Migraine (including retinal migraine)
    Uhthoff phenomenon (demyelination)

Intracranial tumor

Nonorganic visual loss

Adapted from Ahmed R, Foroozan R. Transient monocular visual loss. *Neurol Clin.* 2010;28:619-629.[2]

Table 16-3

CLINICAL ASPECTS OF COMMON RETINAL EMBOLI

Type	Appearance	Source
Cholesterol	Yellow-orange or copper color	Common or internal carotid artery
	Refractile	Rarely from aorta or innominate artery
	Rectangular	
	Usually located at bifurcations of retinal vessels	
Platelet-fibrin	Dull gray-white color	From wall of atherosclerotic vessel
	Long, smooth shape	Heart valves
	Concave meniscus at each end	
	Lodge along course of vessel	
Calcium	Chalky white	From heart or great vessels
	Large	Rheumatic heart disease
	Round or ovoid	Calcific aortic stenosis
	Lodge at first or second vessel bifurcation, often overlying disc	

Adapted from Ahmed R, Foroozan R. Transient monocular visual loss. *Neurol Clin.* 2010;28:619-629.[2]

C. Retinal arterial occlusion
   1. Types:
      a. CRAO
      b. Branch retinal artery occlusion (BRAO)
   2. Central retinal artery has narrowest diameter at lamina cribrosa, where it is most vulnerable to occlusion
   3. Five major causes of CRAO:
      a. Embolization
      b. Localized atheromatous stenosis
      c. Arteritic obliteration
      d. Reduced vascular perfusion
      e. Vasospasm
   4. Patient with CRAO reports painless loss of vision
   5. Experimental CRAO persisting > 100 minutes leads to permanent loss of vision
   6. Clinical findings with CRAO
      a. Segmentation of blood in retinal arterioles—"boxcarring"
      b. Visible emboli in 11% to 20% of patients
      c. Axoplasmic flow stasis with retinal edema or "whitening"
      d. "Cherry-red" spot in the macula
      e. After several days, retinal swelling subsides; loss of retinal NFL; optic disc pallor (4 to 8 weeks)
      f. Arteries may demonstrate both narrowing and sheathing
   7. Clinical findings in BRAO
      a. Segmentation of blood in involved branch retinal arteriole—"boxcarring"
      b. Visible emboli in around 60% of patients
      c. Retinal edema localized to area of involved arteriole
      d. With resolution of retinal swelling, area of NFL atrophy and inner retinal thinning; segmental optic disc pallor
      e. Susac syndrome: triad of microangiopathy involving the brain, retina, and cochlea. Consider in a young patient with otherwise unexplained retinal arterial occlusive disease
   8. Emergency treatment of CRAO
      a. Immediate goal is to increase perfusion and preserve flow in the central retinal artery:
         i. Lower intraocular pressure
         ii. Vasodilation
      b. Lower intraocular pressure: anterior chamber paracentesis, ocular massage, topical beta-blocker, topical carbonic anhydrase inhibitor
      c. Vasodilation: breathe into paper bag, inhalation of carbogen (95% O_2, 5% CO_2), intravenous aminophylline, retrobulbar anesthesia
      d. Intravascular injection of tissue plasminogen activator (TPA): no evidence of benefit and greater risk of adverse events in patients treated with intra-arterial TPA compared to conservative therapy in a multicenter randomized trial (European Assessment Group for Lysis in the Eye [EAGLE] study)
      e. Hyperbaric oxygen
      f. All treatment modalities are empiric; none proven due to lack of efficacy in controlled studies

9. Around 25% of patients with acute retinal artery occlusion will have concurrent (imaged within 7 days of the onset of visual symptoms) evidence of acute stroke on diffusion-weighted imaging (DWI) (see also Chapter 20)

    a. Consider hospital admission or emergency room evaluation with MRI of brain and evaluation for stroke for patients with acute retinal artery occlusion

    b. Urgent evaluation is warranted after a stroke or transient visual loss because many recurrent events occur early

10. Survival time of 5.5 years following CRAO versus expected survival of 15 years in age-matched population

11. Three percent to 10% of patients older than 50 years of age with CRAO have giant cell arteritis. Remember to consider a Westergren sedimentation rate STAT!

D. Evaluation and therapy for patients with TMVL and retinal arterial occlusions

  1. Careful history searching for vascular risk factors:

    a. Hypertension

    b. Diabetes mellitus

    c. Hypercholesterolemia/hyperlipidemia

    d. Tobacco use

    e. Cardiac disease: ischemic, valvular, arrhythmia, patent foramen ovale

  2. Physical examination focusing on the eye, neck, and heart

  3. Diagnostic studies are summarized in Table 16-4

  4. Treatment

    a. Medical:

      i. Reduction of vascular risk factors

      ii. Exercise

      iii. Aspirin

      iv. Dipyridamole-aspirin (Aggrenox)

      v. Clopidogrel (Plavix)

      vi. Warfarin (Coumadin)

      vii. Dabigatran (Pradaxa), an anticoagulant for nonvalvular atrial fibrillation

    b. Surgical:

      i. Cardiac—if source of emboli

      ii. Carotid revascularization—North American Symptomatic Carotid Endarterectomy Trial (NASCET): endarterectomy recommended for all patients with symptomatic extracranial stenosis of 70% to 99% whose medical condition does not preclude surgery (Table 16-5)

      iii. **Remember:** consider the surgical perioperative morbidity/mortality rate of your patient versus the natural history of the disease (see Table 16-1) when considering surgical intervention

      iv. Retrospective analysis of the NASCET data found, in patients with TMVL, 6 factors increased stroke risk:

        1. Age > 75 years

        2. Male sex

        3. History of hemispheric transient ischemic attack or stroke

        4. Intermittent claudication

        5. Eighty percent to 94% internal carotid artery stenosis

        6. No collateral circulation (cerebral angiography)

      v. Table 16-6 summarizes impact of these risk factors in patients experiencing TMVL

Table 16-4

EVALUATION OF TRANSIENT MONOCULAR VISUAL LOSS BASED ON SUSPECTED ETIOLOGY

Suspected Cause	Testing to Consider
Embolic	
Atherosclerosis	Ultrasonography, angiography, imaging of aortic arch, fasting serum lipids, blood glucose
Dissection	MRI, MRA
Cardiac thromboemboli	Echocardiography, electrocardiography
Hypercoagulability/hyperviscosity	Coagulation screen (may include protein C, S; Factor V Leiden; antithrombin III; antiphospholipid antibodies; G20210A mutation; homocysteine level; prothrombin time; partial thromboplastin time)
Hyperviscosity syndromes	CBC, serum protein electrophoresis, hemoglobin electrophoresis, blood smear
Hemodynamic	
Primary postural hypotension	Standing blood pressure, autonomic tests
Secondary postural hypotension	Assess blood pressure and medication use
Malignant hypertension	Blood pressure
Preeclampsia/eclampsia	Blood pressure, urinalysis
Reduced ocular perfusion	Ultrasonography/angiography, central retinal artery perfusion pressure
Vascular	
Vasculitis (including giant cell arteritis) and rheumatologic conditions	Urgent erythrocyte sedimentation rate, laboratory tests, angiography, temporal artery biopsy, ANA, syphilis serology antibody, antiphospholipid antibodies
Arteriovenous fistula	Angiography
Vasospasm	Funduscopy, intravenous fluorescein angiography during attack
Drug abuse (eg, cocaine)	Urine drug screen
Optic Nerve and Brain	
Migraine	History and neurological examination, neuroimaging
Epilepsy	Neurological examination, electroencephalography, brain imaging
Optic disc edema (transient visual obscurations)	Funduscopy, brain imaging, LP with opening pressure
Optic disc anomalies (eg, drusen)	Funduscopy, ancillary funduscopic imaging (eg, OCT)
Gaze evoked	Orbital imaging
Cortical ischemia	MRI brain

Adapted from Petzold A, Islam N, Hu HH, Plant GT. Embolic and nonembolic transient monocular visual field loss: a clinicopathologic review. *Surv Ophthalmol.* 2013;58:42-62.[3]

Table 16-5

HIGH-RISK FACTORS FOR CAROTID ENDARTERECTOMY PERIOPERATIVE STROKE/DEATH

Age over 70 years
Refractory hypertension
Severe coronary disease
Severe obstructive pulmonary disease
Marked obesity
Recent or multiple strokes
Bilateral carotid stenosis
Distal ipsilateral carotid stenosis

Adapted from Carter JE. Carotid artery disease and its ocular manifestations. *Ophthalmol Clin North Am.* 1992;5:425-443.[4]

Table 16-6

IMPACT OF RISK FACTORS ON TRANSIENT MONOCULAR VISUAL LOSS

3-Year Risk of Ipsilateral Stroke

Risk Factors	Medical (%)	Surgical (%)	Stroke Risk Reduction (medical minus surgical)
0 to 1	1.8	4.0	–2.2*
2	12.3	7.4	4.9
3 or more	24.2	9.9	14.3

*Negative sign indicates increase in risk.

     vi. Carotid artery stenting:
       1. The Carotid Revascularization Endarterectomy Versus Stenting Trial (CREST): showed stenting and surgery to be equivalent in terms of the composite end point of stroke, myocardial infarction, or death within 30 days, as well as for the rate of ipsilateral stroke up to 10 years
     vii. Extracranial-intracranial arterial bypass surgery: if there is complete carotid stenosis
       1. No proven benefit compared to medical therapy
       2. Remains controversial
     viii. The treatment of asymptomatic patients with carotid occlusion remains controversial
  E. Ocular ischemic syndrome
    1. Chronic hypoperfusion of the globe from ipsilateral (typically marked) or bilateral carotid occlusive disease

Table 16-7

FINDINGS IN OCULAR ISCHEMIC SYNDROME

Conjunctiva

Injected vessels
Dilated episcleral vessels

Cornea

Edema

Anterior chamber

Cells, flare (ischemic uveitis)

Iris

Neovascularization
± Increased intraocular pressure

Pupil

Sluggish reaction
Relative afferent defect

Lens

Cataract

Retina

Dilated arterioles
Dilated venules
Microaneurysms
Retinal hemorrhages
Neovascularization
Vitreous hemorrhage
Traction retinal detachment
Fluorescein angiography: decreased filling and increased transit time

2.   Subdivide findings (Table 16-7)
 a.   Anterior segment ischemia
  i.   Changes in intraocular pressure, elevated from neovascular glaucoma, lower intraocular pressure from chronic hypoperfusion of the ciliary body
 b.   Hypoperfusion retinopathy
3.   Ischemic uveitis is nonresponsive to topical corticosteroid drops
4.   Hypoperfusion retinopathy, also known as *venous stasis retinopathy* with dilated but not torturous retinal veins, occurs 3 to 4 times more commonly than anterior segment ischemia
5.   Retinopathy: dot-and-blot hemorrhages typically located in midperiphery
6.   Treatment
 a.   Ocular neovascularization: intravitreal anti–vascular endothelial growth factor (VEGF) agent; panretinal photocoagulation
 b.   Injection of anti-VEGF into the anterior chamber for anterior segment neovascularization
 c.   Medical:
  i.   Therapy to treat the underlying vascular risk factors
 d.   Surgical therapy:
  i.   Carotid endarterectomy
  ii.   Carotid artery stenting
  iii.   Extracranial-intracranial arterial bypass
 e.   Occasionally intraocular pressure may become markedly elevated after improved carotid blood flow
7.   Five-year mortality: 40% leading cause of death is myocardial infarction
8.   May rarely occur from other causes of carotid stenosis (eg, giant cell arteritis, Takayasu arteritis, Moyamoya syndrome)

    F.   Internal carotid artery dissection

        1.   Leads to ischemia due to decreased blood flow or distal embolization

        2.   Responsible for around 2% of all ischemic strokes

        3.   Cause of stroke in 10% to 25% of younger patients 15 to 49 years of age

        4.   Etiology:

            a.   Spontaneous

            b.   Traumatic

            c.   Arterial wall disease (pseudoxanthoma elasticum, fibrous dysplasia, Ehlers-Danlos syndrome, syphilis)

        5.   Ocular involvement:

            a.   Horner syndrome (see Chapter 8)

            b.   TMVL

            c.   ION

            d.   CRAO

            e.   Ocular motor cranial nerve palsies

        6.   Associated symptoms:

            a.   Headache

            b.   Eye pain

            c.   Neck pain

            d.   Tinnitus

            e.   Dysgeusia

         7.   Diagnostic studies:

            a.   MRA of head and neck may show vessel narrowing "string sign" and hemorrhage within the vessel wall

            b.   CTA of head and neck

         8.   Treatment: controversial

            a.   Medical: generally anticoagulation of some form until recanalization occurs (typically within 6 months)

            b.   Surgical: carotid artery stenting and flow diversion

    G. Moyamoya syndrome

        1.   Condition, more common in Asians, that causes progressive stenosis of the intracranial internal carotid arteries and their proximal branches and predisposes to stroke

        2.   Associated conditions:

            a.   Radiotherapy to the head and neck

            b.   Down syndrome

            c.   Sickle cell disease

            d.   Neurofibromatosis type 1

            e.   Congenital optic disc anomalies (eg, morning glory anomaly)

        3.   Neuroradiologic studies:

            a.   Angiographic appearance characterized by stenosis of the distal intracranial internal carotid artery, extending to the proximal anterior and middle cerebral arteries

            b.   Development of an extensive collateral network at the skull base along with the classic "puff of smoke" appearance on angiography

        4.   Treatment

            a.   Medical: antiplatelet agents and anticoagulation

            b.   Surgical: vascular bypass

H. Ocular motor cranial nerve palsies
1. Very rare association with carotid thrombosis or dissection
2. Ocular pain
3. Ipsilateral visual loss
4. III, IV, VI nerve palsies last 6 to 24 hours
5. Thrombosis of branches of ophthalmic artery supplying orbital branches of III, IV, VI nerves causes ophthalmoplegia; transient because collateral flow is able to restore perfusion to ocular motor nerves (see Figure 16-1)

REFERENCES

1. Trobe JD. Carotid endarterectomy: who needs it? *Ophthalmology*. 1987;94:725-730.
2. Ahmed R, Foroozan R. Transient monocular visual loss. *Neurol Clin*. 2010;28:619-629.
3. Petzold A, Islam N, Hu HH, Plant GT. Embolic and nonembolic transient monocular visual field loss: a clinicopathologic review. *Surv Ophthalmol*. 2013;58:42-62.
4. Carter JE. Carotid artery disease and its ocular manifestations. *Ophthalmol Clin North Am*. 1992;5:425-443.

BIBLIOGRAPHY

Alim-Marvasti A, BI W, Mahroo OA, Barbur JL, Pland GT. Transient smartphone "blindness". *N Engl J Med*. 2016;374:2502–2504.

Benavente O, Eliasiw W, Streifler JY, et al. Prognosis after transient monocular blindness associated with carotid-artery stenosis. *N Engl J Med*. 2001;345:1084-1090.

Biousse V. The coagulation system. *J Neuroophthalmol*. 2003;23:50-62.

Biousse V. Cerebrovascular diseases. In: Miller NR, Newman NJ, eds. *Walsh and Hoyt's Clinical Neuro-Ophthalmology*. 6th ed. Vol 7. Baltimore, MD: Williams & Wilkins; 2005:1967-2168.

Biousse V, Trobe JD. Transient monocular visual loss. *Am J Ophthalmol*. 2003;140:717-722.

Brott TG, Howard G, Roubin GS, et al. Long-term results of stenting versus endarterectomy for carotid-artery stenosis. *N Engl J Med*. 2016;374:1021-1031.

Burde RM, Savino PJ, Trobe JD. Transient visual loss. In: Burde RM, Savino PJ, Trobe JD, eds. *Clinical Decisions in Neuro-Ophthalmology*. 3rd ed. St Louis, MO: Mosby-Year Book; 2002:94-113.

Davis SM, Donnan GA. Clinical practice. Secondary prevention after ischemic stroke or transient ischemic attack. *N Engl J Med*. 2012;366:1914-1922.

Engelter ST, Traenka C, Von Hessling A, Lyrer PA. Diagnosis and treatment of cervical artery dissection. *Neurol Clin*. 2015;33:421-441.

Executive Committee for the Asymptomatic Carotid Atherosclerosis Study. Endarterectomy for asymptomatic carotid stenosis. *JAMA*. 1995;275:1421-1428.

Grotta JC. Clinical practice. Carotid stenosis. *N Engl J Med*. 2013;369:1143-1150.

Lawlor M, Perry R, Hunt BJ, Plant GT. Strokes and vision: the management of ischemic arterial disease affecting the retina and occipital lobe. *Surv Ophthalmol*. 2015;60:296-309.

Lee J, Kim SW, Lee SC, et al. Co-occurrence of acute retinal artery occlusion and acute ischemic stroke: diffusion-weighted magnetic resonance imaging study. *Am J Ophthalmol*. 2014;157:1231-1238.

Mendrinos E, Machinis TG, Pournaras CJ. Ocular ischemic syndrome. *Surv Ophthalmol*. 2010;55:2-34.

Schumacher M, Schmidt D, Jurklies B, et al. EAGLE-Study Group. Central retinal artery occlusion: local intra-arterial fibrinolysis versus conservative treatment, a multicenter randomized trial. *Ophthalmology*. 2010;11:1367-1375.

Scott RM, Smith ER. Moyamoya disease and moyamoya syndrome. *N Engl J Med*. 2009;360:1226-1237.

Trobe JD. Carotid endarterectomy for transient monocular visual loss and other ocular ischemic conditions. *J Neuroophthalmol*. 2005;25:259-261.

Winterkorn J, Kupersmith MJ, Wirtschafter JD, Forman S. Treatment of vasospastic amaurosis fugax with calcium-channel blockers. *N Engl J Med*. 1993;329:396-398.

CHAPTER 17

Nonorganic Visual Disorders

Richard H. Fish, MD, FACS; Rod Foroozan, MD; and Michael S. Vaphiades, DO

I. **DEFINITIONS AND HISTORICAL PERSPECTIVE**
   A. Nonorganic visual disorders
      1. No physiologic or organic basis
      2. *Nonorganic* has been suggested as the best term. Multiple other terms have been used: *functional, nonphysiologic*
      3. Classically divided into 2 main groups:
         a. Hysteria
         b. Malingering
      4. These 2 groups cannot always be differentiated; rather form a spectrum of disease
      5. Accounts for 1% to 5% of patient visits in a general ophthalmic practice
   B. Malingering: willfully misleading the existence or seriousness of a disease or disability for the purpose of a consciously desired end
      1. Duke-Elder[1]: "Common manifestation of human weakness…wicked or lazy"
      2. Keltner and colleagues[2]: California syndrome—economic gain from visual loss. Estimated $300 million paid in 1982 for fraudulent workers' compensation claims
      3. During Fiscal Year 2009-2010, Fraud Division of California Department of Insurance identified and reported 5728 suspected fraudulent claims, made 269 arrests, and referred 280 submissions to prosecuting authorities. Potential loss amounted to $1.15 billion
   C. Hysteria (Greek: "condition of the womb"): also known as *conversion disorder.* Subconscious expression of symptoms without demonstrable organic findings, usually involving loss or alteration of sensorimotor functions. Symptoms may have underlying symbolic meaning and are often precipitated by psychological stress or physical trauma
      1. Referred to in Egyptian papyri, writings of Hippocrates, and in the New Testament of the Bible
      2. "Ancient (Greeks)…traditionally believed that bodily symptoms we now call hysterical were caused by a womb which wandered throughout the body."[3] These ideas had been incorrectly ascribed to Plato for 2 millennia, but subsequent scholarship and Greek translations have disputed this[4]
      3. Early neurologists Charcot and Babinksi attempted to explain hysterical paralysis and functional vision loss

- 233 -

Foroozan R, Vaphiades MS. *Kline's Neuro-Ophthalmology Review Manual, Eighth Edition (pp 233-245).* © 2018 SLACK Incorporated.

        4.   Freud[5]: sexual pleasure in looking (scopophilia); results in repression of forbidden sights into the unconscious with the eyes now "at the disposal of the repressed sexual instinct and hence unable to function properly"

D. DSM-V[6]

    1.   "Hysteria" is now included in the large category of Somatic Symptom and Related Disorders: "…prominence of somatic symptoms associated with significant distress and impairment" that "have their initial presentation mainly in medical rather than mental health care settings"

        a.   Includes somatic symptom disorder; illness anxiety disorder; psychological factors affecting other medical conditions; other somatic symptom and related disorders

        b.   "Hysteria" would now be properly termed *conversion disorder* (functional neurological symptom disorder). Diagnostic criteria are as follows:

            i.   One or more symptoms of altered voluntary motor or sensory function

           ii.   Clinical findings provide evidence of incompatibility between the symptom and recognized neurological or medical conditions

          iii.   The symptom or deficit is not better explained by another medical or mental disorder

          iv.   The symptom or deficit causes clinically significant distress or impairment in social, occupational, or other important areas of functioning, or it warrants medical evaluation

           v.   Further classified according to symptom type. Here "with special sensory symptoms (eg, visual…disturbance)"

        c.   Ocular Münchausen syndrome (see page 243, IV, H)—now termed *factitious disorder*—is also under the category of Somatic Symptom and Related Disorders

            i.   Falsification of physical or psychological signs or symptoms, or induction of injury or disease, associated with identified deception

           ii.   The individual presents him- or herself (or another individual [formerly "Münchausen's by proxy"]) to others as ill, impaired, or injured

          iii.   The deceptive behavior is evident even in the absence of obvious external rewards

          iv.   The behavior is not better explained by another mental disorder, such as delusional disorder or another psychotic disorder

    2.   "Malingering" is not considered a mental illness. In DSM-V, it receives a V code as one of the other conditions that is the focus of clinical attention. Defined as "intentional production of false or grossly exaggerated physical or psychological symptoms, motivated by external incentives such as avoiding military duty, avoiding work, obtaining financial compensation, evading criminal prosecution, or obtaining drugs." Suspected if the following occurs:

        a.   Medicolegal presentation—attorney referral; self-referral during legal civil or criminal proceedings

        b.   Discrepancy between disability and objective findings

        c.   Lack of cooperation during diagnostic evaluation and in complying with prescribed treatment regimen

        d.   Associated with antisocial personality disorder

E. Differentiating malingering from hysteria

    1.   Malingerer will exaggerate symptoms ("blinder than the blind"), while hysterics are classically described as having "la belle indifference" to their affliction

    2.   Hysterical patients tend to be cooperative; malingerers irritable and combative, especially with prolonged testing

3. Malingering usually involves secondary gain (eg, financial reward or avoiding military service). Hysterics may receive secondary gain in the form of attention

4. DSM-V: "Malingering differs from factitious disorder in that the motivation for the symptom production in malingering is an external incentive, whereas in factitious disorder, external incentives are absent. Malingering is differentiated from conversion disorder and somatic symptom–related mental disorders by the intentional production of symptoms and by the obvious external incentives associated with it. Definite evidence of feigning (such as clear evidence that loss of function is present during the examination but not at home) would suggest a diagnosis of factitious disorder if the individual's apparent aim is to assume the sick role, or malingering if it is to obtain an incentive, such as money"[6]

5. A 2008 study indicated that a "sunglasses sign" or wearing sunglasses in the neuro-ophthalmology clinic, in a patient without an obvious ophthalmic reason to wear sunglasses, is highly suggestive of nonorganic visual loss

6. A 2016 study revealed that 72% of nonorganic or medically unexplained visual loss patients were female. These patients had significantly higher rates of bilateral visual impairment (41%), premorbid psychiatric (27%), as well as functional (24%) diagnoses and psychotropic medication usage (22%) and were significantly more likely to report preceding psychological stress (18%)

II. **EVALUATION: IN ASSESSING PATIENTS WITH NONORGANIC VISUAL DISORDERS, LEARN A FEW TESTS WELL AND BE ABLE TO PERFORM THEM QUICKLY AND NATURALLY. THE DIAGNOSIS OF NONORGANIC VISUAL LOSS REQUIRES THE EXCLUSION OF AN ORGANIC CAUSE FOR THE PRESENTING VISUAL DISTURBANCE AND THE DEMONSTRATION OF NONORGANIC PHYSICAL FINDINGS, THOSE THAT ARE INCONSISTENT OR PHYSIOLOGICALLY INCONGRUOUS ON EXAMINATION**

A. Total binocular blindness

1. Observation: truly blind moves cautiously, bumps into things naturally; hysteric avoids objects, "seeing unconsciously"; malingerer goes out of his or her way to bump into objects

2. Pupillary response: easiest and single most important test

   a. Intact direct and consensual responses exclude anterior visual pathway disease (do not forget about pharmacologic mydriasis in a malingerer)

   b. In patients with vision better than NLP, there may be no consistent relationship between amount of visual loss and pupillary deficit

3. Menace reflex: blinking to visual threat

4. Sudden strong illumination. Difficult to suppress reflex tearing

5. Signature: truly blind patients have no difficulty. Functionally blind patients sign their name with exaggerated illegibility

6. Looking at hand or touching index fingers together depends on proprioception, not vision. Blind patients have no trouble with this; malingerers, thinking that these tasks require good vision, will perform poorly

7. OKN: difficult but possible to suppress. Optimum response obtained when rate of succession of object is 3 to 12 per second

8. Mirror tracking: eyes move in response to the image in a mirror as it is rocked back and forth. Mirror must be large enough to prevent patient from looking around it (approximately 33 × 67 cm)

9. Making sudden ridiculous facial expressions

10. Visual evoked response: flash and pattern-reversal stimuli. Correlation exists between check size and level of acuity. Although difficult, it is possible to consciously alter response to pattern-reversal stimulation with convergence, meditation, and intense concentration

B. Total monocular blindness: more common than binocular. Can use any of the previous with unaffected eyes occluded

1. Pupillary response

    a. The swinging flashlight test provides valuable objective evidence of monocular prechiasmal (retina or optic nerve) damage. An RAPD is often present if a patient has a monocular optic neuropathy or an extensive retinal disorder. The absence of an RAPD in a patient reporting monocular blindness does not confirm a nonorganic disorder but greatly increases suspicion of one. Patients with true monocular blindness and bilateral optic nerve dysfunction may not have an RAPD. Also, the patient may state, "My right eye is blind" and have no RAPD, when in reality the patient is erroneously lateralizing a right homonymous hemianopia to the right eye because of the fact that the field loss of the right temporal hemifield is larger than that of the left nasal hemifield

2. The prism dissociation test

    a. The prism dissociation test utilizes a 5 or 6-diopter base-down prism (some patients have fusional amplitudes up to 4-diopters) placed in front of the normal eye and a ½ diopter prism placed in any direction over the "impaired" eye (so the patient will not become suspicious). A 20/20 Snellen letter is projected and the patient is asked if he or she can see 2 vertically placed letters. If the patient can read both letters, the acuity in the "impaired" eye is 20/20

    b. A variation of this test uses an 8-diopter base-down prism placed in front of the normal eye and no prism in front of the "impaired" eye. The patient is then asked if he or she can see the top and bottom line and then asked to read each line. A vertical refixation movement of the eyes is observed when the patient shifts fixation from the lower to the higher image. The higher image represents visual acuity in the eye with the prism (normal eye) and the lower image represents visual acuity in the "impaired" eye. However, to prove normal acuity, the patient must read both (doubled) 20/20 lines. A report of diplopia also provides evidence of binocular visual function

3. Fixation tests

    a. Ten-diopter base-out test: relies on refixation movements to avoid diplopia. Ten-diopter base-out prism in front of a normal eye produces shift of both eyes with a refixation movement of the other eye. A truly blind eye will not refixate, and a prism placed before this eye should result in no movement of either eye

    b. Vertical bar: ruler held 5 inches from the nose in between the eyes while the patient reads at near. Overlap of visual fields allows a binocular person to read across the bar without interruption. A truly monocular patient will pause to shift fixation across the bar. If the patient reads without interruption, functional blindness is confirmed. Can also use a prism in front of the suspected eye, resulting in diplopia that should interrupt reading

4. Fogging tests

    a. Both eyes are open in a phoropter; the patient begins reading the eye chart. Examiner progressively adds more plus to the good eye while the patient keeps reading. Final line read is the patient's acuity in the suspected eye

    b. Crossed cylinder technique: 2 strong cylindrical lenses of equal power—plus and minus—are placed at the same axis in the trial frame over the good eye. Patient reads with both eyes open and the examiner rotates one lens 45 degrees, fogging the good eye

    c. Instill a cycloplegic agent into the unaffected eye; have the patient read at near

5. Color tests
   a. Red/green duochrome in the projector, red/green glasses worn such that the red lens covers the suspected eye. Eye behind the red lens sees letters on red and not green side of the chart; eye behind the green lens sees only letters on the green side. If the patient reads the entire line, the suspected eye is being used
   b. Red/green glasses and Worth 4-dot test. Patient should see appropriate number of dots
   c. Polaroid glasses and vectographic slides: each eye sees different portions of the eye chart. If the patient reads the entire line, both eyes are being utilized
6. Stereoscopic tests
   a. Titmus stereoacuity was traditionally felt to be directly proportional to Snellen acuity (eg, 40 seconds of arc stereoacuity is compatible with no worse than 20/20 Snellen acuity OU). However, Titmus stereoacuity cannot definitively establish normal Snellen acuity. It can suggest, but not fully establish, the diagnosis of nonorganic visual loss. Thus, other conformational tests of normal acuity should also be considered

C. Diminished vision: simulation of visual acuity < 20/20. More difficult to detect. May be binocular or monocular. Can use most of the tests discussed previously, plus the following:
   1. "Bottom-up" acuity method: start with 20/10 line and then proceed up the chart until the patient reads
   2. Near vision: a discrepancy between distance vision and near vision can be suggestive of nonorganic visual loss
D. Electrophysiologic testing
   1. May be helpful to exclude organic causes of visual loss
      a. Full-field ERG
      b. Multifocal ERG
      c. VEP
      d. Multifocal VEP
   2. Erroneous results may occur with ERG and VEP testing, especially in patients who are inattentive or intentionally defocus
   3. Visual angle: varying test distances with eye chart, Landolt C rings, or Tumbling E block such that the patient sees a smaller visual angle or demonstrates inconsistencies (eg, reading 20/20 letters at 10 feet is equivalent to 20/40 acuity)
   4. Move the patient back and forth slightly in the chair, helping him or her "get into focus" or place combinations of lenses adding up to plano in a trial frame to help magnify the vision

III. CONDITIONS MISDIAGNOSED AS NONORGANIC VISUAL LOSS

A. Keratoconus: biomicroscopy, keratometry readings, corneal topography
B. Amblyopia: look for strabismus, anisometropia
C. Early Stargardt disease: macular examination, fluorescein angiography
D. Retinitis pigmentosa sine pigmento: ERG
E. Central serous chorioretinopathy: macular examination, OCT, fluorescein angiography
F. Cystoid macular edema: ophthalmoscopy, fluorescein angiography, OCT
G. Cone dystrophy: ERG
H. Paraneoplastic retinopathy: ERG, systemic evaluation
I. Bilateral occipital lobe infarctions: MRI

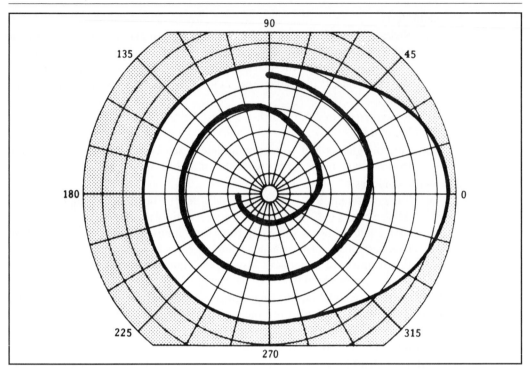

Figure 17-1. Spiraling isopters.

IV. OTHER NONORGANIC EYE DISEASES
  A. Visual field loss
    1. Monocular visual field defects
        a. Concentric contraction with no expansion of the field at an increasing test distance (tunnel vision, see Figure 1-25 and Chapter 1 for differential diagnosis)
        b. Spiraling isopters (Figure 17-1)
        c. Crossing isopters (Figure 17-2)
        d. These same visual field defects have also been reported in patients with frontal lobe tumors
        e. Monocular temporal hemianopia that persists on binocular testing (Figure 17-3)
    2. Binocular visual field defects
        a. Normal binocular perimetry: visual field performed with both eyes open measures approximately 180 degrees in width with no blind spots due to overlap of monocular fields
        b. Monocular visual field subtends approximately 150 degrees, with a greater field temporally due to unpaired temporal crescent (see Chapter 1)
        c. True monocular blindness: binocular perimetry demonstrates blind spot of a normal eye with loss of the temporal crescent of the blind eye (Figure 17-4)
        d. Nonorganic monocular blindness: binocular perimetry reveals a full visual field (Figure 17-5)
        e. Nonorganic bitemporal hemianopia: patients with true bitemporal hemianopia have a binocular field composed of 2 nasal hemifields (Figure 17-6). With nonorganic bitemporal hemianopia, the patient claims inability to see temporally, with only a thin island of vision straddling the vertical midline (Figure 17-7)

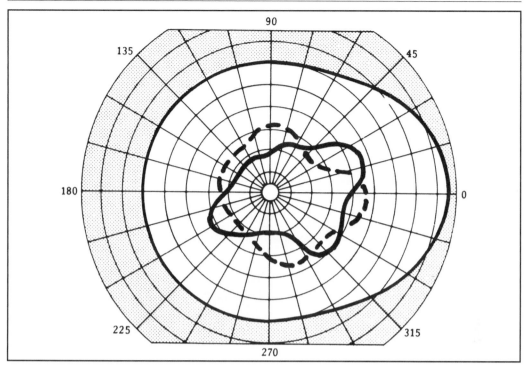

Figure 17-2. Crossing isopters.

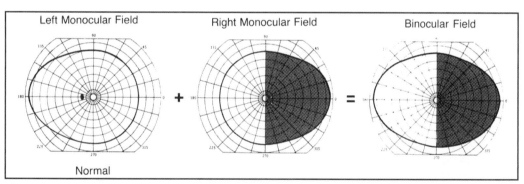

Figure 17-3. Nonorganic hemianopia.

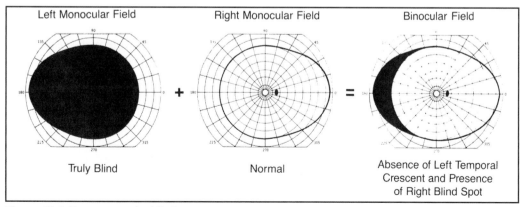

Figure 17-4. True monocular blindness.

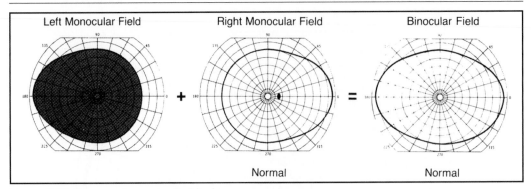

Figure 17-5. Nonorganic monocular blindness.

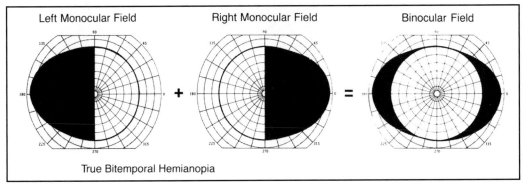

Figure 17-6. True bitemporal hemianopia.

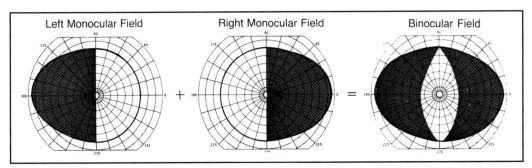

Figure 17-7. Nonorganic bitemporal hemianopia.

      f.   Binasal hemianopia: rare. Usually due to optic nerve or retinal disease (glaucoma, disc drusen, chronic papilledema, retinoschisis, retinal detachment, chorioretinal degeneration). Intracranial causes include basilar skull fracture, neurosyphilis, chiasmal arachnoiditis, and neoplasm. Binasal defects of organic etiology are seldom complete and rarely respect the vertical midline. If defects are complete, there is "prefixation blindness" (Figure 17-8)

      g.   Caution: automated perimetry can be suggestive but typically cannot differentiate nonorganic from organic visual field loss. Malingerers can simulate neurologic field defects when tested with an automated visual field machine

B. Voluntary nystagmus

    1. Irregular brief bursts of rapid frequency, low amplitude, horizontal pendular eye movements; actually back-to-back saccades

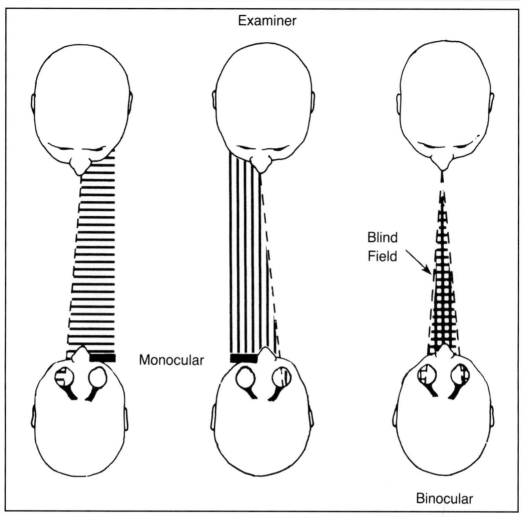

Figure 17-8. Binasal hemianopia. Monocular testing reveals hemianopic field defects nasal to the visual axis in each eye. With an organic etiology, binocular testing confirms blindness in the area where the 2 nasal hemifields overlap (prefixation blindness). An object moving through this area will suddenly disappear and reappear. (Adapted from Thompson HS. Binasal field loss. In: Thompson HS, ed. *Topics in Neuro-Ophthalmology.* Baltimore, MD: Williams & Wilkins; 1979:84.)[7]

2. Up to 8% of normal individuals can produce this
3. Usually bilateral and conjugate
4. May be associated with convergence, fluttering eyelids, blinking, or strained facial expression
5. Oscillopsia common
6. The initiation of nystagmus is under voluntary control, while rate, amplitude, and duration of nystagmus are not
7. Difficult to maintain longer than 10 to 20 seconds
8. May be familial

C. Accommodative spasm
1. Relatively common
2. Intermittent episodes of convergence associated with miosis, accommodation, and induced myopia

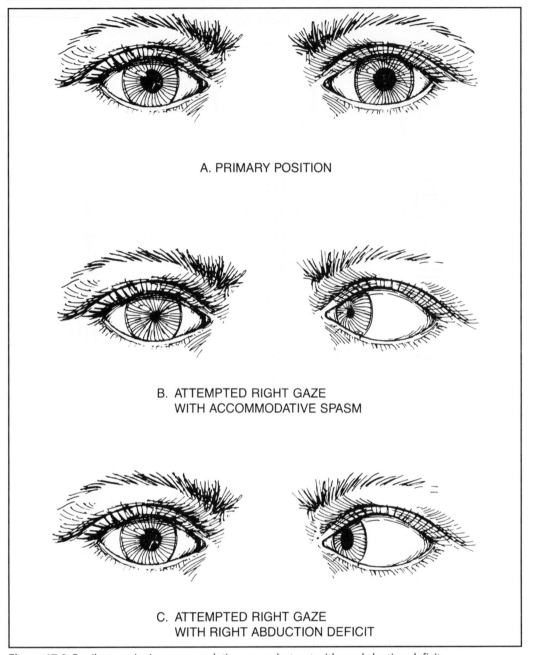

A. PRIMARY POSITION

B. ATTEMPTED RIGHT GAZE
WITH ACCOMMODATIVE SPASM

C. ATTEMPTED RIGHT GAZE
WITH RIGHT ABDUCTION DEFICIT

Figure 17-9. Pupils constrict in accommodative spasm but not with an abduction deficit.

3. Pupils constrict on attempted lateral gaze (Figure 17-9)
4. No abduction deficit with oculocephalic (doll's head maneuver) or caloric testing
5. May have diplopia and micropsia
6. May be interrupted by patching or cycloplegia
7. Differential diagnosis includes VI nerve palsy and other conditions causing limited abduction (see Chapter 4)
8. Treatment is difficult; may involve atropine drops and bifocals; medial rectus injection with botulinum toxin

D. Monocular diplopia: usually nonorganic cause but occasionally organic
   1. External causes: chalazion; eyelid tumor at ridge of corneal epithelium; mucus strand, vegetable fiber, or oil droplet in tear film
   2. Optical causes: irregular astigmatism; keratoconus; tilted or subluxed lens; lens clefts, vacuoles, or cataracts; gas bubbles, glass, crystals, parasite larvae in vitreous; macular cysts; epimacular membrane, central serous chorioretinopathy, diabetic macular edema causes distortion, not diplopia
   3. Neurologic causes: rare. Reported in pituitary tumor, tumor or hemorrhage of occipital cortex, lesions in FEF controlling voluntary eye movement
   4. Transiently seen following strabismus surgery in patients with anomalous retinal correspondence
   5. Diagnosis:
      a. Pinhole usually eliminates optical causes
      b. Careful retinoscopy and biomicroscopy is essential
      c. Contact lenses may be useful in correcting about 60% of cases of monocular diplopia
      d. Corneal topography can be helpful, especially when irregular astigmatism is present
E. Voluntary blepharospasm
   1. May be unilateral or bilateral
   2. May resemble ptosis or true blepharospasm
      a. Assess finding in upgaze as nonorganic ptosis with brow depression seen with forced eyelid closure will typically be more difficult to maintain in upgaze
   3. Isolated or associated with nonorganic decreased vision or accommodative spasm
F. Nonorganic asthenopia
   1. Complaints of painful sensations in and around the eyes, lacrimation, photophobia
   2. Inability to read without headache or eyestrain despite correction of refractive error and normal muscle balance
G. Voluntary gaze palsy
   1. Infrequently seen
   2. Limitation of upgaze
      a. Lack of cooperation
      b. Normal aging phenomenon
      c. Nonorganic etiology
      d. Rule out dorsal midbrain syndrome (see Chapter 2)
   3. Paralysis of horizontal gaze: one case report of a patient unable to make saccadic or pursuit movements to the left. Examiners were unable to overcome "paralysis" with oculocephalic (doll's head maneuver) testing, OKN, or mirror tracking. Also noted were convergence and miosis on attempted left gaze
H. Ocular Münchausen syndrome
   1. Deliberate deception by a patient involving fabricated medical histories, self-inflicted physical abnormalities, and self-mutilation
   2. Reported ocular manifestations include voluntary nystagmus; subconjunctival hemorrhage; conjunctivitis; pharmacologic mydriasis; corneal erosion, repeated foreign bodies, ulcer, and alkali burn; self-induced chronic orbital cellulitis requiring exenteration; and chronic periorbital abscess
   3. Psychiatric evaluation suggested, but treatment is frequently unsuccessful
I. Nonorganic chromatopsia or micropsia

V. NATURAL HISTORY OF NONORGANIC VISUAL LOSS

A. One-quarter of patients have been noted to have a chronic course with no improvement of visual acuity

B. Prior series, especially before institution of multifocal ERG, have noted frequency of maculopathy in patients thought to be nonorganic

C. Just over 50% of patients have been noted to have continued functional visual loss when followed for months to years. Few were socially or economically impaired despite persistent visual loss

D. Seventy-two percent of 46 patients younger than 21 years of age in one series showed improvement in nonorganic visual field loss

E. Beware of the patient with both organic and nonorganic disease. A follow-up study of 85 patients with a variety of conversion disorders found the following:

   1. Twenty-two patients were found to have coexistent organic diseases, including generalized disease of the CNS

   2. Two patients subsequently developed schizophrenia

   3. Four patients committed suicide

   4. Eight patients died of organic disease that was present at the time of diagnosis of "hysteria"

F. Children tend to have a good prognosis (85% with complete resolution by 1 year in one series)

G. Consider abuse as an underlying contributing factor for the development of symptoms

VI. TREATMENT OF NONORGANIC EYE DISEASE

A. Reassurance that the problem will get better, emphasizing positive things that the eye does well—peripheral vision, normal pupils, optic nerve, retina, etc

B. Eye drops, orthoptic exercises, or spectacles may draw attention to the eyes and undermine reassurance

C. Confrontation is rarely productive

D. Psychiatric consultation as these patients may have underlying psychiatric disorders and a preceding strong emotional event leading to the current symptoms, and may be more likely to develop depression and anxiety

REFERENCES

1. Duke-Elder S, ed. *System of Ophthalmology*. Vol V. London, UK: Henry Kimpton; 1970:487-501.

2. Keltner JL, May WN, Johnson CA, et al. The California syndrome. Functional visual complaints with potential economic impact. *Ophthalmology*. 1985;92:427-435.

3. Adair MJ. Plato's view of the 'wandering uterus'. *Classical J*. 1996;91:153-163.

4. Adair MJ. Plato's lost theory of hysteria. *Psychoanalytic Quarterly*. 1997;66:98-106.

5. Freud S. The psycho-analytic view of psychogenic disturbances of vision. In: Freud S, ed. *The Standard Edition of the Complete Psychological Works of Sigmund Freud*. Vol XI. London, UK: The Hogart Press; 1957:211-218.

6. American Psychiatric Association. *Diagnostic and Statistical Manual of Mental Disorders*. 5th ed. Arlington, VA: American Psychiatric Publishing.

7. Thompson HS. Binasal field loss. In: Thompson HS, ed. *Topics in Neuro-Ophthalmology*. Baltimore, MD: Williams & Wilkins; 1979:84.

Bibliography

Bengtzen R, Woodward M, Lynn MJ, Newman NJ, Biousse V. The "sunglasses sign" predicts nonorganic visual loss in neuro-ophthalmologic practice. *Neurology.* 2008;70:218-221.

Dattilo M, Biousse V, Bruce BB, Newman NJ. Functional and simulated visual loss. *Handb Clin Neurol.* 2017;139:329-341.

Goldstein JH, Schneekloth B. Spasm of the near reflex: a spectrum of anomalies. *Surv Ophthalmol.* 1996;40:269-278.

Lessell S. Nonorganic visual loss: what's in a name? *Am J Ophthalmol.* 2011;151:569-571.

Lim SA, Siatkowski RM, Farris BK. Functional visual loss in adults and children. *Ophthalmology.* 2005;112:1821-1828.

Massicotte EC, Semela L, Hedges TR 3rd. Multifocal visual evoked potential in nonorganic visual field loss. *Arch Ophthalmol.* 2005;123:364-367.

McIntyre A. Spasm of the near reflex: a literature review. *Br Orthopt J.* 2001;58:3-11.

O'Leary ÉD, McNeillis B, Aybek S, Riordan-Eva P, David AS. Medically unexplained visual loss in a specialist clinic: a retrospective case-control comparison. *J Neurol Sci.* 2016;361:272-276.

Reynolds EH. Hysteria, conversion and functional disorders: a neurological contribution to classification issues. *BJP.* 2012;201:253-254.

Scott JA, Egan RA. Prevalence of organic neuro-ophthalmologic disease in patients with functional visual loss. *Am J Ophthalmol.* 2003;135:670-675.

Sitko KR, Peragallo JH, Bidot S, Biousse V, Newman NJ, Bruce BB. Pitfalls in the use of stereoacuity in the diagnosis of nonorganic visual loss. *Ophthalmology.* 2016;123:198-202.

Stewart JFG. Automated perimetry and malingerers. *Ophthalmology.* 1995;102:27-32.

Toldo I, Pinello L, Suppiej A, et al. Nonorganic (psychogenic) visual loss in children: a retrospective series. *J Neuroophthalmol.* 2010;30:26-30.

Wandling LJ, Wandling GR Jr, Faith Marshall M, Lee MS. Truth-telling and deception in the management of nonorganic vision loss. *Can J Ophthalmol.* 2016;51:390-392.

CHAPTER 18

Disorders of Higher Visual Function

JASON J. S. BARTON, MD, PHD, FRCPC;
CHRISTOPHER A. GIRKIN, MD, MSPH, FACS; AND MICHAEL S. VAPHIADES, DO

I. **ANATOMIC OVERVIEW**

   A. Visual information is sent from the retina to striate cortex through the retino-geniculo-striate relay, which has 3 subcortical divisions: the parvocellular, the magnocellular, and, to a lesser extent, the koniocellular pathways

   B. After striate cortex, visual signals are distributed into a large hierarchical network of extrastriate visual areas in the occipital, temporal, and parietal lobes

   C. These extrastriate areas are organized into 2 main cortical processing streams: a ventral occipitotemporal stream (the "what stream"), and a dorsal occipitoparietal stream (the "where stream"; Figure 18-1)

   D. As one proceeds higher in the visual hierarchy, regions become less concerned with the specific retinotopic location of visual stimuli and more concerned with their specific properties, like color, form, and motion

   E. Damage to extrastriate areas leads to loss of specific types of perception, causing distinctive visual syndromes that have localizing value for where the lesion is (Table 18-1)

II. **COMPONENTS OF THE VISUAL SYSTEM**

   A. Retinogeniculate pathways

   1. More than 22 types of ganglion cells exist in the primate retina. While many project to subcortical areas for functions, such as the pupil light reflex, diurnal rhythms, and reflexive eye movements, 3 project via the LGN to striate and extrastriate cortex to support conscious visual perception

   2. Parvocellular pathway

      a. Originates in midget ganglion cells in the retina, which have small receptive fields and thus high spatial resolution

      b. Projects to parvocellular layers of the LGN

      c. Conveys red-green color opponency

      d. Parvocellular cells sustain firing as long as a light is present and have low temporal resolution (ie, cannot keep up with rapidly changing stimuli)

      e. High-pass resolution perimetry, contrast sensitivity at high spatial frequencies, and color tests probe this pathway

Foroozan R, Vaphiades MS. *Kline's Neuro-Ophthalmology Review Manual, Eighth Edition* (pp 247-259).
© 2018 SLACK Incorporated.

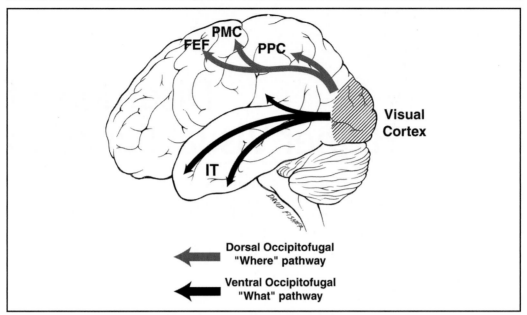

Figure 18-1. Parallel visual pathways in the human. The ventral ("what") pathway involves the medial inferotemporal cortex (IT) for object recognition. The dorsal ("where") pathway involves lateral occipital and PPC for spatial analysis, and projects to the FEF and premotor cortex (PMC).

Table 18-1

CEREBRAL VISUAL SYNDROMES

Area V1

      Cerebral blindness

      Anton syndrome

      Syndrome of agitated delirium and hemianopia

      Blindsight

Intermediate Visual Cortex

      Cerebral achromatopsia

      Cerebral akinetopsia

Dorsal Stream High-Level Cortex

      Bálint syndrome

      Simultanagnosia

      Optic ataxia

      Acquired ocular motor apraxia

      Hemineglect

Ventral Stream High-Level Cortex

      General visual agnosia

      Prosopagnosia

      Alexia (without agraphia)

      Topographagnosia

3. Magnocellular pathway
   a. Originates in parasol ganglion cells in the retina, which have large receptive fields and low spatial resolution
   b. Projects to magnocellular layers of the LGN
   c. Magnocellular cells fire transiently with onset and offset of stimuli and have high temporal resolution
   d. Frequency-doubling perimetry and motion-automated perimetry probe this pathway
4. Koniocellular pathway
   a. Originates from the bistratified ganglion cells in the retina, which have large receptive fields and low spatial resolution
   b. Conveys blue-yellow color opponency
   c. Short-wavelength automated perimetry (SWAP) probes this pathway

B. Early and intermediate visual cortical areas
   1. Macaque monkeys have more than 30 cortical areas with visual responsivity, comprising almost 50% of the entire cortex
   2. Area V1 is primary visual cortex, also known in humans as *striate cortex* (named for the stria of Gennari that can be seen in cross-section), calcarine cortex (as it occupies the calcarine sulcus and its banks), or Brodmann area 17
   3. Areas V2 and V3 are early visual areas that surround area V1 (Figure 18-2)
   4. Areas V4 and V4a are intermediate visual areas in the lingual gyrus, involved in color processing (Figure 18-3)
   5. Areas V5 and V5a, also known as the *MT and MST areas*, are intermediate visual areas in the lateral occipital lobe, involved in motion perception (see Figure 18-2)

C. High-level visual processing
   1. These can be grouped into a dorsal and a ventral stream of processing (see Figure 18-1)
      a. Dorsal occipitoparietal stream ("where" pathway)
         i. Includes the lateral intraparietal area and regions in the inferior parietal lobule
         ii. Involved in localizing objects in space, motion processing, stereopsis, and guidance of eye or reaching movements
         iii. Projects to parietal and frontal regions involved in motor control and subcortical regions like the SC
      b. Ventral occipitofugal pathway or "what" pathway
         i. Includes areas in medial occipitotemporal region and anterior temporal lobe
         ii. Involved in processing object color, shape, and texture
         iii. Such information interacts with memory and semantic (meaning) systems to support object recognition

III. SYNDROMES ASSOCIATED WITH DAMAGE TO STRIATE CORTEX (AREA V1)

A. Cerebral blindness
   1. Definition: loss of all conscious vision after damage to striate cortex and/or optic radiations
   2. Distinguished from ocular blindness by preserved pupil light reflexes; normal funduscopy and other signs of cerebral dysfunction can help
   3. VEPs may not be helpful, as they can be present in cerebral blindness or abnormal in healthy subjects for technical reasons

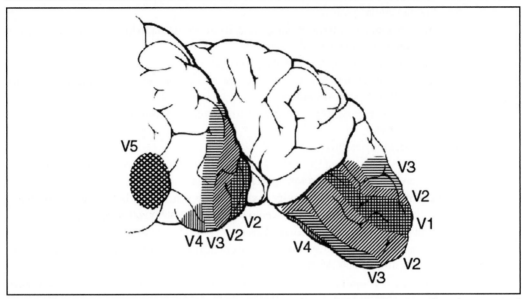

Figure 18-2. Posterior lateral view of the human visual cortex showing the clinically relevant visual associative areas. The cerebellum has been removed and the hemispheres have been separated and displaced to display medial and lateral occipital regions. V1 corresponds to the primary or striate visual cortex.

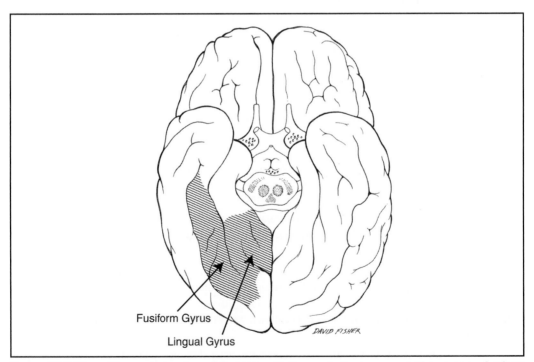

Figure 18-3. View of the ventral surface of the brain with the cerebellum removed. The posterior fusiform and lingual gyri contain the human color processing areas.

  4. Persistent cerebral blindness: common causes are embolic stroke and prolonged hypotension

  5. Transient cerebral blindness: common causes are postictal state, posterior reversible encephalopathy (PRES) from hypertension or chemotherapy, trauma, eclampsia, and venous thrombosis

  6. Post-traumatic cerebral blindness is a syndrome mainly of children and young adults, complicating 1% of closed head injury, with recovery often within 24 hours

  7. Normal MRI is a good prognostic sign for recovery from cerebral blindness

B. Anton syndrome

  1. Definition: denial of blindness, in the absence of dementia and delirium

  2. Occurs in 10% of patients with bilateral damage to striate cortex or optic radiations

  3. Patients with ocular blindness may also deny visual loss, but these usually have dementia or confusion and hence do not meet the strict definition

  4. If denial occurs in a nondemented patient with ocular blindness, he or she likely has bilateral frontal lobe disease

  5. Possible causes:

   a. Damage to higher cognitive centers mediating awareness

   b. Psychiatric denial

   c. Disconnection of visual experience from cerebral regions involved in awareness (eg, between thalamus and parietal lobes)

C. Syndrome of agitated delirium and hemianopia

  1. An acute confusional state may occur with sudden hemianopia

  2. It is linked to lesions that involve the medial occipital lobe, parahippocampus, and hippocampus

D. Blindsight

  1. Definition: unconscious visual abilities remaining in blind patients

  2. Mainly reported for patients with postchiasmal visual loss (ie, lesions of optic radiations or striate cortex)

  3. Proving blindsight in a patient requires careful exclusion of artifacts such as light scatter and unstable fixation

  4. A taxonomy

   a. Action blindsight: residual manual and saccadic localization of visual targets. This is the most studied type

   b. Attention blindsight: residual motion perception

   c. Agnosopsia: residual form and color perception

  5. Blindsight may depend on residual function of the following:

   a. The SC

   b. A pathway from the colliculus through the pulvinar to extrastriate cortex

   c. Surviving projections from the LGN to extrastriate cortex

  6. Not all patients with hemianopia or cerebral blindness have blindsight; a major challenge is to determine why some do and some do not

  7. It is unclear whether blindsight improves with practice, helps in rehabilitation from hemianopia, or is of any practical benefit to those who have it

IV. **SYNDROMES CAUSED BY DAMAGE TO EARLY VISUAL CORTEX (V2 AND V3)**

A. The effects of V2/V3 lesions are not well characterized, as most lesions will also affect V1 or the optic radiations

B. It is said that they may cause quadrantanopia, but this is debatable. Problems with figure-ground segregation and perception of illusory contours are predicted from neurophysiology

V. SYNDROMES CAUSED BY DAMAGE TO INTERMEDIATE VISUAL CORTEX

    A. Cerebral achromatopsia

       1. Definition: selective loss of color perception due to cerebral damage

       2. Caused by lesions of posterior lingual and fusiform gyri

       3. Bilateral lesions cause complete achromatopsia; unilateral lesions cause contralateral hemiachromatopsia, which is often asymptomatic

       4. Often associated with superior visual field defects and disorders of the ventral occipitotemporal stream, such as prosopagnosia

       5. Best diagnosed with tests of color sorting, such as the Farnsworth-Munsell 100-hue test

    B. Cerebral akinetopsia

       1. Definition: selective loss of visual motion perception due to cerebral damage

       2. Caused by bilateral lesions of the lateral occipital gyri, unilateral lesions may cause asymptomatic deficits in the contralateral hemifield

       3. Rare, with only 2 well-documented cases, due to cerebral infarctions following sagittal sinus thrombosis

       4. Requires special computerized tests of motion perception for diagnosis

VI. HIGH-LEVEL VISION: SYNDROMES OF THE DORSAL OCCIPITOTEMPORAL PATHWAY

    A. Bálint syndrome: a triad of simultanagnosia, optic ataxia, and ocular motor apraxia, with bilateral parietal lesions

       1. These 3 elements are only loosely associated and can occur independent of each other, as they result from damage to different networks for attention, manual motor control, and saccadic eye movements

       2. Diagnosing Bálint syndrome requires exclusion of extensive field defects and general cognitive impairment

    B. Simultanagnosia

       1. Definition: inability to interpret complex multi-element scenes, despite intact perception of individual elements

       2. This is an attentional deficit in that subjects cannot pay attention to more than one or a few objects at a time

       3. Often, patients see a few trees but not the forest, which is called *local capture*. If the big picture is compelling and vivid, though, they may show global capture, seeing the forest without being aware of the trees

       4. Due to bilateral lesions of Brodmann areas 18 and 19, in lateral occipital cortex

       5. Tested with multi-element displays, such as the Cookie Theft Picture: patients report only fragments of the display and cannot derive the overall meaning of the picture (Figure 18-4)

    C. Optic ataxia

       1. Definition: inaccurate guidance of reaching movements to visual objects, despite preserved visibility of the objects, and preserved sensation and movement of the reaching limb

       2. Related phenomenon is "visual disorientation," a defect in judging spatial position and distance of objects

       3. In some patients, this is not just a visuospatial problem. With unilateral lesions, optic ataxia may affect the contralateral arm only, while in other patients, reaching to somatosensory targets (ie, to their own body parts with their eyes closed) is also affected

       4. Optic ataxia is most evident when reaching to objects in the peripheral visual field, rather than to foveated targets

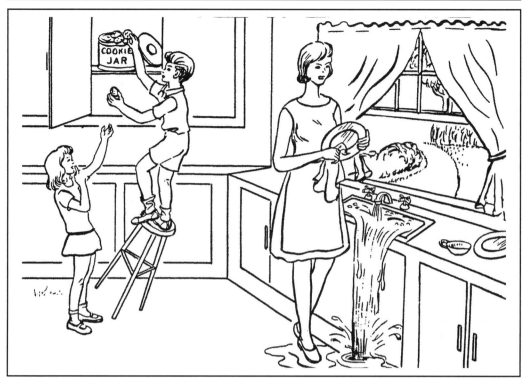

Figure 18-4. The "Cookie Theft Picture," adapted from the Boston Diagnostic Aphasia Examination. This picture contains a balance of information among the 4 visual field quadrants. A patient is asked to describe the events in the picture, a task that requires assimilation of the entire visual scene.

5. Due to lesions of inferior parietal lobule, occipitofrontal white matter tracts, or premotor cortex
6. Tested by having the patient reach with either arm for objects seen in one and then the other hemifield, then contrasting this with reaching with eyes closed to his or her own body parts

D. Acquired ocular motor apraxia
1. Definition: difficulty initiating voluntary saccades
2. Most evident for saccades to command; reflexive saccades to suddenly appearing targets may be preserved
3. Related phenomenon is spasm of fixation, in which subjects have trouble making a saccade to a second object if the current object at which they are looking remains visible
4. Subjects may also have inaccurate saccades. Their eyes may wander in search of the target, even though it is visible
5. Due to bilateral lesions of parietal eye fields (also known as *lateral intraparietal cortex*), FEF, or both
6. Tested by having the subject make saccades on command to visible targets, to suddenly appearing targets, or to a sudden noise

E. Hemispatial neglect
1. Definition: inability to pay attention to stimuli located in the space contralateral to the lesion
2. Far more common with damage to the right hemisphere, which plays the dominant role in spatial attention

3. Often multimodal: patients may ignore sounds from contralateral space or touch on the contralateral side of the body. They may even believe that their contralateral body parts do not belong to them

4. Due to damage to a predominantly right-sided attentional network, including PPC, FEF, thalamus, and the white matter tracts between these

5. While hemineglect is often associated with hemianopia, patients with chronic hemianopia but not hemineglect show an opposite, compensatory effect, paying more attention to the region of space on their blind side

6. Occurs with acute unilateral hemispheric lesions and often improves with time

7. Tested with the following:

    a. Having patients draw clocks or objects, in which they may fail to include one side

    b. Bisecting lines, in which they place the halfway point toward the side of their lesion

    c. Cancellation tasks, in which they have to circle or cross out all elements on a display. This is most sensitive, particularly if the display contains distractors. Patients fail to circle many items on the side opposite to their lesion

VII. High-level vision: lesions of the ventral occipitotemporal pathway in humans

A. General visual agnosia

1. Definition: inability to recognize previously known objects by sight, with preserved recognition by other modalities

2. Teuber's[1] famous definition: a percept stripped of its meaning. Also popularized as Oliver Sack's[2] "the man who mistook his wife for a hat"

3. Types:

    a. Shape (or visual form) agnosia: inability to perceive elementary properties such as curvature, surface, and volume; instead, patients make inferences about object identity from color or texture. Classic cause is carbon monoxide poisoning

    b. Integrative agnosia: inability to piece together elementary features into a perceptual whole. This can be seen with bilateral peristriate infarcts or Alzheimer disease

    c. Associative agnosia: inability to access stored information about objects because of disconnection or destruction of those memories. This occurs with left or bilateral lesions of the parahippocampal, fusiform, and lingual cortex

B. Prosopagnosia

1. Definition: loss of the ability to recognize familiar faces or learn new ones

2. Linked to bilateral or right-sided lesions of the fusiform gyrus and/or anterior temporal lobe

3. Functional MRI in healthy subjects shows a network of face-responsive areas, including the occipital face area, fusiform face area, and anterior inferior temporal area

4. Types:

    a. Apperceptive prosopagnosia: inability to perceive with precision the shape of faces, mainly with fusiform lesions

    b. Associative prosopagnosia: loss of facial memories or a disconnection that prevents linkage of the face being seen to facial memories, mainly with anterior temporal lesions

5. Ability to perceive other facial information such as age, gender, and expression may be preserved

6. Many but not all prosopagnosics also have trouble with fine distinctions for other object categories so that they cannot distinguish between different types of cars, flowers, etc

7. Developmental prosopagnosia is prosopagnosia that has been present since birth, and there may be an absence of any visible or known brain damage. It may have a genetic basis with familial transmission, associated with early cranial trauma, anoxic encephalopathy, medial occipital polymicrogyria, posterior cerebral atrophy, and epilepsy.

C. Pure alexia

1. Definition: pure alexia, also known as *alexia without agraphia*, represents an inability to read while maintaining the ability to write or loss or reduction in reading ability in a previously literate person

2. Spectrum:

   a. Mild: letter-by-letter reading in which the time needed to read a word is proportional to the number of its letters

   b. Severe: global alexia in which subjects may not be able to read single letters, numbers, music notation, or map symbols

3. If due to a visual problem, subjects can still write. Alexia with agraphia, in contrast, is a linguistic disorder

4. Some represent a selective visual agnosia from left fusiform damage. Functional MRI in healthy subjects shows a visual word form area in the left fusiform gyrus

5. Some are a disconnection syndrome. A left-sided lesion may cause right hemianopia and also interrupt callosal fibres transmitting information from right striate cortex to reading processors in the left hemisphere (Figure 8-5)

D. Topographagnosia

1. Definition: loss of the ability to orient and navigate in familiar surroundings

2. Types:

   a. Landmark agnosia: inability to recognize familiar buildings and scenes, linked to right occipitotemporal lesions, affecting the parahippocampal place area, often associated with prosopagnosia

   b. Impaired cognitive map formation: subjects cannot form a mental image of their environment. Functional MRI shows that this ability is linked to the hippocampi bilaterally and the precuneus

   c. Heading disorientation: subjects cannot represent direction with respect to cues in the environment

VIII. **VISUAL HALLUCINATIONS, ILLUSIONS, AND PERSEVERATIONS**

A. Definitions:

1. Hallucination: visual experience without a corresponding external stimulus

2. Illusion: misinterpretation of an existing external stimulus

3. Perseveration: abnormal persistence or recurrence of a previously seen visual image

B. Many neurologic, psychiatric, or toxic states can cause hallucinations, but almost always with abnormal mental states. Of the conditions with hallucinations and a lucid mind, the following are most important:

1. Release hallucinations (Charles Bonnet syndrome)

   a. Definition: hallucinations related to bilateral visual loss that usually overlaps in some portion of the field

   b. This can occur with ocular or cerebral causes of visual loss

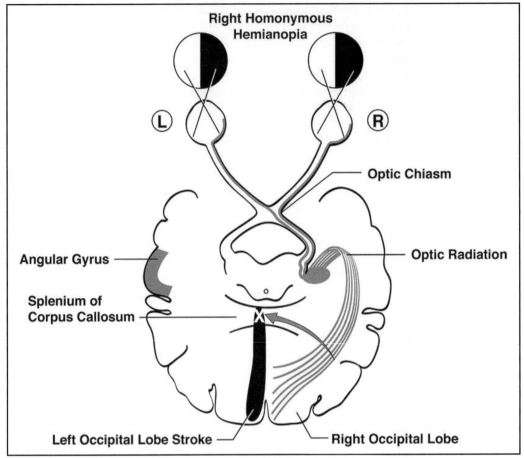

Figure 18-5. Patient with a left occipital stroke and right homonymous hemianopia. Visual information enters the right hemisphere through the intact left hemifield. However, with damage to both the left occipital lobe and the splenium of the corpus callosum, the left hemispheric language centers are deprived of all visual input.

c.   Visual hallucinations are operationally defined as follows: phosphenes, which are unstructured lights such as flashes, sparkles, zig-zag lines or rainbows, black and white or colored, static or moving; photopsias, which are structured images such as geometric figures (triangle, cubes, pyramids, etc) or other simple pictures often occurring in a repetitive pattern (resembling wallpaper with flowers, leaves, or other objects on a uniform plain background); and formed visual hallucinations, which are complex scenes including people, animals, furniture, landscapes, vehicles that may be stationary or mobile, colored or black and white, and perceived, at least temporarily, as real

d.   Occurs in 11% to 13% of blind patients; up to 40% of patients with hemianopia admit to this if asked

e.   Positive spontaneous visual phenomena (PSVP) in the blind hemifield may be noted in nearly half of patients with ischemic infarctions of the retrochiasmal visual pathways. These PSVP were subdivided into phosphenes, photopsias, visual hallucinations, palinopsia, and agitated delirium with hemianopia. PSVP were never associated with auditory or other sensory positive phenomena, except in patients with agitated delirium. Patients who experience PSVP may be more likely to be aware of their visual loss.

      f.   No treatment is needed if the patient has insight and hallucinations are not threatening. Reassurance that the patient is sane and increased socialization and activity may help. A number of medications such as carbamazepine have been tried

      g.   Hemianopic anosognosia (HAN) is defined as the unawareness of visual loss in the homonymous hemifield or hemiquadrant defect. It occurs in 62% of patients with homonymous visual field defects due to ischemic infarcts. Patients with phosphenes, photopsias, or visual hallucinations are usually aware of their visual field loss

  2. Visual migraines (see Chapter 15)

  3. Visual seizures

      a.   Often occurs with occipital or temporal lobe lesions

      b.   Content can be simple or complex and is of uncertain localizing value. Possibly the type of hallucination right at onset may point to the lesion site, but epileptiform discharges can spread rapidly to adjacent cortex

      c.   Characteristics of visual seizures:

          i.   Usually lack the typical history of migraines

          ii.   Duration is short, whereas release hallucinations are highly variable, sometimes lasting hours. If visual seizures are prolonged, they usually will turn into a generalized seizure

          iii.   Content is often stereotypical (ie, the same visual experience each time it occurs), whereas release hallucinations can differ from one episode to another

          iv.   There may be other seizure phenomena during a spell, such as eye deviation, head turn, rapid blinking, or nystagmus

  4. Peduncular hallucinations

      a.   Similar in visual aspects to release hallucinations, except that they do not have visual loss

      b.   Associated with inverted sleep-wake cycles and midbrain signs such as III nerve palsy, Parkinsonism, or hemiparesis

      c.   Due to lesions of the substantia nigra pars reticulata or perhaps the ascending reticular activating system

  5. Childhood abuse/trauma has been associated with visual hallucinations

C. Visual perseveration:

  1. Localizing value and mechanisms of perseverative phenomena are not known

  2. Types:

      a.   Palinopsia

          i.   Definition: preservation in time of a previously viewed image

          ii.   Patients report seeing a previously viewed image either immediately after it was seen, much like an abnormally persistent afterimage, or minutes to days later (delayed type)

          iii.   Usually associated with hemifield defects, and sometimes as a transient feature in their evolution

          iv.   It can occur with a variety of cerebral lesions, or as a toxic effect of street drugs such as LSD and mescaline, or medications such as clomiphene, trazodone, and nefazodone

      b.   Cerebral polyopia

          i.   Definition: preservation in space of a currently viewed image (ie, seeing 2 or more images)

  ii. Unlike diplopia from ocular motor defects, this is a monocular diplopia, or can be a polyopia

  iii. Unlike monocular diplopia due to optic aberrations, the diplopia is present and identical in both eyes and is not eliminated by pinhole

  iv. Rare, usually accompanied by field defects or other cerebral visual disorders

IX. **POSTERIOR CORTICAL VISUAL LOSS ASSOCIATED WITH DEMENTIA**

  A. Posterior cortical atrophy (PCA)

  1. A form of Alzheimer disease, presents with preserved memory and language, but with a progressive, dramatic, and relatively selective decline in vision and/or literacy skills such as spelling, writing, and arithmetic. These patients also present with visual agnosia, visual neglect, and visual hallucinations and often have a homonymous hemianopia.

  B. The Heidenhain variant of Creutzfeldt-Jakob disease (CJD)

  1. A rare, degenerative, invariably fatal brain disorder. The Heidenhain variant of CJD manifests with isolated visual manifestations, including homonymous hemianopia and a normal brain MRI. Diffusion-weighted and FLAIR MRI may demonstrate early cortical abnormalities and a CSF assay for the 14-3-3 protein may be normal, even in pathologically confirmed cases

REFERENCES

1. Teuber HL. Alteration of perception and memory in man. In: Weiskrantz L, ed. *Analysis of Behavioral Change.* New York, NY: Harper & Row; 1968.

2. Sacks O. *The Man Who Mistook His Wife for a Hat and Other Clinical Tales.* New York, NY: Summit Books; 1985.

BIBLIOGRAPHY

Aguirre G, D'Esposito M. Topographical disorientation: a synthesis and taxonomy. *Brain.* 1999;122:1613.

Barton JJS. Structure and function in acquired prosopagnosia: lessons from a series of ten patients with brain damage. *J Neuropsychol.* 2008;2:197-225.

Barton JJS. Disorders of higher visual processing. In: Aminoff MJ, Boller F, Swaab RF, eds. *Handbook of Clinical Neurology.* 3rd series. 2011;102:223-261.

Barton JJS, Rizzo M, eds. *Vision and the Brain, Vol 21, Part 2: Neurologic Clinics of North America.* Philadelphia, PA: WB Saunders; 2003.

Bisiah E, Vallar G. Unilateral neglect in humans. In: Boller F, Grafman J, eds. *Handbook of Neueropsychology.* 2nd ed. Vol 1. New York, NY: Elsevier; 2000:459-502.

Celesia GG, Brigell MG, Vaphiades MS. Hemianopic anosognosia. *Neurology.* 1997;49:88-97.

Danckert J, Rossetti Y. Blindsight in action: what can the different sub-types of blindsight tell us about the control of visually guided actions? *Neurosci Biobehav Rev.* 2005;29:1035-1046.

Dobel C, Bolte J, Aicher M, Schweinberger SR. Prosopagnosia without apparent cause: overview and diagnosis of six cases. *Cortex.* 2007;43:718-733.

Duchaine BC. Developmental prosopagnosia with normal configural processing. *Neuroreport.* 2000;11:79-83.

Farah MJ. *Visual Agnosia.* 2nd ed. Cambridge, MA: MIT Press; 2004.

Gersztenkorn D, Lee AG. Palinopsia revamped: a systematic review of the literature. *Surv Ophthalmol.* 2015;60:1-35.

Haque S, Vaphiades M, Lueck CJ. The visual agnosias and related disorders. *J Neuroophthalmol.* 2017. [In press].

Jacobs DA, Lesser RL, Mourelatos Z, Galetta SL, Balcer LJ. The Heidenhain variant of Creutzfeldt-Jakob disease: clinical, pathologic, and neuroimaging findings. *J Neuroophthalmol.* 2001;21:99-102.

Johnen A, Schmukle SC, Hüttenbrink J, Kischka C, Kennerknecht I, Dobel C. A family at risk: congenital prosopagnosia, poor face recognition and visuoperceptual deficits within one family. *Neuropsychologia.* 2014;58:52-63.

Kanwisher N, McDermott J, Chun MM. The fusiform face area: a module in human extrastriate cortex specialized for face perception. *J Neuroscience.* 1997;17:4302-4311.

Manford M, Andermann F. Complex visual hallucinations. Clinical and neurobiological insights. *Brain.* 1998;121:1819-1840.

Menon GJ, Rahman I, Menon SJ, et al. Complex visual hallucinations in the visually impaired: the Charles Bonnet syndrome. *Surv Ophthalmol.* 2003;48:58-72.

Shevlin M, Dorahy M, Adamson G. Childhood traumas and hallucinations: an analysis of the National Comorbidity Survey. *J Psychiatr Res.* 2007;41:222-228.

Stoerig P, Cowey A. Blindsight in man and monkey. *Brain.* 1997;120:535-559.

Rizzo M, Barton J. Central disorders of visual function. In: Miller NR, Newman, NJ, eds. *Walsh and Hoyt's Clinical Neuro-Ophthalmology.* 6th ed. Vol 1. Philadelphia, PA: Lippincott Williams & Wilkins; 2005:575-645.

Tzekov R, Mullan M. Vision function abnormalities in Alzheimer disease. *Surv Ophthalmol.* 2014;59:414-433.

Vaphiades MS, Celesia GG, Brigell MG. Positive spontaneous visual phenomena limited to the hemianopic field in lesions of central visual pathways. *Neurology.* 1996;47:408-417.

CHAPTER 19

The Phakomatoses
Neurocutaneous Disorders

ANGELA R. LEWIS, MD AND ROD FOROOZAN, MD

I. **THE PHAKOMATOSES DEFINED**

    A. The phakomatoses are a group of disorders characterized by hamartomas of the skin, CNS, eye, and visceral organs

    B. Hamartomas are abnormal proliferations of mature cells normally found in the involved organ

II. **NEUROFIBROMATOSIS TYPE 1 (NF1)**

    A. Also known as *von Recklinghausen neurofibromatosis* or *peripheral neurofibromatosis*

    B. NF1 occurs in approximately 1 in 2500 to 3000 persons

    C. Decreased life expectancy. Mean age at death is 54.4 years

    D. Genetics

        1. NF1 may be inherited as an autosomal dominant trait; 50% of cases are due to spontaneous mutations

        2. The NF1 gene is located on chromosome 17 (17q11.2). The gene has 100% penetrance but is highly variable in its expression

        3. The NF1 gene, a tumor suppressor gene, produces a protein called *neurofibromin*, which negatively regulates the ras oncoprotein. Neurofibromin accelerates the conversion of active guanosine triphosphate (GTP) bound ras to its inactive guanosine diphosphate (GDP) form

        4. Mutations of the NF1 gene result in a loss of neurofibromin, which leads to an increase in cell growth and tumor formation

    E. Cutaneous lesions

        1. Café-au-lait spots are found in 99% of patients with NF1

            a. Flat hyperpigmented lesions

            b. Present at birth and increase in size and number with time

            c. Distributed randomly over the body but do not occur on the scalp, eyebrows, palms, or soles

            d. Histology: hyperpigmentation of the basal cell layer of the epithelium

        2. Freckles are found in 81% of patients with NF1

            a. Hyperpigmentation of the groin, axilla, inframammary regions, and other intertriginous areas

            b. Usually present by age 6 years

Foroozan R, Vaphiades MS. *Kline's Neuro-Ophthalmology Review Manual, Eighth Edition* (pp 261-271).
© 2018 SLACK Incorporated.

3. Neurofibromas are benign tumors of the peripheral nerves
   a. Composed of axons, Schwann cells, and fibroblasts
   b. Localized (isolated) neurofibromas develop in 99% of patients with NF1
      i. Circumscribed lesion
      ii. Uncommon before age 6 years; will increase in size and number with age
   c. Plexiform neurofibromas develop in 60% of patients with NF1
      i. Congenital
      ii. Extensive interdigitation into surrounding tissue
      iii. Associated with soft tissue hypertrophy
      iv. Ten percent risk of undergoing malignant transformation
4. Glomus bodies
   a. Small dermal arteriovenous anastomoses that control body temperature
   b. Usually located in the skin of the fingers and toes under the nail bed
   c. Frequency unknown
   d. They cause pain and sensitivity to cold

F. Ocular lesions
   1. Lisch nodules
      a. Melanocytic hamartoma
      b. Tan, brown, or yellow dome-shaped lesions that protrude from the iris surface
      c. Uncommon prior to age 6 years, but increase in number with age
      d. Do not cause visual symptoms
   2. Eyelid
      a. Café-au-lait spots
      b. Neurofibromas—both isolated and plexiform. Plexiform neurofibromas of the upper eyelid are associated with defects of the sphenoid bone and with congenital glaucoma
   3. Orbit
      a. Orbital neurofibromas
      b. Defects in the sphenoid wing; may cause pulsating proptosis
   4. Optic nerve glioma (see Chapter 10)
      a. Predominant intracranial neoplasm in NF1. Occurs in 15% of patients with NF1
      b. Grade 1 pilocytic astrocytoma
      c. Occurs predominantly in young children; most optic nerve gliomas are diagnosed by age 6 years. Fifty percent to 75% are asymptomatic at the time of diagnosis
      d. Fifty percent of patients with optic nerve and chiasmal gliomas will experience ophthalmologic problems: proptosis, strabismus, loss of visual acuity, papilledema
      e. Gliomas may involve the hypothalamus, leading to endocrine abnormalities (eg, precocious puberty, diabetes insipidus)
      f. Orbital fat-suppressed gadolinium-enhanced MRI is essential in demonstrating optic nerve, chiasm, optic tract, and gadolinium-enhanced MRI of the brain for thalamic/basal ganglia/cerebellar involvement. Optic nerve and chiasmal gliomas are diagnosed by MRI. On T_2 images, one sees a fusiform enlargement of the optic nerve
      g. Few patients with symptomatic gliomas will require treatment, whether by chemotherapy, surgery, or radiation
      h. Visual pathway gliomas may remain stable, enlarge, or regress (post-biopsy or spontaneously)

     5. Corneal nerves may be enlarged in NF1

     6. Retinal lesions are uncommon and nonspecific. Patients may have a combined hamartoma of the retina and retinal pigment epithelium (RPE) or an astrocytic hamartoma

G. CNS lesions
1. Tumors of the CNS are common
   a. Optic pathway glioma
   b. Brainstem glioma
   c. Schwannoma
   d. Meningioma
2. Aqueductal stenosis
3. Macrocephaly
4. Headaches
5. Seizures
6. Cognitive impairment

H. Visceral lesions
1. Increased risk for malignancies
   a. Neurofibrosarcoma
   b. Malignant myeloid disorders
   c. Rhabdomyosarcoma
   d. Wilms tumor
   e. Pheochromocytoma
   f. Breast cancer
2. Skeletal abnormalities
   a. Short stature
   b. Pseudarthrosis
   c. Scoliosis
3. Hypertension may be secondary to a pheochromocytoma or renal artery stenosis
4. Gastrointestinal stromal tumors: mainly in the small bowel and are indolent

I. Diagnostic criteria: must have at least 2 of the following to make a diagnosis of NF1:
1. Six or more café-au-lait spots: must measure at least 5 mm in prepubertal individuals and at least 15 mm in postpubertal individuals
2. Two or more neurofibromas of any type or one plexiform neurofibroma
3. Axillary or inguinal freckling
4. Optic nerve glioma
5. Two or more Lisch nodules
6. Distinctive osseous lesions, such as sphenoid dysplasia or cortical thinning
7. A first-degree relative with NF1 by the criteria listed previously

III. NEUROFIBROMATOSIS TYPE 2 (NF2)

A. Also known as *bilateral acoustic neurofibromatosis* or *central neurofibromatosis*
B. NF2 is seen in 1 in 25,000 persons
C. Genetics
1. NF2 is inherited as an autosomal dominant trait
2. The NF2 gene is located on chromosome 22 (22q11.2). It is a tumor suppressor gene
3. The NF2 gene produces a protein called *schwannomin* or *merlin*, which negatively regulates Schwann cell production. Loss of this protein allows overproduction of Schwann cells

D. Cutaneous lesions are uncommon. Rarely, patients will have a few (less than 6) café-au-lait spots or peripheral neurofibromas

    E. Ocular lesions
1. Posterior subcapsular cataract
2. Epiretinal membrane
3. Combined hamartoma of the RPE and retina
4. Optic nerve sheath meningioma

    F. CNS lesions
1. Bilateral vestibular schwannomas are the hallmark of this syndrome
    a. Typically present in the third decade of life
    b. Symptoms include progressive hearing loss, tinnitus, and vertigo
    c. Histology: schwannomas are benign tumors arising from Schwann cells
2. Schwannomas of other cranial nerves and spinal and peripheral nerves
3. Meningiomas: optic nerve sheath, intracranial, intraspinal
4. Gliomas
5. Ependymomas

    G. Revised criteria for diagnosing NF2
1. Definite NF2: must have one of the following:
    a. Bilateral VIII nerve schwannomas
    b. A first-degree relative with NF2 and a unilateral VIII nerve mass
    c. A first-degree relative with NF2 and 2 of the following lesions: neurofibroma, meningioma, glioma, schwannoma, or a posterior subcapsular lenticular opacity
2. Presumptive or probable NF2
    a. Unilateral VIII nerve mass and meningioma, glioma, schwannoma, or posterior subcapsular lenticular opacity
    b. Multiple meningiomas and unilateral VIII nerve mass, glioma, schwannoma, or posterior subcapsular lenticular opacity

IV. ALTERNATE FORMS OF NEUROFIBROMATOSIS

    A. Conditions showing some of the classic features of either condition (NF1 or NF2), but not in a typical manner

    B. Alternate forms of NF1
1. Segmental neurofibromatosis: patients have manifestations of NF1 limited to one or more areas of the body
2. Familial café-au-lait spots: patients only have café-au-lait spots
3. Familial spinal neurofibromatosis: patients have multiple neurofibromas along the spinal canal and café-au-lait spots

    C. Schwannomatosis is an alternate form of NF2. The schwannomas are confined to the skin and spine. The VIII cranial nerves are spared

V. TUBEROUS SCLEROSIS COMPLEX (TSC)

    A. Syndrome also known as *Bourneville disease*

    B. Incidence is estimated at 1 in 6000 persons

    C. Genetics
1. TSC is inherited as an autosomal dominant trait, but 66% of cases represent spontaneous mutations
2. Two distinct genes can cause TS: TSC1 and TSC2
    a. The TSC1 gene is on chromosome 9 (9q34) and encodes a protein called *hamartin*
    b. The TSC2 gene is on chromosome 16 (16p13.3) and encodes the protein tuberin
    c. Inactivation of both alleles of either TSC1 or TSC2 is required to produce TSC

        d.   Mutations in TSC2 are more common (50%) and associated with a more severe phenotype than mutations in TSC 1 (20%)

D. Cutaneous lesions

    1. Adenoma sebaceum appears in 75% of patients with TSC

        a.   Reddish-brown papular rash in the malar region

        b.   Histologically, these lesions are angiofibromas. They consist of vascular, fibrous, and dermal tissue elements

    2. Mountain ash leaf spots are seen in 90% of patients with TSC

        a.   Hypomelanotic macules

        b.   Can be present at birth

        c.   Best seen with ultraviolet light (Wood lamp)

    3. Subungual/periungual fibromas are seen in 25% of TSC patients

        a.   Angiofibromas of the nail

        b.   More common on toenails than fingernails

    4. Shagreen patches are seen in 20% of TSC patients

        a.   Connective tissue hamartoma

        b.   Gross appearance: area of thickened skin, usually over the lumbosacral region

E. Ocular lesions

    1. Retinal astrocytic hamartoma

        a.   Present in 75% of TSC patients

        b.   Multiple lesions are often found in one eye

        c.   Twenty-five percent of patients will have bilateral lesions

        d.   Rarely affects vision

        e.   Three types of astrocytic hamartoma

           i.   Type 1: flat, smooth, and semitranslucent

           ii.   Type 2: most common; opaque, nodular, elevated, and calcified

           iii.   Type 3: central calcification with peripheral semitranslucent rim

    2. Patches of RPE depigmentation

    3. Angiofibroma of the eyelids and conjunctiva

F. CNS lesions

    1. Cortical tubers (hamartomas)

        a.   Alterations in cerebral cortex pattern; affected gyri are enlarged and hardened

        b.   Disruptions in cerebral cortical cellular pattern lead to seizures and intellectual disabilities. Size and number of tubers positively correlate with the level of cognitive impairment and severity of seizures in patients

    2. Subependymal nodules

        a.   Irregular nodules that protrude into the ventricles from the subependymal layer and often calcify

        b.   Often enlarge and are then referred to as *giant cell astrocytomas*

        c.   May enlarge to cause obstructive hydrocephalus

G. Visceral lesions

    1. Lymphangiomyomatosis affects the lung parenchyma

        a.   Occurs in 1% to 6% of cases and only in women with TSC

        b.   Can cause spontaneous pneumothorax and respiratory failure

        c.   Treatment includes hormonal therapy and lung transplantation

    2. Renal system

        a.   Angiomyolipomas are composed of abnormal blood vessels, smooth muscle, and adipose tissue. These renal tumors are seen in 80% of patients with TSC

      b.   Renal cysts are seen 15% to 20% of the time

      c.   Renal cell carcinoma occurs in 2% of patients

   3.   Rhabdomyomas of the heart are common, seen in 67% of patients

      a.   Rhabdomyomas are usually clinically silent

      b.   These lesions decrease in size and may disappear over time

   4.   Sclerosis of the calvarium and spine occur in 40% of TSC patients

   5.   Pitting of tooth enamel is common

H.   Diagnostic criteria

   *Genetic diagnostic criteria: identification of either a TSC1 or TSC2 pathogenic mutation is sufficient to make a definite diagnosis of TSC

   *Clinical diagnostic criteria:

- Definite TSC: either 2 major features or 1 major feature plus 2 minor features
- Possible TSC: 1 major feature plus 1 minor feature
- **Note:** A combination of the 2 major clinical features lymphangioleiomyomatosis and angiomyolipomas without other features does not meet criteria for a definite diagnosis

   1.   Major features

      a.   Facial angiofibromas ≥ 3 or fibrous cephalic plaques

      b.   Nontraumatic ungual or periungual fibroma ≥ 2

      c.   Hypomelanotic macules (3 or more) at least 5-mm diameter

      d.   Shagreen patch

      e.   Cortical dysplasias (includes tubers and cerebral white matter radial migration lines)

      f.   Subependymal nodules

      g.   Subependymal giant cell astrocytoma

      h.   Multiple retinal hamartomas

      i.   Cardiac rhabdomyoma

      j.   Lymphangiomyomatosis

      k.   Renal angiomyolipoma ≥ 2

   2.   Minor features

      a.   Dental enamel pits ≥ 3

      b.   Intraoral fibromas ≥ 2

      c.   Nonrenal hamartoma

      d.   Retinal achromic patch

      e.   "Confetti" skin lesions

      f.   Multiple renal cysts

VI. Von Hippel-Lindau disease (VHL)

A.   Also known as *angiomatosis* of the retina and cerebellum

B.   VHL neoplasms are hypervascular and overproduce angiogenic peptides such as VEGF

C.   VHL occurs in 1 in 36,000 persons

D.   Genetics

   1.   VHL is inherited as an autosomal dominant trait

   2.   VHL is associated with a mutation of both alleles of the vhl gene (3p25-26). It is a tumor suppressor gene

E.   There are no cutaneous lesions

F.   Ocular lesion—retinal hemangioblastoma

   1.   Usually the first manifestation of VHL; can be missed in its early stages due to peripheral location and small size

2. Stages of a retinal hemangioblastoma
   a. Stage 1—preclassical: lesion is small and without feeder vessels
   b. Stage 2—classical: lesion takes on a globular shape and feeder vessels are evident
   c. Stage 3—marked by extravasation of lipid and plasma
   d. Stage 4—reached if a retinal detachment occurs
   e. Stage 5—marked by blindness secondary to retinal detachment, glaucoma, or persistent uveitis
3. Fifty percent of patients will have bilateral eye disease; 60% will have multiple lesions in one eye; 50% will have severe visual loss
4. Histologically, hemangioblastomas are composed of capillaries and glial cells
5. This lesion can be treated with photocoagulation, cryotherapy, or intravitreal injection of anti-VEGF agents

G. CNS lesions
   1. Hemangioblastoma
      a. Most often located in the cerebellum (52%), but can occur in the spinal cord (44%) and brainstem (18%)
      b. Usually asymptomatic until the third decade of life. Patients present with signs of raised intracranial pressure—headache, nausea, papilledema, and VI nerve paresis. May also have vertigo, nystagmus, and ataxia
   2. Syrinx
      a. May be located in the spinal cord or brainstem
      b. Symptoms include weakness and atrophy of the hands and arms, pain, and nystagmus
   3. Endolymphatic sac tumors
      a. Have been found to have the same genetic defects as other VHL tumors
      b. Patients present with hearing loss, tinnitus, vertigo, and facial weakness

H. Visceral lesions
   1. Renal cell carcinoma
   2. Pheochromocytoma
   3. Benign cysts of the kidneys, pancreas, liver, and epididymis
   4. Polycythemia: the CNS hemangioblastoma produces erythropoietin

I. Diagnostic criteria
   1. A single hemangioblastoma of the CNS or retina and a visceral manifestation (multiple renal, pancreatic, or hepatic cysts; pheochromocytoma, renal carcinoma)
   2. Definite family history and any of the previously mentioned manifestations
   3. Presence of VHL gene mutation

VII. STURGE-WEBER SYNDROME (SWS)

A. Also known as *encephalotrigeminal angiomatosis*: characterized by capillary-venous vascular malformations of the brain, meninges, and skin
B. Rare syndrome. Estimated frequency of 1 in 50,000
C. Hereditary pattern is unknown
D. It is caused by a somatic mosaic mutation in G protein alpha subunit q (GNAQ)
E. Facial lesion—facial angioma
   1. This lesion is also referred to as a *port-wine stain* or a *nevus flammeus*
   2. Present at birth
   3. The reddish-purple lesion is usually unilateral and follows cutaneous distribution of V^1 and V^2. V^3 is less often affected. One, 2, or all 3 dermatomes may be involved simultaneously

        4.   Facial angiomas can be bilateral. Some patients have extensive lesions that involve the trunk and limbs

        5.   Port-wine stain is associated with hemihypertrophy of the face

  F.   Ocular lesions

        1.   Glaucoma is seen in 60% of patients with SWS. Sixty percent of patients will develop glaucoma prior to age 2 years

           a.   Glaucoma is usually ipsilateral to the facial angioma

           b.   More common in patients with facial angiomas involving the upper eyelid

           c.   Glaucoma is believed to be secondary to an anterior chamber angle anomaly and/or elevated episcleral venous pressure

           d.   Glaucoma difficult to control

        2.   Choroidal hemangioma

           a.   Seen in 40% of patients with SWS

           b.   Ipsilateral to the facial angioma

           c.   Two types:

               i.   Diffuse choroidal angioma is the most common—"tomato ketchup fundus"

               ii.   Localized angiomas

           d.   Can cause hyperopia and retinal degeneration

        3.   Heterochromia iridis: the iris ipsilateral to the facial angioma may be deeply pigmented

        4.   Angiomas of the conjunctiva and sclera

  G.   CNS lesion: leptomeningeal hemangioma

        1.   The angioma is located between the pia and arachnoid

        2.   Ipsilateral to the facial angioma; 15% of lesions are bilateral

        3.   Most often located over the parieto-occipital cortex

        4.   Underlying cortex is maldeveloped and hypoplastic

           a.   Cortical veins are absent or nonfunctional

           b.   Calcium deposited within the blood vessels and superficial layers of the cortex. Produces "tram-track" appearance on CT scanning

        5.   Consequences of cortical and meningeal lesions

           a.   Seventy-five percent will have contralateral seizures

           b.   Fifty-five percent to 85% of patients will have some form of learning disability

           c.   Hemiplegia

           d.   Homonymous visual field defect

           e.   Headaches/migraines

           f.   Growth hormone deficiency

  H.   No visceral lesions

  I.   Diagnostic criteria: patients must have 2 of the following criteria:

        1.   Facial angioma with ipsilateral intracranial hemangioma

        2.   Ipsilateral choroidal hemangioma

        3.   Congenital glaucoma

VIII. WYBURN-MASON SYNDROME (WMS)

  A.   Also known as *retinocephalic vascular malformation*

  B.   Incidence and hereditary pattern unknown. Rare syndrome

  C.   Cutaneous lesions are rare; some patients have a facial angioma

D. Ocular lesions
   1. AVM of the retina
      a. This lesion is also known as a *racemose angioma*
      b. It is unilateral and most often located in the posterior pole
      c. Visual acuity can range from 20/20 to NLP
   2. Orbital AVM
   3. Optic nerve AVM
E. CNS lesion—AVM of the CNS
   1. Ipsilateral to the retinal AVM
   2. Fifty percent will be symptomatic
F. Visceral lesions: patients may have AVMs of the ipsilateral maxilla, pterygoid fossa, mandible, and spine
G. Diagnostic criteria: the classic WMS consists of an intracranial AVM and separate retinal AVM

IX. **Ataxia-telangiectasia**
   A. Also known as *Louis-Bar syndrome*
   B. A-T occurs at a frequency of 1 in 40,000 to 100,000 live births
   C. Genetics
      1. Inherited as an autosomal recessive trait
      2. The A-T gene is on chromosome 11 (11q22-23)
      3. The A-T gene encodes a protein called *ATM*, which plays an important role in DNA damage repair
   D. Cutaneous lesion—telangiectasias of the skin
      1. Occurs on exposed areas of skin—ears, nose, neck, antecubital fossae
      2. Usually presents around age 4 years
   E. Ocular lesions
      1. Bilateral bulbar conjunctival telangiectasia
         a. Appears between the ages of 3 and 6 years
         b. Becomes more prominent with age
      2. Ocular motility disturbances
         a. Patients first develop ocular motor apraxia
         b. Later, impairment of smooth pursuit
         c. Eventually, complete supranuclear ophthalmoplegia
   F. CNS lesion—atrophy of the cerebellum
      1. Atrophy particularly prominent in the cerebellar cortex and vermis
      2. Clinical consequences of cerebellar atrophy
         a. Cerebellar ataxia becomes evident when the patient begins to walk; progressive; patients are wheelchair bound by age 10 years
         b. Dysarthria
         c. Chorea
         d. Dystonia
         e. Regression of intellectual milestones
   G. Visceral lesions
      1. Respiratory infections are frequent
         a. Hypoplastic thymus
         b. Hypoplasia of tonsils, adenoids, and lymphoid tissue
         c. Deficiency of IgG2, IgG4, IgA, and IgE

   2. Patients with A-T have poor auto-DNA repair after exposure to ultraviolet light and radiation. This leads to a 100-fold increased cancer rate. They often develop leukemia and lymphoma
   3. Elevated alpha-fetoprotein level
   4. Male and female hypogonadism
H. Diagnostic criteria
   1. Definitive diagnosis: Increased radiation-induced chromosomal breakage in cultured cells or progressive cerebellar ataxia with mutations on both alleles of ATM
   2. Probable A-T: Progressive cerebellar ataxia with 3 of the following 4 features:
       a. Ocular or facial telangiectasia
       b. Alpha-fetoprotein at least 2 SD above normal for age
       c. Serum IgA at least 2 SD below normal for age
       d. Increased radiation-induced chromosomal breakage in cultured cells
   3. Possible A-T: Progressive cerebellar ataxia with at least 1 of the following 4 features:
       a. Ocular or facial telangiectasia
       b. Alpha-fetoprotein at least 2 SD above normal for age
       c. Serum IgA at least 2 SD below normal for age
       d. Increased chromosomal breakage after exposure to radiation

X. **KLIPPEL-TRÉNAUNAY-WEBER SYNDROME (KTWS)**
A. KTWS is a sporadic disorder. Incidence and mode of inheritance is unknown
B. KTWS is characterized by the following triad:
   1. Cutaneous capillary malformations
   2. Varicosities
   3. Bony and soft tissue hypertrophy
C. Most common site is leg, followed by arm, trunk, and rarely head and neck
D. Cutaneous lesion—port-wine stain
   1. Present at birth
   2. Found in 98% of patients with KTWS
   3. Darkens and thickens with age
E. Ophthalmologic manifestations
   1. Port-wine stain of the face
   2. Orbital varix
   3. Heterochromia irides
   4. Varicosities of the retina
   5. Choroidal angioma
F. CNS lesions uncommon
G. Visceral lesions
   1. Varicose veins
       a. May be present at birth, but usually obvious during childhood
       b. Complications: lymphedema, stasis ulceration, pulmonary embolism
   2. Hypertrophy of bone and soft tissues
       a. Causes an increase in both length and girth of affected extremity
       b. Progressive during first several years of life
       c. Disproportionate enlargement of a single extremity can cause scoliosis and gait abnormalities
H. Diagnostic criteria—patient must have 2 of the following criteria:
   1. Cutaneous vascular abnormality
   2. Soft tissue and/or bony hypertrophy
   3. Varicose veins

Bibliography

Chan JW. Neuro-ophthalmic Features of the neurocutaneous syndromes. *International Ophthalmology Clinics*. 2012;52:3, 73-85.

Comi AC. Current therapeutic options in Sturge-Weber syndrome. *Semin Pediatr Neurol*. 2015;22:295-301.

Crino PB, Nathanson KL, Henske EP. Medical progress: the tuberous sclerosis complex. *N Engl J Med*. 2006;355:1345-1356.

Ess KC. Tuberous sclerosis complex: a brave new world? *Curr Opin Neurol*. 2010;23:189-193.

Ferner RE. The neurofibromatosis. *Pract Neurol*. 2010;10:82-93.

Gihiczak GG, Meine JG, Schwartz RA, et al. Klippel-Trenaunay syndrome: a multisystem disorder possibly resulting from a pathogenic gene for vascular and tissue overgrowth. *Int J Dermatol*. 2006;45:883-890.

Goutagny S, Kalamarides M. Meningiomas and neurofibromatosis. *J Neurooncol*. 2010;99:341-347.

Kaye LD, Rothner AD, Beauchamp GR, et al. Ocular findings associated with neurofibromatosis type II. *Ophthalmology*. 1999;99:1424-1429.

Kerrison JB. Phacomatoses. In: Miller NR, Newman NJ, eds. *Walsh and Hoyt's Clinical Neuro-Ophthalmology*. 6th ed. Vol 2. Baltimore, MD: Williams & Wilkins; 2005:1823-1898.

Lewis RF, Lederman HM, Crawford TO. Ocular motor abnormalities in ataxia-telangiectasia. *Ann Neurol*. 1999;46:287-295.

Perlman SL, Boder E, Sedgewick RP, Gatti RA. Ataxia-telangiectasia. *Handb Clin Neurol*. 2012;103:307-332.

Shields JA, Shields CA. Systemic hamartomases. In: Manis MJ, Macsai MS, Huntley AC, eds. *Eye and Skin Disease*. Philadelphia, PA: Lippincott-Raven; 1998:367-380.

Taylor AMR, Byrd PJ. Molecular pathology of ataxia telangiectasia. *J Clin Pathol*. 2005;58:1009-1015.

Theos A, Korf BR. Pathophysiology of neurofibromatosis type 1. *Ann Intern Med*. 2006;144:842-849.

Tsipursky MS, Golchet PR, Jampol LM. Photodynamic therapy of choroidal hemangioma in Sturge-Weber syndrome, with a review of treatments for diffuse and circumscribed choroidal hemangiomas. *Surv Ophthalmol*. 2011;56:68-85.

Waele L, Lagae L, Mekahli D. Tuberous sclerosis complex: the past and the future. *Pediatr Nephrol*. 2015:30:1771-1780.

Ward BA, Gutmann DH. Neurofibromatosis 1: from lab bench to clinic. *J Ped Neurol*. 2005;32:221-228.

Yohay K. Neurofibromatosis types 1 and 2. *Neurology*. 2006;12:86-93.

CHAPTER 20

Neuroimaging

ROD FOROOZAN, MD

I. **GENERAL CONSIDERATIONS**

    A. Optimal results of a neuroimaging study often result from the following:

        1. Selection of the correct study

        2. The study correctly performed

        3. The study interpreted correctly

    B. Interpretation of images is often facilitated by precise and accurate information submitted by the clinician and discussed with the interpreting radiologist. This clinical information may include the following:

        1. Suspected location of pathology

        2. Suspected causes and differential diagnosis

II. **IMAGING MODALITIES**

    A. Magnetic resonance imaging (MRI)

        1. Radiofrequency pulses transiently change the magnetic movements of nucleons (protons and neutrons). As relaxation occurs, specific signals are generated depending on the sequence and tissue consistency. Sequences include the following:

            a. T-1 better for anatomy

                i. Air, fluid, bone appear hypointense (dark)

                ii. Fat appears hyperintense (bright)

                iii. Brain gray matter is relatively hypointense compared to white matter

            b. T-2 better for inflammatory, ischemic, neoplastic lesions

                i. Fluid appears hyperintense

                ii. Brain gray matter appears hyperintense compared to white matter

            c. Gradient echo imaging

                i. Susceptible to magnetic field inhomogeneities

                ii. Detects: blood products, iron, calcium, manganese

            d. Fluid-attenuated inversion recovery (FLAIR)—good for white matter disease

                i. T-2 weighted effects preserved while keeping cerebrospinal fluid (CSF) dark

                ii. Especially good for identifying periventricular changes

                      1. Ischemic foci

                      2. Multiple sclerosis plaques

Foroozan R, Vaphiades MS. *Kline's Neuro-Ophthalmology Review Manual, Eighth Edition* (pp 273-279).
© 2018 SLACK Incorporated.

        e. Diffusion-weighted imaging (DWI)—good for acute stroke

           i. Areas of acute infarction appear hyperintense with corresponding hypointensity on apparent diffusion coefficient imaging

          ii. Detects cerebral ischemia within minutes

        f. Diffusion tensor imaging (DTI) uses MRI techniques to provide information about water mobility and tissue organization in white matter

           i. DTI enables fiber tract mapping

          ii. May also be helpful in brain maturation, demyelination, ischemia, trauma, and neoplasia

  2. Images can be easily generated in multiple planes without the need to reposition the patient

  3. Intravenous contrast shows areas of contrast-enhancement from a disturbance of the blood-brain barrier

        a. Systemic fibrosis syndrome is a concern with intravenous contrast agents, especially in patients with renal insufficiency

        b. With repeated imaging, contrast agents have been shown to be deposited in brain tissue with uncertain clinical consequences

  4. Fat suppression technique helps eliminate the hyperintense signal of orbital fat on T1-weighted images

B. Magnetic resonance angiography (MRA)

  1. Creates images due to intensity differences between flowing blood and stationary tissue

  2. MRA pulse sequences:

        a. Time-of-flight

        b. Phase contrast

  3. Often enhanced with intravenous contrast

  4. May overestimate degree of vascular stenosis >2 mm

C. Magnetic resonance venography (MRV)

  1. Particularly helpful in imaging the cerebral venous sinuses in patients with papilledema suspected of having venous sinus thrombosis

D. Computed tomography (CT)

  1. Differences in X-ray attenuation by tissue result in images with different densities (bone is hyperdense, air and water hypodense)

  2. Rapid image acquisition and widely available

  3. Uses ionizing radiation

  4. Iodinated contrast dye delineates areas of blood-brain barrier breakdown

        a. Iodine contrast reactions and renal insufficiency are concerns

E. Computed tomographic angiography (CTA)

  1. Sensitive in the detection of cerebral aneurysms greater than 2 mm

  2. Prone to artifact from adjacent bone

F. Computed tomographic venography (CTV)

  1. Particularly helpful in imaging the cerebral venous sinuses in patients with papilledema suspected of having venous sinus thrombosis

G. Cerebral angiography

  1. Flowing blood can be imaged to demonstrate stenosis, aneurysm, vascular malformations, arteriovenous fistula, vasculitis, and dissection

        a. Digital subtraction helps remove signal from surrounding tissue, often helpful when trying to determine true vascular abnormalities from artifact (eg, bone)

      2.   Still the gold standard for vascular lesions

          a.   Flow from arteriovenous shunts only detected with cerebral angiography

      3.   Morbidity of 2% to 5% dependent on the institution and underlying vascular risk factors

  H. Ultrasonography

      1.   Color Doppler imaging

          a.   Helpful in detecting carotid artery stenosis

          b.   Helpful in detecting reversal of blood flow in the superior ophthalmic vein due to carotid-cavernous sinus fistula

      2.   A and B scan ultrasonography

          a.   Demonstrates hyperechoic signal of optic disc drusen

          b.   Demonstrates fluid within the optic nerve sheath in patients with papilledema

      3.   Ultrasound biomicroscopy (UBM)

          a.   Helpful for anterior segment abnormalities

  I. Functional imaging

      1.   Provides information about tissue function, particularly helpful when typical structural imaging studies appear normal

          a.   Positron emission tomography (PET)

             i.   Decay of radioisotope detected in areas of high brain metabolism

             ii.   Able to distinguish brain tumor recurrence versus cerebral radionecrosis

          b.   Single-photon emission CT (SPECT)

             i.   Employs iodinated radioactive tracers to assess cerebral blood flow and metabolism

             ii.   Used in cases of stroke, epilepsy, dementia

             iii.   Poor spatial resolution

          c.   Functional MRI (fMRI)

             i.   Depends on changes in regional blood flow with changes in brain metabolism

             ii.   Limited clinical use: may aid in preoperative planning of brain tumor resection

          d.   Magnetic resonance spectroscopy (MRS)

             i.   Provides information on tissue composition based on 5 principal spectra including N-acetylaspartate, choline, creatine, lipid, and lactate

             ii.   Different disorders (eg, neoplasm, abscess) produce differences in the pattern of these spectra

  J. Retina, optic disc, and retinal nerve fiber layer (NFL) imaging

      1.   Particularly helpful in distinguishing retinopathy as the cause of visual loss

      2.   To diagnose and follow retinal NFL and ganglion cell thickness in patients with optic neuropathy (like optic neuritis and glaucoma)

          a.   Scanning laser polarimetry

          b.   Scanning laser ophthalmoscopy

          c.   OCT

III. CHOICES IN IMAGING

  A. The choice of an imaging modality depends on the clinical scenario and suspected pathology (Table 20-1)

  B. The choice between CT and MRI may also depend on advantages and disadvantages of the selected modality and individual patient characteristics (Table 20-2)

Table 20-1

GENERAL GUIDELINES FOR NEUROIMAGING STUDIES DEPENDING ON CLINICAL SCENARIO

Clinical Scenario	Imaging Study	Clinical Remarks
Acute hemorrhage	CT	CT better for acute subarachnoid hemorrhage
Aneurysm	MRA, CTA, catheter angiography	May be missed by MRI and CT
Arteriovenous malformation (AVM)	Catheter angiography	Helps show feeding and draining vessels
Calcification	CT	CT better for bone and calcium
Carotid cavernous fistula	Catheter angiography	Shows orientation of fistula and can be used to help treat lesions
Carotid dissection	MRI, MRA, CTA, catheter angiography	Many lesions can be detected without catheter angiography
Carotid stenosis	Doppler, MRA, CTA, catheter angiography	Catheter angiography still the gold standard for vascular lesions
Cerebral venous disease	MRI, CT, MRV, CTV	MRV and CTV may show evidence of clot that may be overlooked with MRI and CT
Cerebral visual loss	MRI, fMRI	fMRI particularly helpful in showing loss of cortical function when MRI is normal
Chiasmal syndrome	MRI	MRI better for soft tissue and better in the coronal plane
Demyelination/multiple sclerosis (MS)	MRI	MRI better for soft tissue and white matter disease; FLAIR
Evolving hemorrhage	MRI, CT	MRI can help date hemorrhage
Foreign body	CT	MRI contraindicated with ferromagnetic foreign bodies such as vascular clips
Infarct	MRI	DWI able to detect acute infarction
Infection	MRI	Abscess, meningitis
Meningitis	MRI	With contrast enhancement better for soft tissue
Neoplasm	MRI, CT	MRI better demonstrates edema and full extent of tumor
Orbitopathy	MRI/CT	Include fat suppression with MRI
Parasellar/sellar lesion	MRI	Can help delineate pituitary gland from surrounding tissue MRI better for soft tissue
Optic neuritis	MRI	Better for soft tissue Include contrast and fat suppression

(continued)

Table 20-1 (continued)

GENERAL GUIDELINES FOR NEUROIMAGING STUDIES DEPENDING ON CLINICAL SCENARIO

Clinical Scenario	Imaging Study	Clinical Remarks
Paranasal sinus disease	CT, MRI	CT shows bony details better than MRI
Pediatrics	CT, MRI	MRI may be preferable but may require sedation
Posterior fossa	MRI	CT limited by bony artifact
Radiation damage	MRI	Often contrast enhancement with radiation necrosis
Thyroid eye disease	MRI, CT, US	Iodine contrast generally avoided with CT
Trauma	CT	CT is faster, shows acute blood and bone disease
White matter disease	MRI	FLAIR sequences best on MRI Poorly seen on CT

Adapted from *Basic and Clinical Science Course Section 5: Neuro-ophthalmology.* San Francisco, CA: American Academy of Ophthalmology; 2011:82.[1]

Table 20-2

COMPARISON OF NEUROIMAGING WITH MAGNETIC RESONANCE IMAGING AND COMPUTED TOMOGRAPHY

	Advantages	Disadvantages	Contraindications
MRI	Better for soft tissue, including optic nerve and orbital apex	Typically greater cost Contrast dye reactions and systemic nephrogenic fibrosis	Ferromagnetic implants/ metallic foreign body Pacemakers Metallic cardiac valves Non–MRI-compatible intracranial aneurysm clips Cochlear implants
CT	Can be better for trauma to the globe and orbit, especially when foreign body suspected Better for bone and calcium Better for acute hemorrhage	Exposure to ionizing radiation dose Iodine-based dye contrast reactions Limited resolution in the posterior fossa	

Adapted from *Basic and Clinical Science Course Section 5: Neuro-ophthalmology.* San Francisco, CA: American Academy of Ophthalmology; 2011:82.[1]

IV. IMAGING OF SELECTED CLINICAL SCENARIOS

A. Optic neuropathy. Imaging entire optic nerve, including orbital, canalicular, cranial portions

1. MRI of brain and orbits with fat suppression and contrast. Fat suppression techniques help eliminate hyperintense signal of orbital fat on T1-weighted images

2. Can be helpful to distinguish between inflammatory (typically with optic nerve enhancement) and ischemic (typically without optic nerve enhancement) optic neuropathies

B. Chiasmal/sellar lesions. Soft tissue imaging is typically best performed with MRI

1. MRI of the brain with contrast and attention to the optic chiasm and sella

2. Obtain direct coronal views that show the relationship of the sellar structures, including the pituitary gland, to the intracranial optic nerves and optic chiasm

3. Particularly helpful with suprasellar masses that have cystic components (such as craniopharyngioma and cystic pituitary tumors) and multiple signal intensities (such as pituitary apoplexy)

C. Pupil-involving III nerve palsy

1. Imaging should exclude a compressive lesion involving the III nerve

   a. Soft tissue lesions involving the III nerve (tumors, infiltration, enhancement) are typically best seen with contrast-enhanced MRI

   b. Aneurysms (most commonly posterior communicating artery) often require specific vascular studies

      i. Less invasive studies MRA and CTA. There remains controversy about which modality is better suited to detect clinically important aneurysms. The choice often is dependent on the institution, available technology, and the radiologist interpreting the study

      ii. Catheter angiography. Remains the gold standard for the detection of vascular lesions. If clinical suspicion is high, catheter angiography may be required even with negative MRA and/or CTA studies

D. Thyroid eye disease

1. Orbital study with CT or MRI

2. Able to detect the following:

   a. Enlarged extraocular muscles; tendons spared

   b. Increased orbital fat

   c. Proptosis

   d. Inflammation involving the orbit suggestive of active disease

3. Dysthyroid optic neuropathy may be due to the following:

   a. Apical compression of optic nerve by enlarged extraocular muscles

   b. Stretching of optic nerve due to increased orbital fat

E. Papilledema

1. Typically best assessed with MRI for the soft tissue, including the optic nerves, meninges, cerebral venous sinuses, and for the intracerebral ventricles (for hydrocephalus) and CSF pathway (including structural lesions such as Chiari malformations)

   a. Phase contrast cine (PCC) MRI can help assess CSF dynamics

   b. MRV (and CTV) helpful to exclude cerebral venous sinus thrombosis

2. CT often useful for screening in emergency settings to exclude a mass lesion

REFERENCE

1. Katz B. *Basic and Clinical Science Course Section 5: Neuro-ophthalmology*. San Francisco, CA: American Academy of Ophthalmology; 2011:82.

BIBLIOGRAPHY

Chaudhary N, Davagnanam I, Ansari S, Pandey A, Thompson BG, Gemmete JJ. Imaging of intracranial aneurysms causing isolated third cranial nerve palsy. *J Neuroophthalmol*. 2009;29:238-244.

De Wyngaert R, Casteels I, Demaerel. Orbital and anterior visual pathway infection and inflammation. *Neuroradiology*. 2009;51:385-396.

Fang Y, Duong T, Tantiwongkosi B. Advanced MR Imaging of the visual pathway. *Neuroimag Clin N Am*. 2015;25:383-393.

Hess CP, Dillon WP. Imaging the pituitary and parasellar region. *Neurosurg Clin N Am*. 2012;23:529-542.

Jäger HR. Loss of vision: imaging the visual pathways. *Eur Radiol*. 2005;15:501-510.

Kardon RH. Role of the macular optical coherence tomography scan in neuro-ophthalmology. *J Neuroophthalmol*. 2011;31:353-361.

Mallery RM, Prasad S. Neuroimaging of the afferent visual system. *Semin Neurol*. 2012;32:273-319.

Murchison AP, Gilbert ME, Savino PJ. Neuroimaging and acute ocular motor mononeuropathies: a prospective study. *Arch Ophthalmol*. 2011;129:301-305.

Osborn AG, Salzman KL, Jhaveri MD, Barkovich AJ, et al. *Diagnostic Imaging: Brain*. 3rd ed. Philadelphia, PA: Lippincott Williams & Wilkins; 2015.

Tantiwongkosi B, Hesselink JR. Imaging the ocular motor pathways. *Neuroimag Clin Am*. 2015;25:425-438.

Trick GL, Calotti FY, Skarf B. Advances in imaging of the optic disc and retinal nerve fiber layer. *J Neuroophthalmol*. 2006;26:284-295.

Vaphiades MS. Imaging the neurovisual system. *Ophthalmol Clin North Am*. 2004;17:465-480.

Financial Disclosures

Dr. Jason J. S. Barton is on the Scientific Advisory Board for Vycor Corp and on the Executive Board for Medicalogic Corp, and he is a speaker for LAUNCH program, Serono.

Dr. John E. Carter has no financial or proprietary interest in the materials presented herein.

Dr. Richard H. Fish has no financial or proprietary interest in the materials presented herein.

Dr. Rod Foroozan has no financial or proprietary interest in the materials presented herein.

Dr. Christopher A. Girkin has no financial or proprietary interest in the materials presented herein.

Dr. Saunders L. Hupp has no financial or proprietary interest in the materials presented herein.

Dr. Lanning B. Kline has no financial or proprietary interest in the materials presented herein.

Dr. Angela R. Lewis has no financial or proprietary interest in the materials presented herein.

Dr. Jennifer T. Scruggs has no financial or proprietary interest in the materials presented herein.

Dr. Michael S. Vaphiades has no financial or proprietary interest in the materials presented herein.

Dr. Mark F. Walker has no financial or proprietary interest in the materials presented herein.

Index

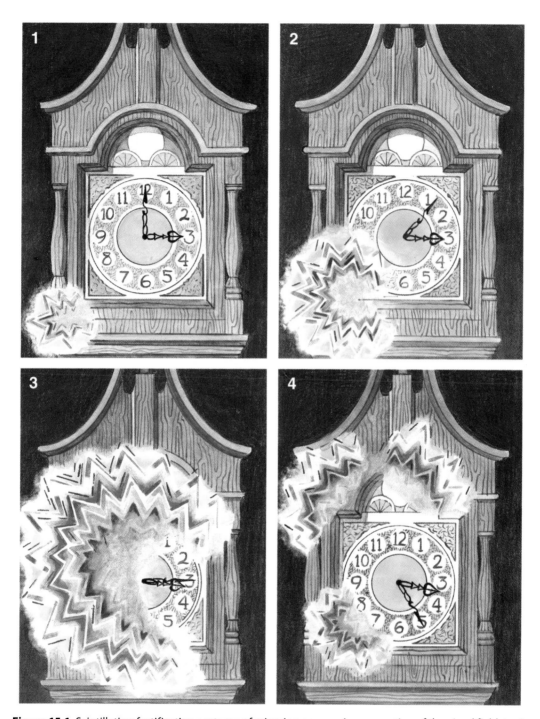

Figure 15-1. Scintillating fortification scotoma of migraine appears in one portion of the visual field, typically enlarges to cover central fixation, then "marches" toward the periphery and breaks apart. The entire phenomenon lasts 15 to 30 minutes. (Reprinted with permission from Hupp SL, Kline LB, Corbett JJ. Visual disturbances of migraine. *Surv Ophthalmol*. 1989;33:221-236.) **Please see original figure on page 211.**

Table

SELECTED NEURO-OPHTHALMIC EMERGENCIES

Condition	Chapter Reference
Giant cell arteritis	Chapter 9, p 153
Tolosa-Hunt syndrome	Chapter 7, p 126
Pituitary apoplexy	Chapter 15, p 216
Wernicke encephalopathy and ophthalmoplegia/nystagmus	Chapter 2, p 80
Aneurysmal compression of the III cranial nerve	Chapter 5, p 104
Carotid dissection with Horner syndrome	Chapter 16, p 231
Rhinocerebral mucormycosis and cavernous sinus syndrome	Chapter 7, p 125
Central and branch retinal artery occlusion	Chapter 16, p 226
Decompensated myasthenia	Chapter 11, p 175
Papilledema	Chapter 9, p 143
Seizures involving the visual pathways	Chapter 18, p 257
Carotid-cavernous fistula	Chapter 7, p 125